NEUROLOGY in
OUR MIDST

NEUROLOGY in OUR MIDST

A Primer to Neuroanatomy and
Clinical Neurology

Dr. Amado M. San Luis

Copyright © 2019 by Dr. Amado M. San Luis.

Library of Congress Control Number:		2018914207
ISBN:	Hardcover	978-1-9845-6960-8
	Softcover	978-1-9845-6961-5
	eBook	978-1-9845-6959-2

All rights reserved. No part of this book may be reproduced or transmitted in any form or by any means, electronic or mechanical, including photocopying, recording, or by any information storage and retrieval system, without permission in writing from the copyright owner.

Any people depicted in stock imagery provided by Getty Images are models, and such images are being used for illustrative purposes only.
Certain stock imagery © Getty Images.

Print information available on the last page.

About the Cover
Title: "HUMANSCAPE" in acrylic on canvas. It speaks of the body's (humanscape's) link with reality—how it is perceived and reacted to, how our everyday responses (individually or socially) are affected or shaped by sensitive neural links.

International Visual Artist (Sculptor, Painter, Performance Art): Sam Penaso, Guindulman,Bohol, Philippines. Had 26 solo exhibits: Japan, Austria, Germany, Singapore, New York & Abu Dhabi. Recepient of multiple international grants and international awards.
e-mail: samuelpenaso@yahoo.com
website:www.facebook.com/sampenaso
www.instagram.com/sampenaso
Tel: (632)4147921 or 09989989899

About the Illustrations
Drawings: by the author
Digital Conversion: Ryan D. Abainza
facebook.com/ryanabainza
ryanabainza@gmail.com

Rev. date: 05/08/2019

To order additional copies of this book, contact:
Xlibris
1-888-795-4274
www.Xlibris.com
Orders@Xlibris.com
551799

CONTENTS

Dedication ix
Acknowledgments xiii
Foreword xvii
Preface xix
Introduction 1
Anatomic Orientation 3
Chapter I 7
The Physiology or Mechanism of Neural Transmission
Chapter II 13
General Anatomy of the Central Nervous System
Chapter III 17
The Descending Motor or Pyramidal Tract System
Chapter IV 25
The Nociceptive Pain and Associated Spinothalamic Tracts
Chapter V 35
The Other Ascending Sensory Fibers
Chapter VI 43
The Cranial Nerves

    Chapter VI-A 47
    Cranial Nerve I- Olfactory Nerve
        (Function: Sense of Smell)

    Chapter VI-B 53
    Cranial Nerve II- Optic Nerve
        (Function: Vision/Seeing)

Chapter VI-C **67**
Cranial Nerve III- Oculomotor Nerve, Cranial Nerve IV-
Trochlear Nerve, Cranial Nerve VI-Abducens Nerve
    (Functions: Pupillary Constriction, Eye Opening, and Eye
    Movements)

Chapter VI-D **81**
Cranial Nerve V- Trigeminal Nerve
    (Functions: Face Sensation and Mastication)
        Functional Anatomy of CN V Trigeminal Nerve Sensory
        Branches 82
        Functional Anatomy of the Muscles of Mastication 86

Chapter VI-E **89**
Cranial Nerve VII- Facial Nerve
    (Functions: Facial Muscles of Expression, Taste, Eye Closure,
    Lacrimation, Salivation, Sound Modulation)
        The Facial Motor Nerve 92
        The Nervus Intermedius 94

Chapter VI-F **99**
Cranial Nerve VIII- Vestibulocochlear Nerve
    (Functions: Hearing and Balance)
        The Cochlear Nerve. 100
        The Vestibular Nerve. 105

Chapter VI-G **115**
Cranial Nerve IX- Glossopharyngeal Nerve
    (Functions: Taste, Salivation, Baroreflex, Swallowing, Ear & Palatal
    Sensation)
        Glossopharyngeal Nerve-Parasympathetic Nerve to the
        Parotid Gland 116
        Glossopharyngeal Nerve's Role in Swallowing 117
        Glossopharyngeal Nerve for Taste 117
        Pain, temperature, and touch sensation of CN IX 118

Chapter VI-H **123**
Cranial Nerve X- Vagal Nerve
    (Functions: Taste, Salivation, Carotid Sinus Reflex, Hering-Breuer,
    Visceral Organ Control, Swallowing, Phonation, External Canal
    Sensation)

CN X Vagus Nerve-afferent fibers.................................. 125
CN X. Vagus Nerve-efferent Arm 125
CN X. Vagus Nerve Autonomic Reflex arms.................... 127

Chapter VI-I...**131**
Cranial Nerve XI- Accessory Nerve
 (Swallowing and Head Movement)

Chapter VI-J..**135**
Cranial Nerve XII- Hypoglossal Nerve
 (Functions: Swallowing and Sound Formation/Phonation)

Chapter VII **141**
The Spinal Cord and Peripheral Nerves
 (Functions: Sensation, Motor Strength, Reflexes, Autonomics)
   The Topography of the Spinal Cord 142
   The Backbones 144
   The Spinal cord..144
   Descending Fibers of the Spinal Cord 146
   Other Descending Fibers of the Spinal Cord 150
   Ascending Fibers of the Spinal Cord.....................151
   Other ascending fibers of the spinal cord..............153
   Autonomic Nervous System of the Spinal Cord....154
   The Topography of Peripheral Nervous System 158
   The Motor Component of the Peripheral Nerves. 163
   The Sensory Component of the Peripheral Nerves. 170
   The Autonomic Nervous System 173
   Anatomy of the Autonomic Nervous System 174
   Parasympathetic Nervous System (PSNS)............175
   Sympathetic Nervous System (SNS) 176

Chapter VIII..**187**
The Cerebellum
 (Functions: Balance, Voluntary Muscle Coordination, Visio-vestibular-spatial-proprioceptive Coordination, Cognition and Affect)

Chapter IX...**195**
Basal Ganglia
 (Functions: Learning and Modulating Programmed Motor Acts)

Chapter X 203
The Cerebral Cortex
  (Functions: Memory, Learning, Language, Cognition, and Emotion)

Chapter XI 223
The Functional Anatomy of Sleep and Consciousness

Chapter XII 249
Cerebrospinal Fluid Circulation

Chapter XIII 255
Cerebral and Spinal Blood Circulation
  The Heart. 258
  The Branches of the Aortic Arch (Fig. 55). 260
  The Posterior Circulation (Table VI). 261
  The Anterior Circulation. 266
  Special Clinical Correlates for Stroke Recognition: 270
  Spinal Cord Blood Supply 275
  The Venous Drainage of the CNS 277

Summary 282
Bibliography 284
Index 295

DEDICATION

To my lovely wife, Cynthia, mother to our eight beautiful children, astute pediatrician, palliative care expert, caring doctor and nurse, excellent teacher, a superhuman…my inspiration.

Neurology in Our Midst

(A Primer to Neuroanatomy and Clinical Neurology)

ACKNOWLEDGMENTS

Translating and condensing into a book ones long experience in teaching neurology to medical students, nurses and physical therapists is an arduous task made more difficult by the need to address the fears and disinterest of the future health care providers. Dr. Romeo A. Divinagracia, President of UERMMMCI, challenged me to pursue writing a book about neurology. I am grateful for that dare and for providing the milieu to pursue the project. I extend this gratefulness to Dr. Alfaretta Tan-Reyes, Dean of the College of Medicine who provided valuable suggestions and constant reminding of the importance of the book. My special thanks to the Department of Clinical Neurosciences Faculty Staff who freed me from teaching assignments and other tasks that allowed me to research and write. I am sincerely appreciative for the sabbatical leave granted by my alma mater, UERMMMCI, College of Medicine.

The thoughts written in this book are not mine alone but from a thirty-five-year conglomeration of informations shared by various persons who are worthy of my utmost gratitude. Dr. Joven Cuanang, after arriving from his neurology residency at Harvard Medical School-Massachusetts General Hospital, invited me in 1977 to be a pioneer resident in Adult Neurology at UERMMMC which I gladly accepted though it deviated from my interest in child neurology. Together with Dr. Brigido Carandang, who at that time, just arrived from the University of California, Davis, I owe the foundation of my knowledge and skills in neurology and the discipline of inquisitiveness, research, teaching, and organization. My thanks to the Japanese Government for the Monbusho Scholarship Grant. To my *sensei*, Prof. Yoshigoro

Kuroiwa and Prof. Motohiro Kato who allowed me to explore new pursuits in neurology, neurophysiology, and research; and to the other sensei, colleagues, residents and staff of Kyushu University Neurological Institute who catered to my needs during my fellowship, *domo arigato gozaimashita!*

My sincere appreciation to my colleagues at the Philippine Neurological Association (PNA) and Asian and Oceanian Association of Neurology (AOAN) -- two organizations of neurologists dedicated to share knowledge with one another. I am a proud recipient of these academic exchanges. Friendships evolved in these interactions and I am fortunate to have this with Prof. Bhim Singhal who holds my utmost respect. Thank you Bhim for writing the foreword of the book.

Sincere thanks to, Cora Derige, the line editor, who met with me several times to improve the content of the drafts and painstakingly tried to understand medical terms to develop the text; to Josephine Reyes Arce who labored in proofreading the draft that contained strange medical terms; and to Dr. Rene Mendoza who reviewed the initial part of the book and provided encouragement. My appreciation to Ryan Abainza, who transformed my drawings to digital illustrations. Sam Penaso, an International Artist from the picturesque island of Bohol, Philippines, though I had not met personally, willingly permitted to use his beautiful painting, "Humanscape," that coincidentally depicted the very essence of this book. My classmate and good friend, Cooper Resabal, facilitated the link with this great art work. My thanks to both of you.

My daughter Nikki, the real writer in the family is my consultant, who provided valuable insights and suggestions during the writing process and critical guides to help me navigate the nuances of writing. My two daughters who are also neurologists, Hana and Carmela, gave critical recommendations and opinions. To my other children and their partners who provided the cheers in this effort, Caru and Catherine, Fatima and Miko, Patrick, Darren, Miguel, Malou, and Maan. Thanks my valuable kids. My kisses of love to my grandchildren, Cy, Cerrah, Lucy, Franco and Cito who provided comfort when the stresses of writing came my way.

My beautiful and loving wife, Cynthia, patiently prodded, nudged, and pushed me and offered all emotional and material support. She kept on reminding me to be direct and to keep the sentences short. She is my inspiration. Without her this book will not see the light. Thank you dear wife.

Gratitude to the medical students of Class 2014 of St. Luke's College of Medicine Willliam H. Quasha Memorial who gave their time to read the first draft and provided their comments and suggestions. My appreciation to Dr. Annie De Leon, Medical Director of Quirino Memorial Medical Center for granting a sabbatical that allowed me to write. My colleagues who were invited to critique parts of the book provided valuable guides. These are: Dr. Dede Gunawan, Dr. Artemio Roxas Jr, Dr. Arnel Malaya, Dr. Carmelita Divinagracia, Dr. Dada Mesina-Nepomuceno, Dr. John Carlo Timbol and Dr. Deborah Bernardo. To all my students, residents, nurses, physical therapists, neuroscience colleagues, friends and patients, thank you. I learned so much from all of you.

To my parents, Mario and Jesusa, thank you for your prayers, guidance and sacrifices.

Neurology in Our Midst
(A Primer to Neuroanatomy and Clinical Neurology)

FOREWORD

I am indeed honored to have been invited to write the foreword for Professor Amado San Luis' book 'Neurology in Our Midst'—A Primer to Neuroanatomy and Clinical Neurology. Neurology has long been considered as a specialty which 'inspires awe' among the medical fraternity. It is not uncommon for medical students & resident doctors to get cold feet when confronted with a Neurology case in the exam or during ward rounds.

Professor Amado San Luis has written this book with the primary objective of dispelling this 'fear psychosis' surrounding the study of Neurology. This book is a refreshing change from the standard neurology textbooks. Rather than focus on neurological diseases & syndromes, the author discusses the anatomical pathways to explain how a particular symptom & finding originates. While seeing a neurological case, the first and most important step is to determine where the lesion lies. Sound knowledge of neuroanatomy alone can guide us to the precise localization & thus aid the correct diagnosis & management.

The Professor's mastery of the subject is reflected in the way he holds the reader's hand and guides him through the maze of information, consolidating the basic concepts of Neuroanatomy and Neurophysiology along the way. Case studies with clinic-anatomic correlations and a brief review of diagnostic possibilities are to me the stand out feature in each chapter. The several illustrative diagrams further add to the value of the book.

The book has been written in a clear, concise style – easy to read & comprehend. One looks forward to reading the next page and then the next and so on. This is no mean achievement. I must compliment

Professor Amado San Luis who has used his vast experience of teaching for over three decades to write this very informative book. I am sure it will be more than useful for medical students, nursing staff, health care professionals & all those who care for persons with neurological illnesses.

Bhim Singhal MD, D.Sc (Hon.), FRCP (London & Edin), FAMS
Director of Neurology
Bombay Hospital Institute of Medical Sciences
Former Professor & Head of Neurology Grant Medical College & Sir J.J. Group of Hospitals
Mumbai, India

PREFACE

"Neuroanatomy is my most difficult subject in medicine!" doctors' complain.

A family practitioner said, "I hated my rotation in neurology after seeing a comatose patient. I had a dreadful experience."

"I often fear questions that relate to patients with strokes… I am just not confident to answer them." – shared by a physical therapist.

"Every time neurological patients are in our care, there is this constant fear in me that patients might die anytime!" … lamented by a registered nurse in a hospital.

Dread, difficulty, insecurity, helplessness, and fear are everyday experiences shared by doctors, nurses, physical therapists, and caregivers -- health care providers, who are given the inescapable task to meet the demands of patients with neurological diseases. Patients afflicted with sudden or long-term brain diseases or injuries, and their families, experience distressing uncertainty and will demand reliable and understandable answers to questions such as, "What happened?", "How did it happen?", "What should be done?", and "What will happen?" Queries are anxiously repeated as often as clinical changes happen and until a satisfactory response to their questions are met. The responsibilities faced by the healthcare providers look formidable and pre-existing disdain of neurological cases has compounded the situation. These negative feelings had its formative years when medical students, nurses and other care providers studied neuroanatomy and clinical neurology. It was at this stage when neurology, to some extent, was so feared that it led to a condition called neurophobia.

Jozefowicz described Neurophobia in 1994 as fear of the neural sciences and clinical neurology that is due to the students' inability to apply their knowledge of basic sciences to clinical situations [1,2,3]. In the three decades of teaching neurology, I came to notice that medical students, residents, general practitioners, nurses, and physical therapists widely share this fear. I have also observed this attitude of fear create a wide communication gap between patients and their families and health care providers. There is, therefore, a need to lessen, if not eliminate, neurophobia among health care providers. Thus this book.

The book is designed to be read by medical and nursing students and physical therapists before starting their journey to neuroanatomy and clinical neurology and before beginning clinical rotations. The book serves as a "neurology map" that will provide the prospective neuroscience students a view of where one is going and what to expect. The emphasis is to understand how our brain and body usually function during our daily activities and how diseases or injuries can change them. The reader is not expected to memorize functional structures seemingly in preparation for an exam. This primer does not aim to replace the usual medical books prescribed in neuroanatomy and clinical neurology. This strategy provides clinical meanings to boring anatomic structures that students are expected to memorize. Examples of how neuroanatomic functional structures are examined to unravel abnormalities are included. The process will help in localization, diagnosis and, ultimately, to treatment.

The regular activities and functions of people are dissected, as to, how the nervous system weaves its various parts to make them happen. The exploratory journey is punctuated by breaks to mention some diseases or injuries that affect the functions of the nervous system. Examples of case stories based on actual patients are modified to enhance clinical-anatomic correlations. The names of the characters of the stories are creations of the author. Some neurological examinations are described to serve as triggers to pursue the development of these skills which are not purely mechanical but associated with physio-anatomic understanding. Repetitions are liberally used to facilitate comprehension.

Neuroanatomic details of the thalamus and hypothalamus are limited to their participation in some functions. Illustrations were done by the author to emphasize that anybody can do simple drawings to facilitate grasp of functional anatomy. The readers are encouraged to freely trace the directions and connections of neural structures by using different colors that would enhance understanding. Tables are limited and are used to emphasize some points in the discussion. Some contents of the book may catalyze one's mind to understand particular topics. "Google" those topics. Follow the interests of your brain. There might be a neuroscience talent within. The intended beneficiaries of this book are ultimately the patients afflicted with neurological diseases and the medical providers who will be tasked to help.

INTRODUCTION

Everything that we do has its origin, control, termination, and processing in the nervous system, a compelling reason why one should at least get a good idea of how the brain works. Even when sleeping, the mind never stops working. Look at the people around you. See how they walk, the accompanying body movements, the speed, the balance, the directions they set, their decisions to hurry or to stop, their avoidance to bump each other even while some are talking through their I-phones. All these people are in amazing assortments of fluid activities, but not one has a conscious idea about how delicate and precise the brain integrates the complex nervous system to make what you have witnessed happen. Then one person with a limp and pace slower than those of the rest strikes your attention. He makes you wonder why he was different. Could it be that his brain function has been disturbed and has adapted to the need to travel? While reading this and imagining what the text is describing, your brain is integrating all the learned information, as well as the "unlearned" when you were still in your mother's womb, to form a system of communication. When your friend taps you on the shoulder, he recognizes you through his memory; his smile is made possible by the finite control of the muscles of the face while your memory cells likewise influenced your response. Your interpretation of the smile is yours alone, a recognition of friendship, much of which is integrated by your limbic system, the seat of emotion. Neurology, the study of the nervous system, is all around us and within us, in our midst.

The General Plan, Direction and Goals

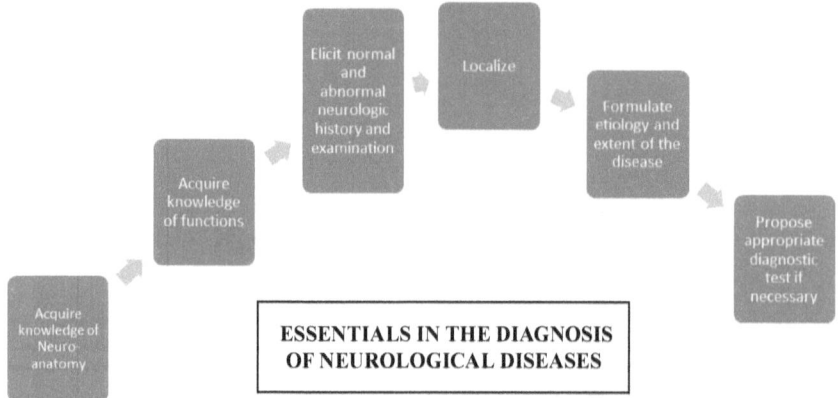

When planning a journey, one has to identify the destination, set the direction, organize the system (needed clothes, accommodation, tickets, maps, budget, etc.) and processes (addresses, time, dates, terminal, schedules, etc.). The same holds when one intends to understand a neurological problem. The goal is to arrive at a neurological diagnosis, the foundation that allows treatment plans. The procedure is to break the journey into six essential steps. This book shall provide the first four steps of acquiring knowledge and processes that will prepare one for the fifth and sixth notches which are the reader's utilization of various information that one will assimilate in clinical neurology. The steps, however, are blurred because to appreciate the application of neuroanatomy to clinical neurology one should look at the process as a continuum of normal and disturbance of functions. What makes neurology different is the emphasis on localization which to some is daunting or merely a "turn-off." You will find out after persevering in reading this book that you do not need a GPS to locate most of the problems. Where signs and symptoms intersect is usually where the lesion is. Establishing symptoms and relevant neurological examination findings are the framework for arriving at a preliminary diagnosis that will guide one to choose the appropriate and the most economical diagnostic tool. Understanding the meaning of abnormal neurological examination findings are very much crucial in establishing clinical parameters that will tell one if the patient is getting worse or getting better -- critical factors in clinical judgment that cannot be replaced by any diagnostic armamentarium.

ANATOMIC ORIENTATION

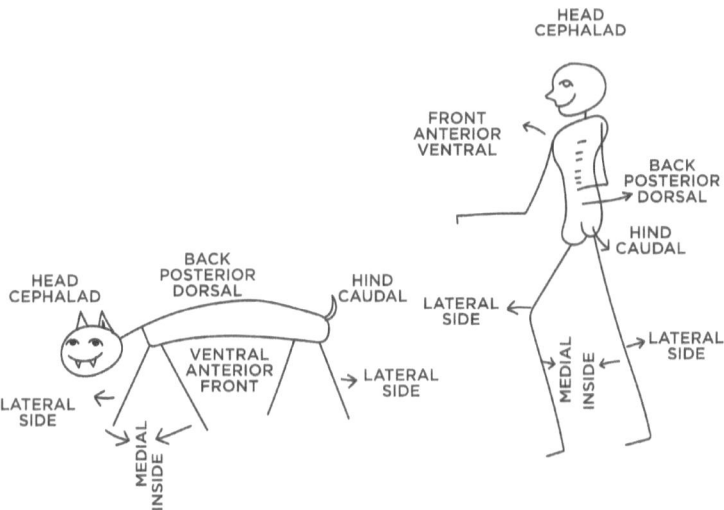

Figure 1. Anatomic terms used relative to the body parts of quadripedal animals and bipedal humans.

Neuroanatomy makes use of anatomic landmarks just like any maps for proper orientation and common language. Maps use the basic north, south, east, and west positions and could be a combination of NE or NW, etc. Human anatomy uses similar combinations. It is interesting to know that in the past, comparative or animal anatomy, particularly on four-legged animals was the basis of the knowledge of human brain structures. It is from this orientation that early anatomists used the term **dorsal** which referred to *the posterior or back part;* **ventral,** *the anterior or front* portion; and **lateral,** to *the outer side; and* **medial**, *to the inner side* (Fig. 1). These were the terms used when describing the *external and internal anatomies* of the four-legged animals. The labels included the *tip of the head or cephalad* or *rostral* and *caudal area* or *towards the tail*. This quadrupedal animal orientation remained through the Renaissance period until human cadaver studies were made possible on two-legged homo sapiens whose ancestor is the Homoerectus in 2,000,000 BC. The shift of quadrupedal posture to bipedal or erect posture can make anatomic orientation confusing. An example is the front or anterior of dogs can be confused as in the front of the face when it is actually cephalad. In humans, the anterior is consistently in the front of the face.

When one reads the **anterior grey horn** of the spinal cord, it refers to the front portion of the grey matter. **Anterolateral-Spino-thalamic fibers** mean that the fiber tracts are located lateral and slightly in front of the spinal cord. An extra clue is that the direction of the thread is from the spine and will end at the thalamus. **Ventroposteromedial thalamus** means the location is at the base, posterior, and central part of the thalamus. (Note that the thalamus is positioned horizontally like a boat in an erect human brain). After a while, as you read the book, you will gradually adopt the language of neuroanatomic landmarks just like how you learned your first language.

"Afferent" and *"efferent"* are terms used to describe the direction of impulses. These are the terms reflex functions often used. There are two arms in the reflex: the *initiating stimuli,* **afferent** *or entering (to the CNS) arm,* and the *transmitting response,* **efferent** *or exiting arm*. An example of this reflex is the pupillary light reflex. The *afferent* or entering arm of the optic nerve transmits the light stimulus while the *efferent* or exiting arm is the parasympathetic fiber of the oculomotor nerve that carries the response and effect a pupillary constriction. It is

a little different inside the brain. The afferent or efferent impulses are inside the nervous system. Examples are the *afferent impulses* from the hypothalamus to the Salivatory nucleus of the medulla, whose *efferent neurons* would send electrical signals through the glossopharyngeal nerve effecting or causing salivary secretion. We will use the terms, afferent and efferent arms, to describe the direction of impulses.

Terms are also used to describe the distance of parts from a central position. The heart is the center of the blood vessels, so arteries or veins near it are described as **proximal vessels** (proximately near) whereas the remote branches are called **distal vessels** (distant vessels). The central station of the peripheral nerves, on the other hand, is the spinal cord, so the nearest branches to the spinal cord are called **proximal nerves** in contrast to the **distal nerves** termed as such because they are the faraway branches or end of the nerves. Distance from the trunk or muscles above describes muscles as **distal or proximal**. Muscles of the hands are distant when related to the forearm. Some diseases involve proximal more than distal parts. Examples are diseases of the muscles, one of which is hypokalemic (low potassium) myopathy. Hypokalemia can manifest as proximal muscle weakness where the person is unable to raise the arms but can give a firm hand grip.

The subway train system where travelers from the central station stop or connect at different substations is like the neural interconnections in the central nervous system. The ganglia are like the substations where interconnections with a group of neurons happen outside the central axis. An example of this is the *sympathetic ganglia* where the sympathetic neurons from the spinal cord interconnect with the ganglionic neurons at the cervical level of the spine. The most prominent of the ganglia is the *dorsal ganglia* where all sensory impulses to the brain and spinal cord pass through. All dorsal ganglia host pseudo-bipolar sensory neurons which are unique because they seemed to have two axons but only one functional unit. One axon transmits sensory stimuli from the periphery of the body while the other pass on the impulses to the spinal cord. Though without synaptic connections, the bipolar neurons transmit impulses to the spinal cord.

There are various "substations" inside the brain and spinal cord where a group of neurons serves as simple relay stations with specific inhibitory or excitatory mechanisms. The spinal cord grey matter has organized islands of neurons called *laminae* with precise functions.

The *cranial nerve nuclei* are a group of neurons that interconnect and participate in cranial nerve functions. The neurons in the thalamus and hypothalamus, on the other hand, have substations named according to their neuroanatomic locations. Examples of the latter are the neurons at the *ventroposterolateral* (VPL) nucleus of the thalamus and *ventrolateral preoptic* (VLPN) nucleus of the hypothalamus.

It will take only a little perseverance, practice, and interest for one to learn the *language of neuroanatomy*.

Chapter I

The Physiology or Mechanism of Neural Transmission

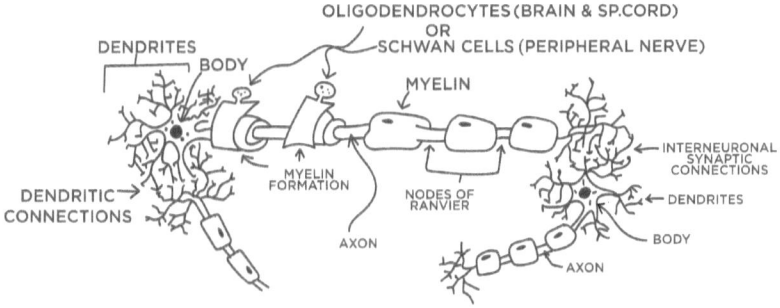

Figure 2. Neuronal structures and dendritic connections that allow transmission of impulses to other neurons and other structures of the body. Cells producing myelin that envelope axons and in between individual myelin are nodes of Ranvier.

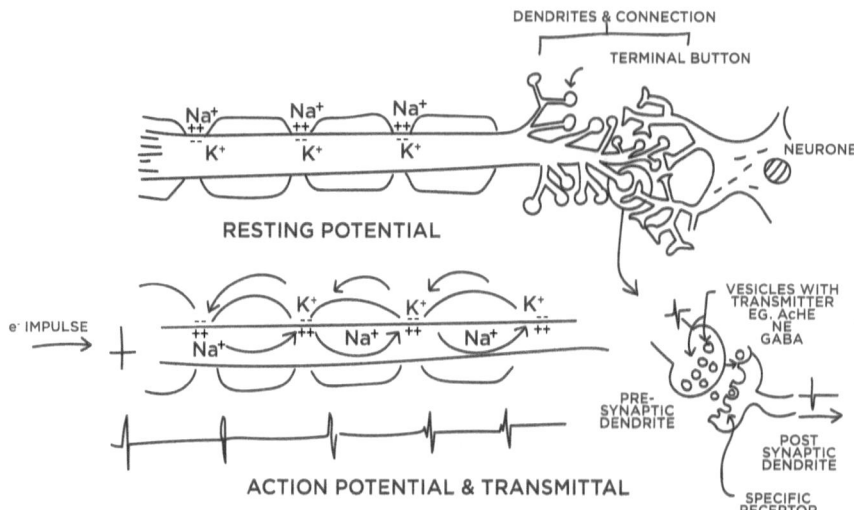

Figure 3. A. Positions of Na+ and K+ at the axonal membrane during resting potential and the negative (-) charge inside and positive (+) charge outside the axon. B. Action potential is marked by shifting of Na+ inside the axon and K+ outside, causing the inside of the axon to become positively charged relative to the negative charge outside. Saltatory conduction of electrical impulses over the myelin and to the nodes of Ranvier (arrows). C. Electrical impulses that reach the terminal pre-synaptic buttons trigger release of transmitters to the post synaptic receptors that results to transfer of impulses and subsequent depolarization.

The leading character in our story is the neuron, the main generator, and a transmitter of electrical impulses in the central nervous system (Fig. 2). The main parts of the neuron are the *body, dendrites, and axon*. The *body* contains the nucleus and organelles which are the main energy source of the neuron. Coming from—and around the walls of the body are several arborized extensions which are called **dendrites,** the receiver of impulses from other neurons or neighboring dendrites. The longest extension or the main arm of the neuron is called the **axon** that transmits impulses and nutrients from the body to its entire length. The axonal lengths vary depending on where it transmits impulses. The nearer the transmission site, the shorter the length. The pyramidal neurons (shaped like the pyramids of Egypt) have the longest axons that extend from the cortex to the last level of the spinal cord. The tip or terminal "buttons" of the axon have fingerlike projections that allow the transmission of electrical impulses to several dendritic receptors of several neurons (Fig. 3). Transmission from one neuronal group to another is just like commuters interconnecting at different subway terminals to reach certain destinations. It is important to appreciate the fact that axonal transmission of impulses is *unidirectional and forward moving*. Also, axons, when bundled as a functional unit in the brain, are called **tracts** and when outside the spinal cord, are called **nerves.** We will use axons interchangeably with tracts or nerves in this book.

How does a living cell, like a neuron, propagate electricity and effect transfer to other neurons? The ordinary electric wire transmits electricity through the inanimate conduction property of the medium which could be copper wire. In live cells, it is riveting and fascinating. There are gates with exclusive locks, doors, and windows in the walls of the axons that allow passive and active entry of chemicals, called ions that will influence conductance. The gates with locks can be likened to specific channels while the windows are like passive pores or doors that need active pumps to open the walls. Shifting movements of chemicals, specifically ions that influence positive or negative charges inside and outside of the axon, create electrical gradients that will determine if there will be conduction of impulses or not. When there is no electrical impulse or at *resting state (Fig. 3, top)*, the axonal wall or membrane keeps the positively charged sodium (Na^+) ion outside along with the negatively charged chloride (Cl^-) ion, while the positively charged potassium (K^+) ion is inside the cell. This gradient maintains a membrane potential of +40 mvolts outside and -60 to -70 mvolts inside the cell. The ionic distribution makes the membrane in a hyperpolarized state. The active process of ion diffusion (likened to windows or pores), K^+ leak channel (like gates), Na^+/K^+ ionic pump (like doors), and carrier protein activities (like doors) determine the polarization of the membrane.

When a propagated electrical discharge from other neurons reaches the axon hillock (the take-off of the axon from the body of the neuron) voltage shift happens. The voltage-gated Na^+ channels (with *electrical potential as the key*), and slow voltage-gated K^+ channel open at the same time. The opening allows entry of Na^+ inside the cell. The result is an increase in positivity, an *action potential or depolarization (Fig. 3, bottom)* that favors transmission of impulses. When the action potential reaches the peak, the voltage-gated Na^+ channel closes while the slow voltage-gated K^+ (potassium) remain open, allowing efflux of K^+ ions that will restore ionic balance in favor of a state of resting potential. This cycle of depolarization and resting state becomes a wave of electrical impulses that is self-propagating, moving forward along the stretch of the axon. As the depolarization waves reach the terminal button, voltage-gated calcium (Ca^{++}) channel opens and allows the pockets of neurotransmitters to go out and interact with receptors of another dendrite, neuron or the muscles. Electrical impulses, therefore, are waves of depolarization transferred to another neuron or muscles upon reaching the synapse. **Pre-synapse** refers to the terminal button while **post-synapse** refers to the receiver of the transmitter.

Neurotransmitters bind at the postsynaptic receptors of dendrites, axons of another group of neurons or receptors of the muscles at the neuromuscular junction. The receptors have very specific or exclusive ligand-gated channels that bind neurotransmitters *(the key to the gate this time is the ligand, a signaling molecule)* and allow specific ions to enter the cell. The type of neurotransmitter will determine if the transmission shall continue or stop (excitatory or inhibitory effect). Neurotransmitter gamma-aminobutyric acid (GABA) ligand-gated channel opens specifically to chloride (Cl), allowing negativity inside the cell, causing inhibition. Glutamine neurotransmitter, on the other hand, opens the ionotropic glutamate channel that allows K^+ and Na^+ passage, causing excitation. The neurotransmitters either block (e.g., GABA) or facilitate transmission (e.g., Norepinephrine or

Acetylcholine). Aside from neurotransmitter-ligand channels coupling, another system operates that would determine the transmission behavior of the cell; this is the coupling with G protein-receptors. The Nobel Prize for Chemistry in 2012 was awarded to Robert Lefkowitz and Brian Kobilka, who detailed the characteristics of G protein-coupled receptors (GPCRs) and described how they interacted with intracellular G protein to create specific intra-cellular behavior [4,5]. These receptors are GPCR doors that open only to a particular key or neurotransmitter. When the door opens, a prolonged process, that may take days of excitation or inhibition, occurs when the neurotransmitter-GPCR couplings interact with intracellular G protein. This slow process invites intriguing speculation that this mechanism might be operant in the storage of information, like storage of memory perhaps and potential sites for therapeutic interventions.

If a wave of action potentials happens, the rate by which it would reach distant targets will still be of creeping speed. So how do electrical impulses travel super-fast?

Schwann Cells of the peripheral nerves and Oligodendrocytes of the brain and spinal cords produce the lipid myelin sheaths that wrapped or enveloped the individual axons in their entire length. The interval of myelin formation made by each Schwann cell or Oligodendrocyte can be likened to train cars connected in series. Myelin serves as an insulator to the entire axonal length. The exposed portions of the axons between myelin are called Nodes of Ranvier (Fig. 2). These bare portions possess voltage-gated channels. This unique arrangement allows electrical impulses to jump on top of the myelin, creating a saltatory or "jumping" conduction of impulses, making transmission faster and efficient (Fig. 3). The speed of conduction depends on the thickness of the myelin. The thicker the myelin, the faster the conduction. The myelin can be affected by diseases and are called, in general, **demyelinating diseases.** The most common of which is multiple sclerosis for brain myelin and polyradiculitis (Guillain-Barre Syndrome) for demyelination of peripheral nerve.

The past two decades have provided us with a better understanding of the functions and molecular structures of the different channels and the ion shifts during electrical conduction of impulses. Correspondingly, more old and new drugs are being discovered to work on the various channels. The earlier medicine against epilepsy, hydantoin, is now known to block sodium channel shifts to prevent seizures while the newer pregabalin is known to block the function of synaptic Ca channels to prevent the release of glutamine in the synapse to control neuropathic pain or to control seizures.

Chapter II

General Anatomy of the Central Nervous System

The *meninges,* which consist of three layers of thick membranous *dura mater* and thin *arachnoid mater and pia mater,* cover the central nervous system until the exit of the nerves. The *pia mater* covers the brain and the penetrating parenchymal vessels (Fig. 4 D). The *arachnoid mater* lies just underneath the *dura mater,* creating a thin *subdural space.* In between the *arachnoid mater* and the *pia mater* is the *subarachnoid space* consisting of cerebrospinal fluid (CSF) and thin attaching fibers called the **trabeculae.** The *dura mater* extends down to the exit of the roots of the peripheral nerves where the external covering changes into *epineurium.*

The major divisions of the central nervous system are the brain or cortex; the brain stem or the trunk which is subdivided into midbrain, pons, and medulla; the cerebellum or the flower; the spinal cord; and the peripheral nerves or the roots that contain efferent motor impulses, afferent sensory impulses and autonomic neural functions (Fig. 4 A & B). On a cross section of the brain, each side will show cerebrospinal fluid-filled triangular-shaped cylinder that runs parallel to the anterior and posterior extent of the cerebrum (Fig. 4 C). These cylinders are called lateral ventricles which will be elaborated when we talk about the cerebrospinal fluid circulation in Chapter 12. The bodies of the neurons are in the gray matter beneath the brain's corrugation or gyri and at various gray islands in the middle areas of the brain, like the basal ganglia, thalamus, and others.

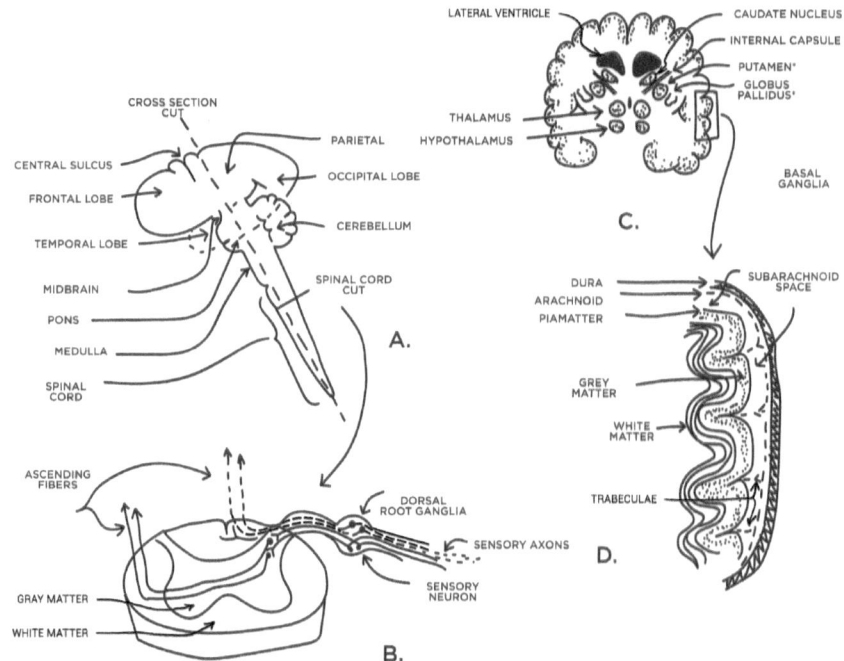

Figure 4. A. Main structures of the central nervous system (CNS). B. Spinal dorsal ganglia and spinal cord connections and sensory ascending fibers. C. Coronal section showing cortical and subcortical structures. D. Three layers of coverings of the CNS and the subarachnoid space.

The butterfly-like gray matter map of the spinal cord also have bodies of neurons. The axons and dendrites are colored cream-white, and their extensions and paths are called the white matter. The gray matter contains relay-neurons that receive or transmit electrical impulses. The white matter consists of "wires" or axons that connect with or arising from the gray matter neurons.

There are neurons outside the spinal cord and the brain that transmit sensations, from many parts of the body and head to neuronal stations in the spinal cord and brain stem respectively that would eventually reach the brain. The dorsal ganglia which are outside the spinal cord houses pseudo-bipolar type of neurons. The neurons do not possess two axons but a single transmitting axon that extends from the sensory receptors in the body to the spinal cord. These dorsal ganglia neurons transmit sensory impulses from the entire body to the neuronal stations in the spinal cord (Fig. 4 B). The neurons outside the brainstem that transmit specialized sensations of smell, taste, hearing, and seeing have their ganglia located near their origin at the skull or head. The nerves that transmit specialized sensations are classified cranial sensory nerves.

The central nervous system admittedly is very complex as it consists of groups of neurons with different functions or purposes and with various circuitries and interconnections. It is, however, mesmerizing to know that it is systematically organized to allow us to identify predictable and repeatable activities which results to a significant degree of uniformity of functions among individuals. This bewildering characteristic will be explored, simplified, and dealt with in this book.

Now that you can visualize how electrical impulses are generated and transmitted, we will now strip them into different functional organizations, or pluck them out from the circuitry, station to station and tract by tract.

Chapter III

The Descending Motor or Pyramidal Tract System

Imagine the routines that we do upon waking up in the morning. We stretch our arms, walk to the bathroom, shower, reach for the shampoo, scrub it over the hair, dry and rub the towel to many directions. We dress up, walk fast to the dining table, reach for and sip the coffee or juice, pour cereals to a bowl of milk, use the spoon and fork to mix them and bring them to the mouth. After breakfast, brush the teeth, then start walking or driving to class or work. Let us stop for a second! Did we ever ask ourselves how it was possible to do all these actions? There are several facets of the nervous system at work here, but we will be conscious only about the movements of the muscles. Where do the actions begin?

The **"little man,"** or **homunculus** [6] is a motor and sensory representation of the human body in the brain that roughly corresponds to the group of neurons at the pre-central gyrus. These motor neurons innervate the corresponding muscles of the body parts. The sensations from various parts of the body that reach the brain have an almost similar body organization at the post-central gyri. (Fig. 5 A).

The *motor or pyramidal neurons* (named as such because they are like the shape of the Pyramids of Egypt) are the initiators of muscle movements. These neurons lie beneath the strip of gray matter called *pre-central gyrus,* and they are arranged approximately to represent specific muscular parts of the body as drawn in the *homunculus model.*

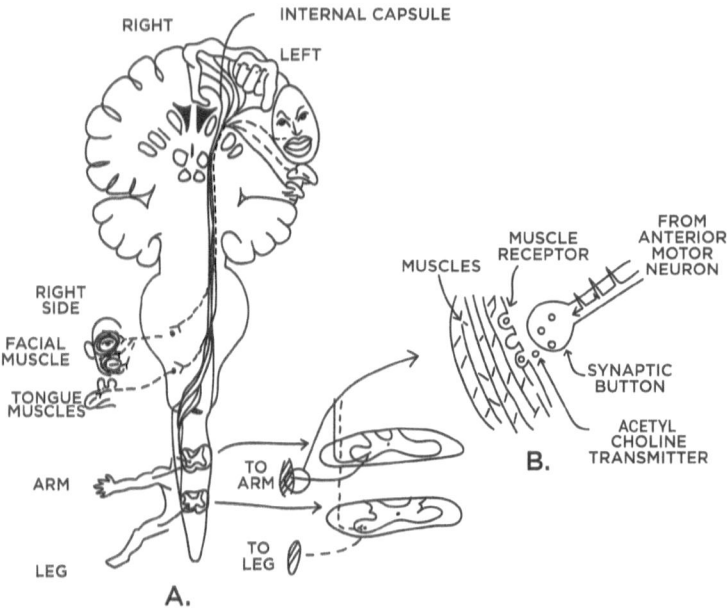

Figure 5. The Pyramidal Tract System. A. The *homunculus* representing pyramidal motor neuronal distribution at the precentral gyrus. Motor neurons send descending and mostly crossing long axons that synapse with opposite motor cells of the brainstem and anterior horn cells of the spinal cord. Subsequently these neurons in turn transmit impulses to the muscle receptors. B. *Neuromuscular junction* where transmitters at the synaptic buttons are released to the muscle receptors after electrical impulses (sharp waves) reach the neuronal terminal.

Try to remember this figure because it tells you which part of the brain is initiating the movements that you are executing. The pyramidal neurons extend their axons all the way to the brainstem and different levels of the spinal cord, making them the neurons with the longest axons in the body. Let us trace the axons as they descend from the cortex. The descending axons of all the pyramidal neurons merge tightly to form the **internal capsule.** The axons continue to descend anteriorly through the brainstem, the so-called, "trunk of the brain." It is here that the descending *axons for the facial and tongue muscles separate from the main bulk to decussate or cross to the opposite side* just before reaching the first station. Connecting motor neurons at the first station will transfer the signals originating from the brain to the muscles of the face and tongue, and because these body parts are in the head, these brainstem neurons are called **cranial nerve motor neurons** for the face and tongue. The rest of the uncrossed axons *(for the rest of the body muscles)* continue to descend until they reach the medulla or the end of the brainstem where the main bulk of the axons cross to the opposite side. Now the crossed axons will continue their way down to synapse with the first station of the motor neurons at various levels of the anterior horn of the spinal cord. Whew! Can you imagine one microscopic thin axon extended this long? It is therefore easy to imagine that the pyramidal axons are vulnerable to diseases or injuries from the brain down to the spinal cord.

Before we continue, let us digest first what we have traced so far. First, the bodies of the neurons are arranged in the gray matter of the pre-motor or pre-central gyrus of the cortex and are arrayed according to the body part location as shown in the homunculus. Second, their axons descend, maintaining an anatomic position as they merge tightly at the internal capsule. Third, as the tracts continue downwards, the face and tongue axons separate from the group to cross before they reach the first station of the corresponding brainstem motor nucleus, while the rest of the axons continue to descend and cross only at the tip of the brain stem (medulla). The crossed-tracts keep the descent to the different spinal cord stations. We have just traced the **cortico-spinal pathway** or the **pyramidal tract**.

Clinical application: The crossing fibers explains why the control to the face and limbs comes from the opposite precentral gyrus. When one has a stroke or another lesion in the *left* internal capsule, one can very well have weakness on the *right* side of the body that includes the right face and tongue muscles.

Let us now look at the first station. It is in this station where the descending pyramidal axons connect with spinal motor neurons at the anterior horn. The spinal motor neurons, in turn, send axons outside the spinal cord as part of the peripheral nerve and at its tips are several finger-like **terminal buttons** or **pre-synapses.** Terminal buttons insert at **muscle receptors or post-synaptic receptors** which are socket-like receptors in the muscles. Varied chemicals or neurotransmitters are released from the pre-synapse and bind with specific muscle receptors (Fig. 5B). The spaces between the synapse and the muscle receptors are called **neuromuscular junctions (NMJ).** When propagated electrical impulses reach the synapse, the neurotransmitters (acetylcholine) inside the vesicles are released to the neuromuscular junction and bind with specific acetylcholine receptors of the muscles. These bindings trigger corresponding chemical and channel shifts that cause fascinating actions of the muscle microfibers seen as a contraction of the muscles. The terminal button's release of neurotransmitters at the NMJ and the binding of the neurotransmitters with the muscle receptors is how electrical signals from the brain reach the muscles to cause muscular contractions. Some diseases can affect specifically these muscle receptors, and the manifestation is a weakness. One typical example is Myasthenia Gravis. **Myasthenia Gravis (MG)** is an autoimmune disease (immune reaction attacking our own body parts) where antibodies attack the muscle receptors (which generally are supposed to protect them). The thymus gland produces the antibodies. Thymectomy or removal of the thymus gland is done commonly in the treatment of MG. The destruction of the muscle receptors fails neurotransmitter-receptor binding, thereby causing motor weakness or fatigue.

The NMJ event, just described, is the final pathway or the story of how the pyramidal neurons move the arms, forearms, hands, and fingers to be able to do many of our morning routines. If we use the right hand to reach out for something, the generated act comes from the left or opposite side of the brain. Got it? Now you know that your morning activities involve the movement of muscles that is initiated from the pre-central motor cortex of the brain. Isn't this interesting?

Case Story:

Engineer Santos was a 50-year-old dedicated manager of an automobile company. He was a very busy person who kept on forgetting his medicine for hypertension and never even considered having his blood pressure checked in the clinic. One day, while having lunch with co-workers, his left hand suddenly became limp, unable to hold the fork while his body started to lean toward the left side. His panicky sentences were so slurred that he could not be understood. When he was about to fall to the left, he was caught by his seatmate just in time. Witnesses claimed that his left leg could not move at all. His companions immediately brought him to a nearby hospital where his blood pressure was found to be very high at 220/110, and CT Scan ordered, showed twenty cubic centimeters of hematoma at the right internal capsule.

Clinical – anatomic Correlation

The most common manifestation of injury to the motor system is weakness or **paresis** and if there is absence of movement, **paralysis**. Disease conditions that involve any of the parts of the pyramidal tract, like the pyramidal neurons, their axons, and myelin; terminal buttons or receptors; spinal motor neurons and their axons (peripheral nerves); and the muscles, can manifest a varied degree of weakness. If the disease affects the motor system *diffusely*, the manifestation is a generalized or bilateral weakness of various degrees. If a *focal* area of the system is involved, like a stroke at the internal capsule (as what happened to Engr. Santos), the expression is a *focal* weakness or hemiparesis at the opposite side of the body. **Focal lesions** involving the central nervous system manifest the symptoms in the body that it correspondingly innervates. **Diffuse or generalized** disease involvement of the brain produces more symptoms than focal lesions to the brain. For example, diffuse brain neuronal involvement could be due to hypoglycemic encephalopathy (involving the entire brain) manifesting as a change in sensorium, cognitive impairment, and generalized weakness. The tempo of the disease manifestations will also provide important clues about the cause of the disease. The acute or sudden left-sided weakness experienced by Engr. Santos is highly suggestive of a stroke – "the weakness appeared like a stroke of lightning." A gradual and progressive right-sided weakness, on the other hand, is indicative of a slow focal involvement of the pyramidal tract at the opposite side of the brain that is often caused by a slow growing mass. The clinical expression of affectations of the pyramidal neurons is not all weakness – a "negative" manifestation. Pyramidal neurons can be electrically irritated by focal diseases, like a mass, expressed as a focal seizure -- a "positive" manifestation. A focal seizure manifest as uncontrollable tonic extensions or tonic-clonic contraction of the muscles of the limbs brought about by electrical discharges coming from the contralateral pyramidal neurons of the pre-motor cortex. Generalized seizures are indicative of uncontrolled electrical discharges involving diffusely the brain manifested as muscle contractions or stiffening of all extremities associated with loss of consciousness and upward rolling of the eyeballs. This episode is a convulsion.

The neurological examination of this system aims at eliciting the presence of weakness and, if present, their distribution; eliciting reflexes and abnormal distribution; and estimating muscle tone. The degree of weakness can be graded at the bedside by this common clinical measure: 0/5 - no movement; 1/5 - trace or flicker of movement; 2/5 - movement is present but unable to raise and overcome the effect of gravity; 3/5 - movement with enough strength to overcome the effect of gravity; 4/5 - movement possible even against mild resistance; 5/5 - normal. Dr. Joseph Babinski discovered that when the lateral aspect of the sole is stroked with a blunt instrument and applying just enough pressure, an "upward movement (extension) of the toe and digits" is elicited when the *pyramidal system is affected above the termination* of the spinal motor neurons (Fig. 6-B). After more than a hundred years, the **Babinski sign** survived the test of time while its mechanism remains an enigma [7, 8]. This sign can be seen generally in infants till two years old and if present after this age, investigation of its cause is warranted. Aside from the Babinski sign, pyramidal tract involvement may also cause an increase in muscle tone *(spasticity)* and cause *clonus* to appear. Flexing the foot suddenly can elicit clonus, and if it is present, a sustained unidirectional flexion-extension tremor or flapping movement can be appreciated (Fig. 6-A). Tapping the patellar joint tendon or knee joint can trigger a knee-jerk. Hyperreflexia is an exaggerated or increased knee-jerk response often associated with

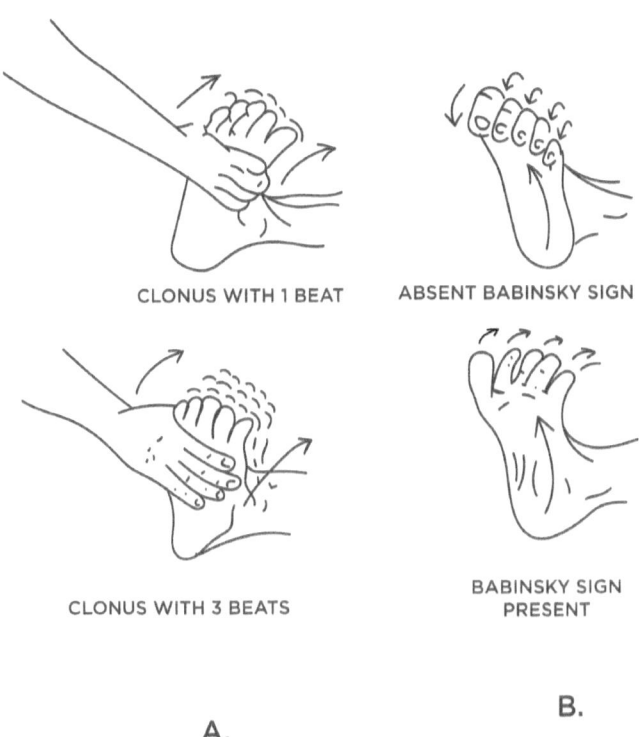

Figure 6. Some features of upper motor neuron signs compared to normal responses. A. Clonus. B. Babinski sign.

increased tone. These are termed **Upper Motor Neuron signs** because the pyramidal tract involvement is *above* the second and fourth lumbar spinal motor level of the spinal cord, the level tested in tapping the knee joint.

Can you predict what will be the neurological examination result of Engr. Santos? There will be a 0/5 left-sided hemiplegia with left facial weakness. Babinski sign will appear on the left. Left-sided hyperreflexia, increased muscle tone and clonus could be seen but sometime may not appear immediately until more than a month from the onset of stroke.

Chapter IV

The Nociceptive Pain and Associated Spinothalamic Tracts

Have you experienced stepping on a burning cigarette butt while frolicking in the beach? Imagine how fast you felt it and how quickly you could lift that foot. This time, pinch yourself at the forearm to cause pain. Did you feel it? How many types of pain did you experience? Imagine if a hated person pinches you with the same degree and location, will you feel the same way? Is pain a friend or a foe?

The external environment provides zillions and infinitesimal good and bad stimuli many of which are picked up by our body senses. The ascending sensory system, including the nociceptive anterolateral spinothalamic tracts, is just one of the body responders necessary for survival.

All parts of our body have sensors specific for different types of stimuli like temperature, touch, pain, vibration, stretch, position in space (a way of feeling where your feet are relative to the ground). We also have special sensors for vision, hearing, taste, and smell that we will cover separately. We will describe first the sensation of pain, a vital and common sensory function that warns and informs us of potential injury or tells us of the presence of a disease.

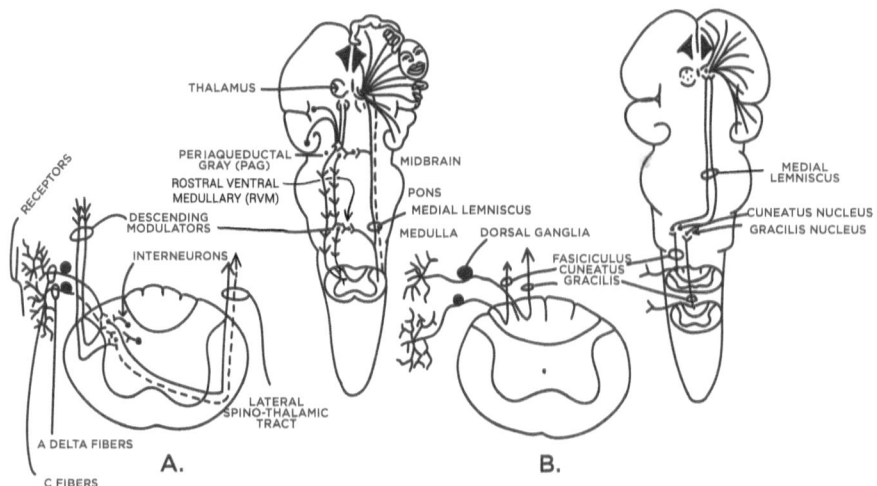

Figure 7. A. Pain (nociceptive), temperature and touch fibers ascending to thalamus where impulses are distributed to the sensory homunculus. Note ascending fibers giving off connections to the descending modulators at the brainstem (arrow line). Cortical and subcortical gray send impulses also to the descending modulators. Descending modulators and interneurons inhibit posterior gray nociceptive neurons. B. Vibratory and position sense fibers ascending through the posterior column and crossing at medulla then to thalamus and cortex.

The nerves that transmit impulses, perceived as pain by the brain, are called **nociceptive fibers** (transmitter of noxious stimuli). Nociceptive sensors that pick-up sensations are distributed in the skin, muscles, tendons, joints, blood vessels, stomach, intestines, and so many other places of the body. These dispersed *sensors are finger-like and thread-like* tips of the axons from pseudo-bipolar neurons that transmit impulses to the neurons of the spinal cord. The pseudo bipolar neurons are located at the dorsal ganglia (Fig. 7-A). The types of nerves that transmit nociceptive stimuli to the spinal cord are **C-fibers and A-delta fibers.** The thinly myelinated C-fibers convey noxious stimuli slowly while the thicker A-delta fibers transmit faster (try to recall the nodes of Ranvier and saltatory conduction of impulses because of the myelin). What is the importance of this? The rapid A-delta transmission allows one to immediately feel the burning cigarette butt, and enable the brain to sense it quickly, and integrates these with the neighboring pyramidal or motor neurons to do something fast and send impulses back down to the muscles to pull the foot from further damage – a defensive mechanism to lessen or avoid tissue injury. Pinch yourself. You will notice and feel two distinct pain sensations. The first is the immediate perception of sharp pain from the stimulus followed a little later by a stinging sensation that lingers. The rapidly- transmitting A-delta myelinated nociceptive fibers convey impulses that explains the instantaneous pain. The lingering sting felt, a hypersensitive area around the injury (hyperalgesia), is transmitted by the C fibers that carry impulses to the second station -- at the posterior horn of the spinal cord. The noxious stimuli eventually will reach the third station of the thalamus [9,10]. It is essential to understand that the neurons at the thalamus distribute the noxious impulses to the limbic system, which is the seat of emotion, and to many areas of the brain for cognition, thus making the noxious stimuli experienced as pain. *Pain is laden with emotion and cognition.*

Pain perception is a gift because it warns us of further injury. It is a gift and not a foe [11]. Lepers lose the sense of pain (anesthesia) in the toes or fingers because the organism, Mycobacterium leprae, propagate inside Schwan cells of the peripheral nerves, destroying the sensation transmitting peripheral nerves. The absence of pain sensation may eventually cause unsightly severance of the toes because of unfelt recurrent injuries or wounds! These ghastly injuries are rare nowadays because of education and advances in the treatment of leprosy. Diabetic neuropathy and vasculopathy have taken over as common causes of lamentable amputation in the modern world.

As you can recall, the C-fibers and A-delta fibers are collectively called **nociceptive fibers**. Impulses from the nociceptive sensors are then transmitted to the neurons at the dorsal ganglia, making this as the *first station*. The extended axons then transmit further the impulses to the *second station* which is the posterior gray nociceptive neurons of the spinal cord (Fig. 7-A.). *Not all harmful pulses reached the brain and perceived as pain.* Important and intriguing activities happen in the second station because it is here where interconnecting influences with neighboring neurons or descending axons from the brainstem will determine if nociceptive impulses will pass through and ascend eventually to the brain (Fig. 7-A). Some nociceptive impulses going to the spinal cord separate and stimulate interneurons (GABA interneurons). These interneurons which are inhibitory, in turn, block the nociceptive neurons in the posterior gray matter of the spinal cord. Descending axonal neurons (descending modulators) from brainstem "non-pain" neuronal groups also prevent the transmission of nociceptive impulses at the spinal posterior gray. Therefore, GABA interneurons and descending brainstem influences are potential blockers of noxious transmission at the spinal cord level. It is important to note that the brainstem "non-pain" neuronal groups that send descending inhibition to the posterior gray of the spinal cord, themselves, can be blocked by other brainstem neurons. When blocking happens, the descending inhibition stops favoring transmission of nociceptive impulses at the spinal cord. The second station at the spinal cord is like a "battleground" of nociceptive impulses and blockers: this is the Gate Control Theory for the transmission of pain [12, 13]. If there is a successful transmission, the spinal nociceptive neurons with its crossing axons will transmit impulses to the opposite white matter where the fibers ascend as the *anterolateral spinothalamic tract.*

Let us digest this again before we proceed. When the dorsal ganglia neurons connect and transmit nociceptive impulses to the spinal neurons at the posterior gray matter, successful transmission of impulses happens only after overcoming the blocking effect of the GABA interneurons within the area and the blocking effect of descending axons from the "non-pain" neurons of the brain stem. Why is understanding of this concept essential? It is necessary because this concept tells us that not all nociceptive sensations are transmitted and reach the brain. Otherwise, we will be living a life in continuous pain. Another importance of understanding this concept is that drugs that control pain work by influencing the blockers or enhancers of pain in this area. A good example is the analgesic opiate drugs that block specific receptors at the second station of the spinal cord resulting in the prevention of the release of nociceptive transmitters, Substance P transmitters.

The axons of the dorsal ganglia neurons will synapse one to two levels with the neurons of the posterior grey horn and if there is a successful transmission of nociceptive impulses, the neurons from this second station will send axons to the opposite side and start its ascent as an anterolateral spinothalamic tract. (Notice the term which tells one where the axon will terminate). This crossing means that if certain diseases or injuries affect the left side of the eighth thoracic level (T8) of the spinal cord, there will be loss of pain sensation at T8 level on the left side (same side of the lesion) and T9-T10 at the opposite right side, about 1-2 levels lower than the left.

Let us follow the ascending nociceptive fibers. The ascending nociceptive fibers have long tracts that reach the thalamus but some exit and connect with "non-pain neurons" in the brainstem. These non-pain neurons are at the Periaqueductal Gray Neurons (PAG), at the Rostral Ventral Medullary Neurons (RVM), and at various brainstem substations. These brainstem neurons receive inhibitory or excitatory impulses from the nociceptive fibers or other neighboring neurons and *even from the brain*. These non-pain neuronal connections are important because these neurons influence pain perception through their descending axons that release inhibitory transmitters to the nociceptive neurons at the second station of the spinal cord, the "battleground" or "Gate control area." We have just described a *long loop reflex* mechanism that moderates pain transmission (Fig. 7-A). These brainstem neurons are also target areas for pain control drugs.

It is now clear that there are two group of neurons that can influence nociceptive transmission, and these are: a) GABA inhibitory interneurons and b) Brainstem non-pain neurons (PAG, RVM, and others) through their descending inhibitory impulses. Can you imagine the ordeal one would experience if these reflexes do not modulate the pain?

Let us trace the nociceptive fibers to the thalamus. Majority of the ascending nociceptive fibers pass through the brainstem as Medial Lemniscus fibers (ML) and connect with Ventroposterolateral (VPL) and Ventroposteroinferior (VPI) thalamic nociceptive neurons. The receiving neuronal groups in the thalamus is the *third station*. These thalamic nociceptive neurons will, in turn, transmit the impulses to two areas of the brain. The first is the Postcentral gyrus which has its homunculus sensory representation. The second consists of the diffuse neurons of the limbic system and their projections and the frontal lobe. The limbic system is a complex system that influences emotion, behavior, motivation, memory, the autonomic nervous system, and the endocrine system. Nociceptive impulses are *experienced as pain* when they reach the different parts of the brain.

Clinical – anatomic Correlation:

The termination of the thalamic nociceptive neuronal axons in the postcentral gray neurons will explain how people can point the location of pain is in the body. The diffuse projections of the thalamic nociceptive neurons, particularly to the limbic system and the frontal lobes, allow the perception of the noxious stimuli as pain, an emotional and cognitive experience. The International Association for the Studies of Pain, define **pain** as an *unpleasant sensory and emotional experience associated with actual or potential tissue damage or describes pain regarding such damage* [14]. The definition means that pain has emotional but underemphasized cognitive components. Many factors (emotional state, finances, loss, spirituality, religious beliefs, etc.) can influence the physiology of pain that impact on their perception and expression. It is for these reasons that most recently, the redefinition of pain is, "*a distressing experience associated with actual or potential tissue damage with sensory, emotional, cognitive and social components* [15]". Tachycardia, dilatation of the pupils and pallor, autonomic sympathetic expression can accompany pain perception. When all these emotional, cognitive, social and other factors are taken into consideration together with physiologic responses in the experience of pain, we call this **Total Pain concept** [16], an idea that one should always remember when evaluating and managing pain. The total pain concept explains why a girl friend's pinch does not feel as bad as the pinch made by a person you hate.

Case Story:

Julia, a 78-year-old widow, who completed a course of radiation for cervical cancer was referred to a hospice team for unrelieved pain despite multiple drug treatments which included three opiate drugs. The hospice team saw her two months after radiation treatment. The patient was dressed appropriately, her beddings were clean, and there were no signs of bed sores. She lied with the thighs flexed and tightly closed. She looked much sedated, almost moribund, but opened her eyes briefly on shaking and on calling her name. A gentle effort to open her legs elicited a distressing moan which triggered verbal concerns from the daughters. Laboratories and imaging studies were all reviewed. Sometimes she was noted to be a little awake, and a little conversant just before the scheduled opiate medicines were to be given, providing an opportunity for the head of the hospice service to whisper to the patient the need to do an internal examination with a promise that the procedure will be gentle and in private. On physical examination, there was an initial resistance and moan, but after a reassuring prodding, the legs opened allowing internal pelvic inspection. The findings revealed local post-irradiation inflammation and very foul-smelling odor that covered the entire room. The leader of the team concluded that the physical results and imaging studies could not explain the pain elicited when the leg was touched. The family described the patient to be sweet, prim and proper. A glamorous lady who was very conscious of the way she dressed and behaved. She loved to play the piano and organ for the choir and hosted small gatherings with friends. The team explained to the family and gently to the patient that the bothersome odor was due to an infection and treatment shall commence. Appropriate treatment treated the foul-smelling discharge entirely. The opiate medications were gradually decreased and subsequently discontinued. She survived for seven more years during which time she enjoyed the company of family and friends and continued to play the piano.

Clinical – anatomic Correlation

Was the patient experiencing pain? Why was it not relieved by multiple pain medicines, including opiate drugs? The team concluded that she had localized pain because of the post-irradiation inflammation with secondary infection. The moaning associated with every movement of the left leg that bothered the patient was more of an expression of embarrassment and an effort to contain the distressing odor coming from the perineum. Her personality and dignity could not accept the "social pain" elicited by the embarrassing odor. Failure to identify factors that could influence the expression of pain can lead to an erroneous conclusion of non-response to pain treatment that may, in turn, lead to an escalation of drug dose. This case emphasizes that in the total pain concept, many factors other than the physical nature of pain can influence the approach and management of pain.

General Classification of Pain:

Julia was suffering from pain due to post-irradiation inflammation and infection in the perineum which is an example of the somatic type of pain. **Somatic pain** is felt typically in the area of injuries or diseases involving the skin, muscles, tendons, and bones. **Visceral pain** is felt after injuries or illnesses affecting the internal organs like the heart, lungs, gastrointestinal tracts, and genitourinary tract. The characteristic of visceral pain is that it is poorly localized and may even feel distant from the area of the disease; this is called **referred pain**. The pain experienced in injury or ischemia to the heart, like a heart attack or angina pectoris, may be felt at the left shoulder or the left jaw. The distribution of the pain, however, is around the area of the organ involved but poorly localized.

Neuropathic type of pain may develop when the peripheral nerve or the central nervous system is injured or affected by diseases. The distribution of the pain is along the neuroanatomic innervation of the involved nervous system. The pain is often described as spontaneous, varied in intensity, and a combination of tingling and fine needle pinches or lightning-like episodes. A perfect example is shingles or herpes zoster infection. The disease involves the dorsal ganglia and corresponding nerves innervating a region of the body. It can affect any part of the body on one side. The inflammatory eruptions of pox vesicles may appear along the T4 to T6 regional distribution of the dorsal ganglia (dermatomal distribution) on either the right or the left side. The distribution is approximately a band-like pain area from the nipple-line to the line at the tip of the sternum. Pain is experienced at the height of herpetic infection or days after the infection, as **post-herpetic neuralgia.**

Temperature, mechanical and chemical sensations have similar receptors and follow the same spinothalamic ascending pathways used by nociceptive fibers. Their interconnections may differ, but their terminations are in nearby post-central gyrus, perhaps allowing needed interactions of neurons with other areas of the brain. The adjacent location is probably for practical reasons. Burning cigarette butt, when stepped upon while barefoot, elicit excruciating pain, but the stimulus is extreme heat or thermal sensation. Warm soup can similarly be felt through the same system but not felt as pain because perhaps the thermal stimulus is not enough to be perceived as pain by the brain. The chemical receptors can be activated by inflammatory mediators when there are musculoskeletal injuries. When somebody hits you solidly in the face, there is an immediate mechanically mediated pain, but when swelling and inflammation set in, a chemically mediated pain comes into the picture.

Neurological examination for pain sensation starts by inspecting the area where there is pain and looking for signs of inflammation like swelling, reddish discoloration, and hematoma. Ask the patient what movements or conditions trigger the discomfort. With the permission and cooperation of the patient, gentle maneuvers are made to test the reproducibility of symptoms based on the different functions of structures that might explain the pain. An example is a movement of joints in and around the area of pain, like rotating the leg to elicit pain at the hip joint in suspected arthritis, sprain, dislocation, or fracture. In a herniated disc, if the protrusion is toward the vertebral foramen, pressure on the exiting nerve may be the cause of the pain. Leg raising test which stretches the pressed nerve can reproduce the pain along the area of its dermatomal distribution. Test the suspected area of the pain for other sensory changes by using a pin and a brush one at a time. With the eyes covered, gently apply the sharp object or if using a brush, stroke lightly the areas of interest; then ask the patient to compare the sensation on both sides and describe the differences in perception if there are any. For the temperature sensation test, the patient is told to identify which is cold or warm when applied along the dermatomal areas. When the nociceptive tracts are affected by a lesion, the manifestation is subjective numbness, and one may elicit different degrees of loss of pain sensation from a pinprick and touch with brush strokes.

Chapter V

The Other Ascending Sensory Fibers

One beautiful sunny morning, while walking in the park, you noticed the smooth pavement changed to a rough multicolored clay tiles and bricks causing you to trip a little, but a rapid adaptation to the new surface allowed the stroll to continue, oblivious of the "balancing" that your body made and the change in your gait. Then entering a theater, the light was suddenly turned off signaling the start of the show. A little bit distressed and unsure of your steps, you stopped and groped for the theater wall. Once the vision adapted to the darkness, you walked but this time with insecure movements and frantic intention to get to a seat. All these actions have a lot of motor participation; but what is noticeable in the first situation are the efforts of the body to maintain fluid movements and balance and in the second situation, the adjustments made while walking in the dark theater, the vision removed. The participation of visual orientation in movements was described and emphasized and was demonstrated by the change in the gait when lights were put off. Removing the influence of optical compensation allows examination of proprioceptive sensation. During the test, the eyes of the patients are closed or blindfolded

The ascending posterior column of the spinal cord transmit the *discriminatory sensations* to the brain. It participates actively in the fluidity of motion and adjustments of the body to different tasks during walking. Some of discriminatory sensations relevant in clinical practice are vibratory sensation, proprioception, position sense, and two-point discrimination. The posterior column that conveys vibratory sensation feeds the muscle spindles that participate in a reflex to keep the tone of the muscles in a "readiness state" that will facilitate muscle contraction—a function essential in rapid muscle movement adjustments associated with posturing when compensating for imbalance. The tuning fork is used to test for vibratory sensation. By letting the patient identify reverberating sensation from a tuning fork applied to various parts of the body is as a way of assessing the functional condition of the posterior column. The posterior column similarly transmit *proprioceptive sensation*. This sensation makes one aware of one's body parts about space. Test proprioception by letting the patient describe, while blinded if the distal digits are being flexed or extended. The maneuver is called *position test*. Proprioceptive sensation allows us to estimate the position of the feet to the floor to allow quick adjustments to maintain smooth, fluid and well-coordinated walking. *Graphesthesia* is another form of discriminatory sensation that enables one to identify numbers written in the palm. *Stereognosis*, is the ability to identify geometrical shapes of objects like the key, coin, cloth texture and recognize rough or pebbled or smooth surfaces. These discriminatory sensations can be disturbed not only with lesions in the posterior column and its ascending pathways but in the parietal cortex too. The parietal lobe participation tells us that much of the motor actions that we do are with wide cortical involvement though we are not much aware of it.

    The peripheral axonal fibers that transmit discriminatory sensory impulses to the spinal cord are the larger fibers, the *Alpha fibers*. The dorsal ganglion neuron, at the *first station*, sends axons to the spinal cord (dorsal column) that will mostly ascend directly to the brainstem's medulla (Fig. 7-B). Note that most of the fibers have *no synaptic connections* at the posterior spinal gray matter. The group of ascending axons is called **fasciculus gracilis** at the lowest level of the spinal cord while the axons that enter in the middle of the spinal cord ascend as **fasciculus cuneatus**. These gracilis and cuneatus axons then synapse with the neurons at the *second station*, the **nucleus gracilis** and **nucleus cuneatus** of the medulla (same root name, easy to remember). The neurons of the gracilis nucleus and cuneatus nucleus at the second station of the medulla, in turn, send their *axons to the opposite side* to join the spinothalamic fibers at the medial lemniscus (ML). The crossed axons then synapse with the neurons at the *third station* or the ventroposterolateral (VPL) nucleus of the thalamus. There are a few branches from the ascending fibers that synapse with the neurons of the spinal posterior gray neurons, and these reflex mechanisms will be discussed when we cover the chapter on the spinal cord.

Let us rest and recapitulate. 1. The nerves for discriminatory sensations are larger and named alpha fibers. 2. The second station is not in the spinal cord but high in the medulla of the brainstem. 3. The first station or the dorsal ganglia neurons from the lower half of the body, send axons to the posterior column of the white matter, as fasciculus gracilis. The ascending fasciculus gracilis is joined later by axons from the upper half of the trunk, as fasciculus cuneatus. 4. The second station is at the medulla where the gracilis and cuneatus nuclei are located still on the same side. 5. The gracilis and cuneatus nuclei send axons *across at the level of the medulla* where they then ascend as a bundle of axons to join the spinothalamic nociceptive fibers at the *medial lemniscus*. 6. These crossed axons then connect or synapse with the VPL nucleus of the thalamus, this is the third station.

Case Story:

Melissa is a 32-year-old music teacher who loves to sing and play the piano, noted slight difficulty walking upon waking up one morning, "I was exerting more effort to walk and direct myself to where I was going." As days passed by, her legs remained strong but clumsy when walking and claimed that she was able to walk better by looking at her steps. There was a mild patch of numbness involving the lateral aspect of her right thigh. The doctor ordered diagnostic tests and Magnetic Resonance Imaging (MRI), but before it was done she was alarmed, "I was missing the keyboards when playing the piano!" Neurological examination revealed decreased sensation over the lateral side of the right upper extremity and left shoulder. There was decreased vibratory sensation in the upper extremity and absent in both legs and feet. She could not identify the upward or downward movement of the toes (position sense) and the right two digits of the hand. She could identify shapes of objects placed on both palms. Her motor function was strong. When standing with her eyes closed and with feet together, she has the tendency to fall which she cannot tolerate. Her gait was slow, and she was noted to slide her feet and slippers when walking. MRI of the entire spine showed small islands of plaques at the thoracic and upper lumbar spine. A bilateral posterior and lateral column T2 weighted hyperdensity at C4-C6 was noted. Strongest consideration was possible multiple sclerosis.

Clinical – anatomic Correlation:

The ascending lateral spinothalamic tract was involved at various levels of the spine in patches to explain the numbness and decreased sensation. The most distressing symptom of Melissa, however, can be caused by a lesion involving the posterior column, particularly the fasciculus gracilis and cuneatus at C4-C6. The pathology caused absence of position and vibratory sensation in both lower extremities manifesting as ataxia (abnormal gait) or difficulty walking, and missing the keyboards of the piano. The lack of position sense resulted in an inability to feel the depth of the feet about the floor resulting in uncertainty in her steps and difficulty in walking. To feel the floor, she needed to slide her feet when walking. To be able to ambulate, she compensated by using her visual system to orient her feet with the floor and the objects around her. The absence of position sense of the fingers of the right hand could result in missing the keys when playing the piano, a problem that alarmed Melissa.

To appreciate the function of the discriminatory senses, enter a very dark movie theater and try to walk. Without being able to see, walking is almost impossible, so one starts to hold on to or touch something to be able to guide the walking including sliding the feet on the floor to maintain body and limb orientation. Now you know that visual and other sensory functions participate in body-environment orientation to provide good motor activities, especially in walking or running. The brainstem reticular formation coordinates the visio-auditory-proprioceptive sensation.

In *tabes dorsalis* due to syphilis, the area commonly affected is the posterior column and this is manifested by position sense abnormality in both legs and absent vibratory sensation. Because of these, the patient is unable to perceive the position of the feet to the ground, resulting in an abnormal "tabetic gait" described as raising the foot and "slapping" the ground while walking. Another disease that can affect the posterior and lateral column is a *B12 deficiency or sub-acute combined degeneration.* These patients use a lot of visual compensation to be able to walk unassisted. It will be difficult for them to walk in a dark theater. The diseases mentioned are commonly referred to as differential diagnoses or important alternative considerations in Melissa's case.

Neurological Examination:

You will notice that the axons for different sensations of the body enter at varying levels of the spinal cord. It is therefore easy to imagine how the body sensations are "mapped" according to the levels of the entry of the nerves into the spinal cord. As mentioned before, the nervous system is complex but organized. The body mapping into the spinal cord levels is called **dermatomes** (Fig. 8.). If you look at the body map, there are too many daunting levels to remember. All you need to know and remember are four patterns which will divide them in an orderly manner.

1. The area between the imaginary line of the upper tip of the clavicle and the shoulder is C5 and above this is the broad base of the head which is C4. The top border of C4 is the line at the level of Adam's apple and between this line, and the base of the skull is C3. The back portion of the head is C2.
2. The nipple line is commonly T4, and the navel is the 10th thoracic level. Just divide the space between T4 and T10 into five equal parts, and this will approximate T5 to T9 levels. Then the space between the navel and suprapubic into two equal parts to give you T11 and T12 levels.
3. With the upper limb extended at a right angle to the body and palm facing the front, divide equally the upper extremity around its diameter. Start the C6 line above the scapula running posterior to upper extremity up to the thumb, and then split this into C7 to T1 around the arm from posterior to anterior side. The index and middle finger are C7 while the ring and small finger C8.

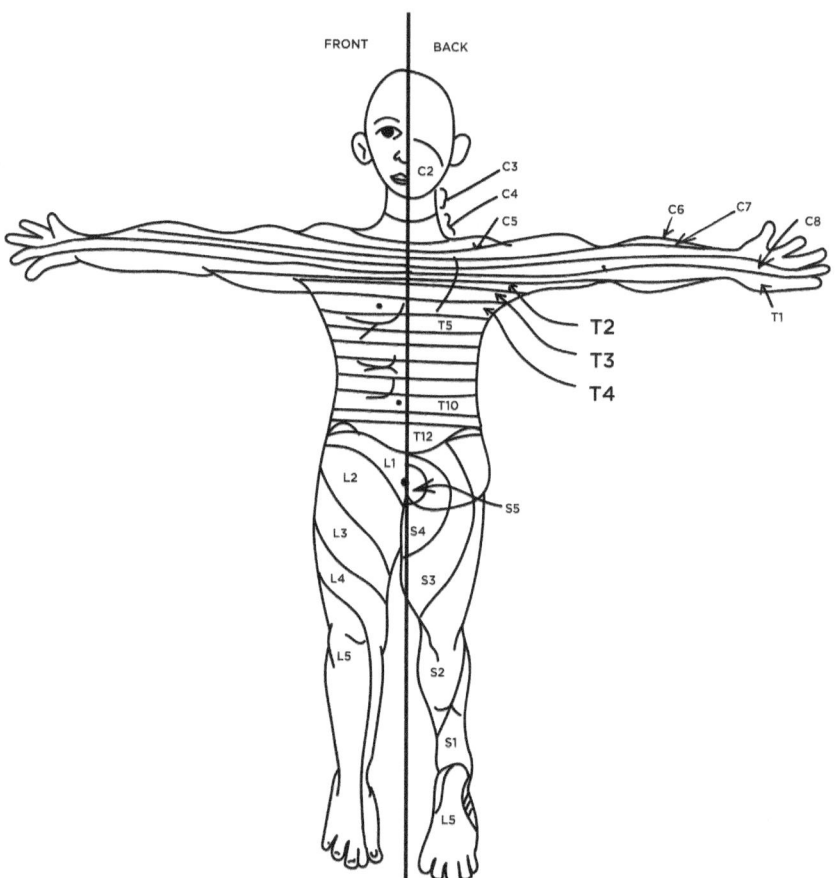

Figure 8. Sensory dermatomal distribution.

4. The anterior thigh is divided diagonally into four following the suprapubic-to-groin-line and the L4-line that extends above the knee, the medial side of the forelimb, and the toe. The diagonal lines will approximate L1, L2, L3, and L4. The L5 level is the lateral side of the foreleg, the lateral portion of the dorsum, and the plantar surface of the feet. Posteriorly, draw a "target" figure with the center as the anal area. Dividing the buttocks into five spaces away from the center will correspond to S5 to S1 innervations. Also, S2 extends below the buttocks downward, to the attachment of Achilles tendon. S1 begins at the lateral most side of the buttocks and extends along the lateral side of S2 and lateral part of the dorsum and plantar surface.

Repeat reading this and refer to the body map about three times, or better still, design your cues to help you remember.

It is best to examine the patient who is blindfolded to remove much of the subjectivity. The different instruments to be used are pins (to test the spinothalamic system and dermatomal level), then painting brush or cotton wisp (to test the anterolateral spinothalamic system and dermatomal level), tuning fork (to test the posterior column gracilis and cuneatus system). Pound the tuning fork (with at least 128 cps) against a firm object to elicit a vibration and apply to bony parts of the extremities and let the patient describe the experience. Compare each side or other parts of the body. Position sense test is done by the examiner flexing the distal digits up or down and letting the patient identify the direction of movements. Position sense test evaluates the function of the posterior column of the spinal cord. These are some of the common bedside maneuvers used in the clinic to save on time. There are other tests that one should be familiar with. Temperature testing use warm and cold water in a small bottle or tube and applied to areas defined in the dermatomal map. The subject then identifies the applied temperature. In the two-point discrimination test, the examiner describes the distance of two points applied simultaneously. The patient is then to determine if only one or two pricks are perceived. Identification and description of objects with varied shapes in the hand of subjects like marble, coin, feather, and cotton are another tests that will evaluate the posterior column of the spinal cord up to the post-central gyrus of the parietal lobe.. Before doing the examination, be sure that you explain to the patient that these are sensory tests and objects would be applied and that they should describe the sensation. Patients must be able to answer the questions in each test correctly. Start the examination on the intact area first and conduct a little trial to get cooperation.

Practical Notes on Descending and Ascending Tracts:

By now, you have a good knowledge of two "vertical neuroanatomic lines" corresponding to the corticospinal tracts and the spinothalamic tracts. This concept is essential for localization. Where the horizontal tracts and vertical lines intersect is usually the location of the lesion. The succeeding chapters will discuss the imaginary "horizontal lines" that help in localization.

Chapter VI

The Cranial Nerves

Cranial nerves are 12 pairs of nerves arising from the brain and the brainstem, exiting and then entering through the different canals or foramina of the skull. Historically, the names, innervations, functions, numbers, nomenclatures, and classifications of these nerves underwent centuries of interesting evolution. It is intriguing to note that the cranial nerves, termed ordinal classifications before, has long been recognized since the time of Galen (2nd century AD) but he mentioned only seven pairs of cranial nerves and this did not include the olfactory tract as part of the cerebrum. He started the cranial nerves with the optic nerve; oculomotor nerve; sensory part of trigeminal nerve; motor part of trigeminal nerve; combined facial and vestibule-cochlear nerves; combined glossopharyngeal, vagus, and accessory nerves; and finally, the hypoglossal nerve. He did not recognize the crossing of optic nerves at the chiasma during that time. The Galenic classification persisted for several centuries and was only challenged in the medieval period when some anatomic details were discovered to have different functions. But the Galenic influence persisted and prevailed until an Englishman, Thomas Willis (1664), who coined the term **Neurology** and described the "Circle of Willis," proposed nine pairs of cranial nerve, which started with the olfactory nerve and considered the accessory nerve a separate cranial nerve. The nine cranial nerves were accepted for about 124 years until, a German physician, Samuel Sommerring (1755-1830), described what we commonly recognize now as the 12 cranial nerves [17]. We should be thankful to these amazing people who contributed and influenced our understanding of the cranial nerves. It took centuries to understand the functions of the cranial nerves, and here we are trying to assimilate all of these in just one sitting!

The cranial nerves are named as such because the location is in the head or cranium, and they supply mostly structures from the tip of the head to the neck, except the glossopharyngeal and vagus nerves that supply the autonomic nerves of the body. The twelve cranial nerve nomenclatures we are going to use are CNI to CN XII. The mnemonics that I used when still a student were <u>O</u>n <u>O</u>ld <u>O</u>regon <u>T</u>ower <u>T</u>op <u>A</u> French <u>V</u>eteran <u>G</u>uard <u>V</u>illages <u>A</u>nd <u>Houses</u>. (You can use your own.)

CN I	O-Olfactory nerve
CN II	O-Optic nerve
CN III	O-Oculomotor nerve
CN IV	T-Trochlear nerve
CN V	T-Trigeminal nerve
CN VI	A-Abducens nerve
CN VII	F-Facial nerve
CN VIII	V-Vestibulo-cochlear nerve
CN IX	G-Glossopharyngeal nerve
CN X	V-Vagus nerve
CN XI	A-Accessory nerve
CN XII	H-Hypoglossal nerve

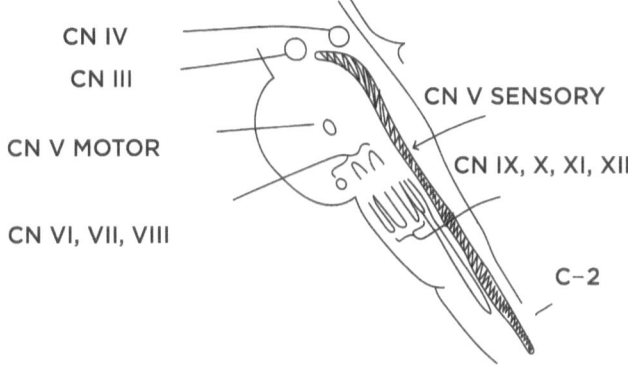

Figure 9. Location of Cranial Nerve Nuclei in the brainstem.

The location of the neurons of the cranial nerves is in the brainstem, except for the first two cranial nerves. Cranial nerves I (Olfactory N) and II (Optic N) send fibers that terminate mostly in the brain. The brain stem is made up of the midbrain, pons, and medulla. There are only two cranial nerve nuclei in the midbrain (Fig. 9). These are CN III (Oculomotor N) and CN IV (Trochlear N). CN IX (Glossopharyngeal N) to CN XII (Vagus N) location are in the medulla. The rest of the cranial nerves are in the pons. See how easy it is to remember? Again! CN III and IV are in the midbrain, CN IX to XII are in the medulla, and the rest are in the pons. CNV has a long and scattered sensory neurons and axons that extends from the upper third of the pons down to the upper cervical C2 level. Hence, the sensory portion of CN V has the longest neuronal and axonal distributions. The motor part of CNV is located in the mid-pons. We will elaborate on this when we discuss this cranial nerves in detail.

Chapter VI-A

Cranial Nerve I- Olfactory Nerve
(Function: Sense of Smell)

Lulled by the ease of social communication through Facebook or Twitter, you were awakened suddenly by a burning baked turkey, and when you opened the oven, it was almost charred. The smoke emanating from the burned turkey was stinging to the eyes and intolerable to breathing. With the turkey gone, the easiest thing to do was to make your favorite pasta with all the herbs in it. Unfortunately, both your nostrils were clogged. Without the scent of the aroma of the herbs, do you think the pasta will taste good?

The primary neurons of CNI-Olfactory Nerve are the only part of the nervous system exposed to the external environment (Fig. 10). The specialized neurons of CNI are the *olfactory receptor cells* which are embedded strategically with the *olfactory epithelium* located at the uppermost mucosa of the nose. The mucosa conveys the air that carries odors (*odiferous substances*). These olfactory receptor cells are neurons with special hair-like dendrites that are like microvilli. These microvilli serve as transducers that transform the chemical interaction with odiferous substances into electricity. The axons of the *olfactory fibers* transmit the transformed electrical impulses to the second olfactory station where it connects with the *mitral neurons and few tufted cells*. This second olfactory station is the *olfactory bulb*, an oval-shaped structure that houses a mixed mass of layered neurons, dendrites and supporting cells that are referred to as the *olfactory glomeruli*. Tufted cells are believed to participate in regulatory feedback mechanism in the transmittal of odor sensation [18].

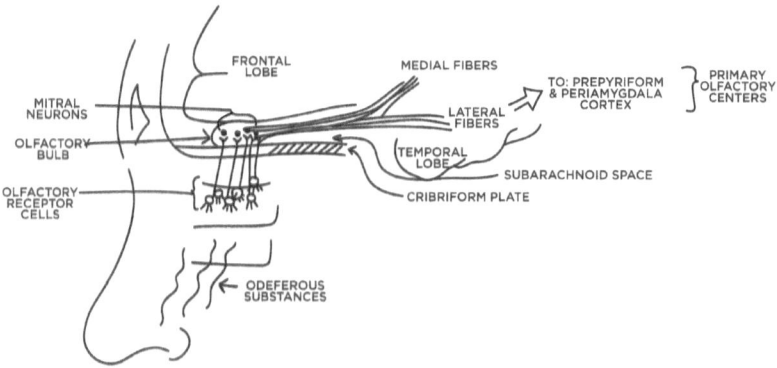

Figure 10. Cranial Nerve I - Olfactory Nerve. Note olfactory receptor cells embedded in the superior nasal wall with synaptic connections to the mitral neurons that send transduced impulses to primary olfactory centers and other areas of the cortex.

The olfactory fibers penetrate the thin bone at the base of the skull, inbetween the eye sockets, which we call *cribriform plate*. Being thin, it can fracture easily in frontal or contrecoup head injuries. The fracture can destroy the passing axons, thereby causing loss of smell (**Anosmia**). The dura at the base of the brain which is firmly attached to the cribriform plate could also be torn, and cause leakage of the brain fluid (**CSF rhinorrhea**), a common accompanying condition with anosmia. CSF rhinorrhea after head trauma opens the brain to the nasal environment and its saprophytic bacteria. The dural leak has a strong predisposition to meningitis, a fundamental reason to give prophylactic antibiotics.

Mitral neurons relay impulses with their axons, bundled and named as an *olfactory tract* that terminates directly at the *olfactory cortex* which is in the medial or inner portion of the *anterior temporal lobes* -- site of the primary olfactory cortex, prepyriform, and periamygdaloid complex (this is near the uncus). Neurons in these areas receive direct and indirect impulses from the hippocampus, amygdala, cingulate gyrus, septate nucleus, and hypothalamus – collectively called the **limbic system**, a critical evolutionary participant in emotion, behavioral reactions and memory formation. These complex cortical interconnections charge the odor with emotion; discriminative sensation; sexual, social and behavioral responses. When the olfactory receptor cells are triggered, the **odor** is the one transmitted. The discriminative and emotional experience is the **scent**.

Case Story:

Mrs. Johnston, a high school principal, was reported to be doing bizarre acts in her house. She was noted to queerly place her shoes inside the refrigerator and her dress in the oven. Two nights before, she was complaining of a headache and inability to sleep. She was still able to eat breakfast but unable to finish half of what she used to consume. The husband tried to talk to her and asked her questions, but the responses were outré of mumbled incomprehensible words. The husband brought her to a neurologist who found her to mutter senseless sounds. The neurologist stroked her palm which elicited an immediate and sustained grasp. When the angle of her lips was touched, she snouted her lips towards the stimuli which were sometimes accompanied by a sucking action. She was able to walk but without direction and purpose. Her motor strength was normal and pinching lightly the arms triggered restless grimace. Her reflexes were hyperactive, and there was no Babinski sign. Electroencephalogram showed abnormal brain waves described as tall delta sharp waves and presence of spikes and wave epileptiform discharges over both posterior frontal and anterior temporal leads. Magnetic resonance imaging with contrast (MRI) showed abnormal enhancement over both anterior temporal and posterior frontal areas. The MRI was interpreted by the radiologist to be possibly Herpes Simplex Encephalitis. Intravenous Acyclovir was given immediately to her. One month after treatment, she recovered her old self to the relief of the loving husband.

Clinical – anatomic Correlation:

We mentioned earlier that the olfactory nerve is the only cranial nerve exposed to the environment because of the location of the olfactory receptor cells in the upper mucosa of the nose. The olfactory receptor cells become potentially an entry point of some infections like herpes simplex virus encephalitis, as in the case of Mrs. Johnston, that characteristically involves the medial temporal and basal part of the frontal lobe -- areas near or connected with the olfactory tract. Other organisms may find entry through the olfactory nerve. There are some suspected cases of rabies infection with no bite exposures but having gone inside a bat cave habitat where some might be rabid. Inhalation of infected bat secretions was suspected. A particular form of amoeba in dirty swimming pools may find entry through the olfactory bulb route [19].

We have reviewed the functional anatomy of the CN I, so now you know why bath and fragrant underarm products are selling well. There are other necessary functions of CN I. If the odor is that of a spoiled or toxic food or burning substances, our nose or the olfactory function *warns us* of poisonous substances. A gourmet experience, a *discriminatory sensation of smell*, is indispensable. When there is no sense of smell, like when you cover your nose or when you have nasal congestion, food does not taste as good because the discriminatory sense of smell is unable to participate in the appreciation of taste. That is why herbs are essential in food because the aromas produced are pleasant scents. People without a sense of smell or with *anosmia* can only appreciate the basic tastes of saltiness, bitterness, sourness, and sweetness. When anosmia is present, the taste is devoid of the effect of the aroma from herbs or scents in the food, depriving the victim of discriminating gustatory experience. Mexican, Italian, and Spanish foods have no taste differences for persons with anosmia who appreciate only simple and monotonous taste of salt or sugar. The experience is emotionally frustrating. Studies have shown that a significant number of patients with anosmia develop depression. Anosmia or decreased smell has been observed to herald the occurrence of Parkinson's Disease and Alzheimer's Disease [20,21].

When neurons in the primary olfactory centers (medial and anterior temporal lobes) spontaneously fire or spark, as in *seizures or epilepsy*, it could initiate an experience related to the neuroanatomic functions for the sensation of smell and the role of the limbic system. When a patient just had a seizure attack, it is necessary to ask, "What was the last thing that you could remember?" The answer will provide a clue to the location of the initiating neurons in the brain. If some would describe a burning tire or difficult-to-describe scent or other odors the experience is called an **uncinate fit** (remember the uncus?) which is an **aura,** an experience just before the loss of consciousness and progression to convulsion. Auras are focal seizure activities usually coming from the temporal lobes that may *not* progress to loss of consciousness or convulsion. An intriguing description of an aura is a feeling called **"déjà vu,"** a strange experience that the place is familiar, or one is in a familiar place yet they remain conscious of the surroundings. The experience may herald the loss of awareness or unconsciousness, and many are witnessed to be doing a simulation of eating or chewing activities. These events are collectively called **temporal lobe seizure** or reclassified as **partial seizure** if there is no loss of consciousness or **complex partial seizure** if there is. There are behavioral patterns that patients manifest in temporal lobe seizures like blank stares, lip smacking, eye roving, the flickering of the eyelids, finger movements, chewing movements and other unusual behavior like raging eyes and running behaviors. Many of these are functions of the limbic system. Patients are unaware of these activities which are called automatisms. It is therefore important to let witnesses of the attack describe in detail the behavior of the patient before generalized convulsions happen. It is equally important to ask the patients what they could remember (the aura) just before they became unaware or unconscious. Ask the patient, "What can you recall just before you lost consciousness?" and to the witness, "Please describe in detail the patient's behavior just before the convulsion." Two simple questions one should remember that will provide a clinical clue that will help us classify the seizure type.

You must have noticed by now that when one loses the sense of smell or experience anosmia, it is described as a **negative manifestation.** On the other hand, if there is an experience of seizures, it is considered a **positive manifestation.**

The sense of smell is highly subjective, so we depend so much on the history to understand the patient's problem. One of the questions to be asked is, "Any problem with smell"? If there is no sense of smell, the term is **anosmia**. If there is a partial decrease of the sense of smell or the person can appreciate odors a little, it is called **hyposmia**. When a patient is unable to discriminate or commits a mistake in identifying the odors, we call it **dysosmia**. A person has **cacosmia** if he continues to smell a foul odor. When there is a perceived odor when there is none, as in **uncinate fit**, it is called **parosmia**. You do not have to memorize these terms, know that this fascinating symptomatology can indeed happen. If on history there is a head injury, ask if there is continuous post nasal drip, especially when standing or sitting because this might not be mucus but CSF fluid or the patient might have CSF rhinorrhea. Patients with this problem need antibiotics prophylaxis to prevent the oral and nasal bacteria from entering through the dural break and cause meningitis. When there is a gradual loss of smell, you should inquire about headaches and visual changes because of a possible olfactory tumor that is pressing on the optic nerve also.

Neurological Examination:

Use coffee, tobacco, peppermint, and other substances, except those that are volatile like alcohol, when testing the olfactory nerve. Using acidic materials stimulates the Trigeminal Nerve (Cranial Nerve V) instead. The test is done with one nostril at a time while blindfolded. The olfactory fibers being near the optic tract, tests for visual acuity and visual field are essential.

Chapter VI-B

Cranial Nerve II- Optic Nerve
(Function: Vision/Seeing)

Sit down in a garden and appreciate the fascinating colors of the grass, the flowers, and the vines. Savor the gift of seeing the multi-colored butterfly, stripes of the bees, the yellow dotted back of the beetle, and the bright colored feathers of the birds. We are unaware that behind this gift is a delicate interplay of neurons that can be disturbed anytime and in so many ways. In our daily lives, our vision is vital. The licensing officer does a quick visual test before getting a driver's license. Do you wonder why the same officer ask if the applicant can see the letter on the right side and the left side? Reading seems to be easy because you can see, but why are some children able to see but unable to read? The inability to read is a condition called **dyslexia**. When the black and white film and television shows progressed to capture the natural color of what our eyes see, it was considered a revolution in the film industry- the entry of Technicolor. But can we see all color ranges?

    The optic nerve is an embryonic out pouching originating from the diencephalon of the fetal brain, making the *retina and the optic nerve part of the brain*. Being such, it shares with the brain the envelope covering of the pia, arachnoid, and dura mater. It also has, for its axonal covering, myelin which is formed in the brain by the *oligodendrocytes,* instead of the *Schwann Cells,* for the peripheral nerves. Have you ever heard the expression "The eye is the window to the brain."? By using the fundoscopy instrument, one can visualize the retina, blood vessels, and the optic nerve head (optic cup) which are "extensions" of the brain

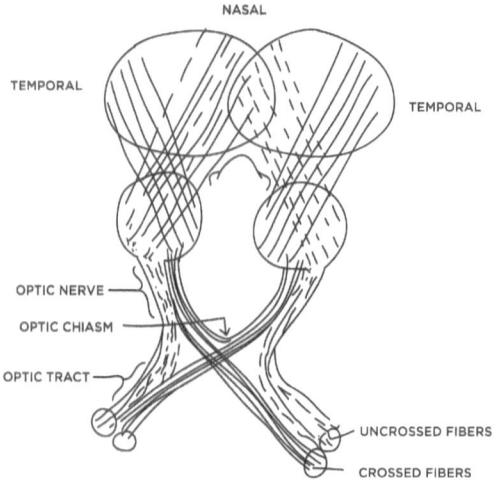

Figure 11. Cranial Nerve II – Visual field with corresponding receiving retinal areas. Retinal ganglion cell projections from both nasal sides cross at the optic chiasm. Temporal side projections from the retina do not cross

structures. There is plenty of disease conditions seen in the retina that is a reflection of what is going on in the brain. An example is *swelling or pallor of the optic disc* which is the exit area of the optic nerve, a finding which could be indicative of *demyelination,* changes that one may see in the brain with multiple sclerosis. Sudden blindness due to ischemic infarction of the ophthalmic artery may show *retinal pallor and hemorrhages* in the retinal floor. Chronic increased intracranial pressure shows swelling of the optic cup and retinal hemorrhages which are characteristic of *papilledema.* Blood from a ruptured aneurysm that diffuses to the subarachnoid space may find its way under the hyaloid membrane of the retina; this is called *subhyaloid hemorrhage.*

The **visual field** is an imaginary ovoid shaped area and an extent that one eye can see when looking straight (Fig. 11). Try focusing on your finger in front. You will notice that there is a limited oval area which the eyes can see. That is your visual field. One can see areas outside the visual field by moving the eyes to the sides or upward and downward. Even while moving the eyes, the field of vision is still the same.

It is fascinating to know that everything that we see or the images that we appreciate are lights with various illuminance. The retinal cells provide varied information, but it is the brain that interprets with finality.

All images and colors that fall on the visual field are perceived as light with different degrees of luminance or **light bands.** The lights are reflected inward through the cornea, the anterior chamber of the eye, the pupils that control the amount of light that enters, the refracting lens, vitreous fluid, and then the retina (Fig. 12).

The retina is the main station for light transduction and transmission. This amazing and wonderful retina hosts several neural elements, fibers, and blood vessels. Two photoreceptors called cones and rods receive the lights with different bands initially. **Cones** process bright light and *green, red, yellow and blue* (GRYB) color bands while **rods** process dim light and black and white bands. It is at these photoreceptors that photochemical reactions with photo pigments happen and transform the light bands into electrical impulses. There are three types of cone photoreceptors based on their sensitivity to color light bands. The L-band which is sensitive to long bands, particularly yellow to the red band; the M-band, for medium bands, particularly to green; and the S-bands,

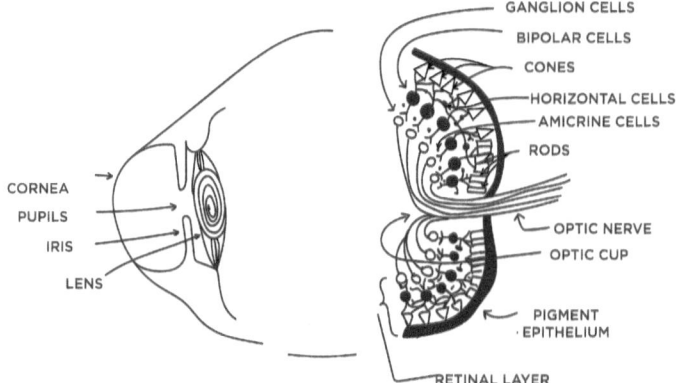

Figure 12. Cranial Nerve II- Parts of the retina including the Ganglion cells (main transmitter of vision) whose axons merge at the Optic Cup and exit as a bundled Optic Nerve.

for short bands, particularly the blue band. The interplay of these photoreceptor types provides the color that your brain finally interprets. Some people experience **color blindness** because of congenital lack or degeneration of one or two of the color cone photoreceptor-types. The most common color blindness that is transferred by the mother to her sons is the red-green blindness which could be due to the absence of the L-type or M-type cones. The absence of cones causes **monochromatic** or total color blindness.

The axons of the rods and cones transmit electrical impulses to adjacent dendrites of the *bipolar cells*. The electrical waves that the bipolar cells receive is modified by *horizontal cells* which have axonal and dendritic connections with them. The modifying influence provides a *dynamic and changing contrast* or *background that sharpens and enhances images* that are eventually transmitted by bipolar cells.

The bipolar cells then synapse with the dendrites of *ganglion cells*. Impulses that the ganglion cells transmit to the visual cortex are influenced by the *amacrine cells* that provide axonal connections with other amacrine cells, bipolar cells, and ganglion cells. The amacrine cells are responsible for *moving sensitive response*; just like the horizontal cells, they *provide contrast background to enhance the image,* and because of their vast connection of bipolar cell types, they *allow the ganglion cells to respond to various ranges of light level* [22,23].

The ganglion cell axons (about a million of them for each eye) merge, and their exit point in the retina is the **optic cup or optic nerve head**. The axons then proceed to exit the eyeball as bundled **optic nerves** which then merge at the **optic chiasma** (Fig. 13). This merging is where ganglion cell axons from medial or nasal parts of the retina cross and join the opposite non-crossing ganglion cell axons from the lateral or temporal side of the retina. This merging is where ganglion cell axons from medial or nasal parts of the retina cross and join the opposite non-crossing ganglion cell axons from the lateral or temporal side of the retina. When these uncrossed and crossed fibers merge after the optic chiasm, they are called the **optic tracts**. The optic tracts now have medial fibers from the opposite retina and lateral fibers from the same side of the retina. The merging of the medial and lateral optic tract fiber means that the right optic tract "sees" the left visual field while the left optic tract "sees" the right visual field (we will elaborate on this later).

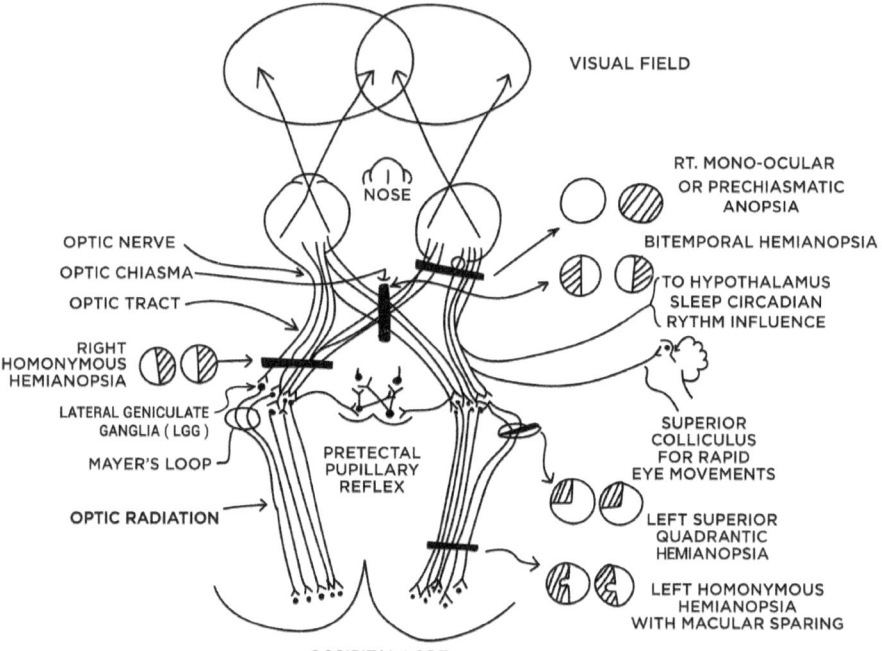

Figure 13. Cranial Nerve II – Visual tract pathway and lesions (heavy line) with corresponding visual field defects. Aside from termination at the Occipital lobe, some Optic nerves terminate to the hypothalamus, superior colliculus and pretectum.

A large part of the ganglion axons terminates at the *Lateral Geniculate Ganglia (LGG)* while some terminate at the *superior colliculi* (the upper, round protrusions at the back of the midbrain). This superior colliculus coordinates rapid eye movement to maintain just one vision. Some ganglion axons terminate at the *hypothalamus* to influence sleep cycle, while some supply the *pretectile* area as the afferent arm of the pupillary reflex (Remember that this is the afferent arm of the pupillary reflex which we will discuss when we tackle the CNIII - Oculomotor nerve).

From the ganglion cells of the retina, the second station is the *LGG* which is a part of the thalamus. The LGG neurons, on the other hand, transmit the visual impulses (this time called **optic radiation**) to the visual cortex of the occipital lobes. It is important to know that the visual impulses from the retina retain their neuroanatomic position after the optic chiasm. The ganglion cell axons at the inferior and superior halves of the retina also retain the same anatomic position after the optic chiasm and even after the lateral geniculate ganglia. It is interesting to note that the inferior fibers of the optic radiation that "sees" the superior or upper portion of the visual field make a detour and loop (this is called **Meyer's loop**) around the anterior horns of the lateral ventricles or at the anterior temporal lobes, then return again to join the optic radiation highways (Fig. 14). These neuroanatomic curious loops explain the **superior quadrantic hemianopsia** when there is a lesion involving the anterior temporal lobe. The superior optic radiation that "sees" the inferior or lower portion of the visual fields goes straight through the parietal white matter to the visual cortex of the occipital lobes.

In summary, light or images reach the retina where photoreceptor rods and cones transform the light bands photochemically into electricity. The *bipolar cells* then transmit the electrical impulses to the *ganglion cells* of the retina. In turn, the ganglion cells transmit the visual impulses through their axons that exit at the *optic disc or optic nerve head* of the retina. Upon exiting the eyeball, the axons are called the *optic nerves. The medial fibers* of the optic nerve merge at the optic chiasm while the lateral fibers maintain their lateral position. The bundling of the lateral and crossing medial fibers after the optic chiasm is now called the optic tract. Most of the *optic tracts* will synapse with the neurons of the *LGG*, whose neurons subsequently send axons, as *optic radiation*, to the *visual cortex* of the occipital lobes.

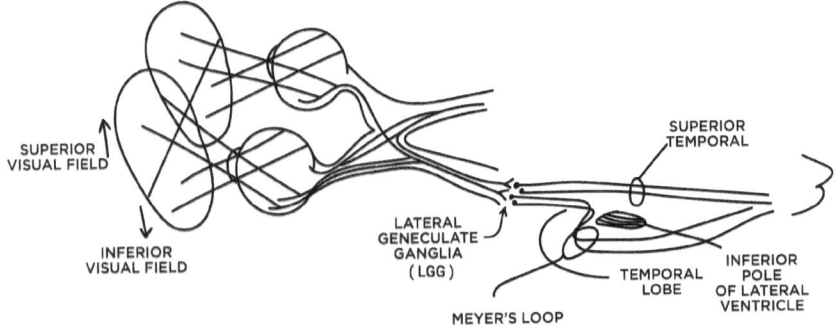

Figure 14. Cranial Nerve II – When viewed from the side, the superior visual field recepient is the inferior retina whose optic nerve fibers position is kept even after the LGG and as the tract curves at the Meyer's loop of the temporal lobe. This explains the superior quadrant hemianopsia shown in fig. 13.

Case Story:

Mr. J. R., 67 years old, gentleman, an art gallery curator, while having lunch experienced sudden dizziness and vomiting followed by numbness of the right side of the face which lasted two minutes. His blood pressure was normal, but his heart was noted to be irregular. He rested in bed for about thirty minutes and then feeling well, he went back to his office. His secretary, however, noted that he keeps bumping objects on his right side, including the doors and tables. The secretary frantically brought him to the emergency room of a nearby hospital where the doctors immediately ordered an MRI that showed a left occipital infarct.

Clinical – anatomic Correlation:

The flows of the axons are maintained from the ganglion cells of the retina to its entire length in the brain (Fig. 15). To appreciate it better, make a closed fist and cross one arm over the other. Now the thumb side will represent the flow of axons from the lateral aspect of the retina. These lateral fibers will keep their course and will NOT CROSS at the chiasma to the opposite side. The thumb fibers will, therefore, remain on the same side. The side of the knuckles will represent the medial fibers of the retina, the axons of which WILL CROSS and join the opposite uncrossed lateral fibers to become the optic tract. The optic tract, therefore, carries axons that "see" the opposite side, i.e., *the right optic tract "sees" the left visual field while the left optic tract "sees" the right visual field.* These crossed knuckle fibers will maintain their course to the occipital cortex connections. The thumb sides of the retina will "see" the middle field of vision. (If you are looking at a portrait picture frame, the field of the face or its center will be the field seen by the thumb side. The knuckle side will see the lateral field of vision or the opposite borders of the frame). The middle field of vision is the nasal field while the lateral field of vision is the temporal field of vision.

The optic chiasm lies in front and a little below the pituitary gland. If there is a pituitary tumor, it can very well compress the chiasm. The effect on the vision is the so-called **bitemporal hemianopsia** because the knuckle sides of the retina that "see" the lateral fields are the ones crossing and therefore get affected first. If one has a lesion affecting the

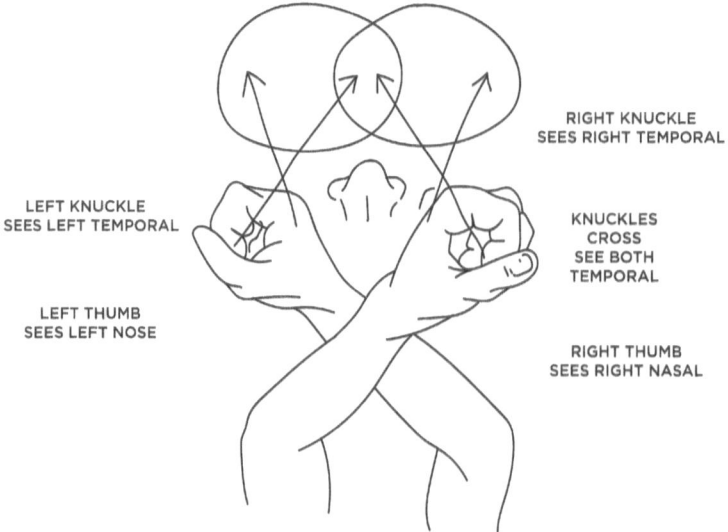

Figure 15. Recall tool for Optic nerve pathway. Thumb side "fibers" remain uncrossed, while the knuckle side "fibers" cross to the opposite side. Thumb side "sees" the nasal side, while knuckle side "sees" the temporal side.

optic tract or forearm after the crossing, an opposite hemifield defect or **homonymous hemianopsia** could happen. The visual field cut was what Mr. J.R. had. The left occipital lobe infarct caused blindness on the right field of vision, causing him to bump all objects on the right side because he could not see this side. He had right homonymous hemianopsia and with this visual field "cut," do you think he should be allowed to drive?

What happens at the visual cortex? Impulses from ganglion cell axons of the retina stimulate lateral ganglionic neurons which in turn transmit neuronal axonal pulses to the occipital visual cortex neurons. These visual cortex neurons synapse with adjacent cells and other non-visual neurons of the brain to allow final interpretation of everything that the eyes see in the visual field. The interconnections with cognitive, memory and psycho-emotional components of the brain provide meaning to what one sees. Disturbing the interconnections with the occipital lobe by lesions, like a stroke, can sometimes cause **visual agnosia** by which one may be able to visualize something but is unable to interpret or recognize its meaning. In **reading dyslexia**, the letter recognition and phonetic association fibers of the occipitotemporal connections on the left side may be disturbed, causing a *"reading disorder"* or inability to read. Seizures due to uncontrolled neuronal electrical discharges involving the temporo-occipital interneuronal connections may manifest as varied visual experiences.

Neurological Examination:

The first important examination is to check how the eyes can see clearly. Traditionally, the Snellen chart or the pocket Snellen chart is used to estimate *visual acuity*. Headlines and subheadlines of newspapers approximate letter sizes in the pocket Snellen chart. Visual acuity is tested with and without corrective lenses. The far distance of about three feet with the pocket Snellen chart can be measured while the near distance is one foot. This test often assesses the anterior chambers of the eyes, i.e., cornea, vitreous, and lens. *The visual field* test is measured usually by an *Octopus perimeter* or manual perimeter. The bedside test is called *confrontation test*. In a cooperative patient, the examiner in a sense confronts the patient because he or she positions the eyes directly about four feet in front of the patient. The examiner's visual field serves as

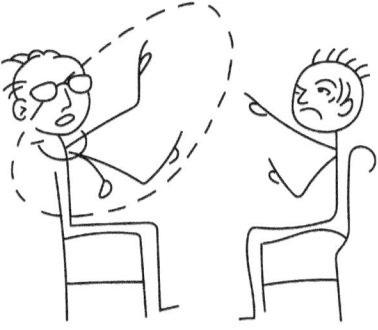

"While focusing your eyes to my nose, I will move my fingers in front of you. What I want you to do is point to the finger that wiggles." One can simulate the visual field examination this way. They termed the examination- confrontation test (unusual threatening term?)

Figure 16. Testing visual field at the bedside by confrontation test.

the control (Fig. 16). The patient is instructed to focus straight without moving the eyes and to point to the examiner's finger that wiggles. The examiner then moves the fingers around an imaginary visual field and wiggles either left or right fingers or even both periodically. The examiner evaluates both visual fields first, then one eye field at a time by covering one eye. Repeating the visual field examination as often is advisable especially when visual field defect is suspected. The examiner also looks for consistency of response. In uncooperative patients *"visual threat"* maneuvers can estimate visual field by suddenly threatening to poke the eyes around the area of the patient's visual field, and a blink or sudden maneuvers to avoid the threat is the normal response. In one to two year-old children, an attractive red ball is passed around the area of the visual field to attract attention. These are *trick maneuvers.-*

Chapter VI-C

Cranial Nerve III- Oculomotor Nerve, Cranial Nerve IV- Trochlear Nerve, Cranial Nerve VI-Abducens Nerve

(Functions: Pupillary Constriction, Eye Opening, and Eye Movements)

Enthralled by the wonderful colors of a butterfly in a garden, you took a picture of its flight with a cell phone camera hoping to capture the expanse of its beautiful wings while on the flight. To your dismay, a blurred picture appears, and the edges doubled -- a big mismatch from the clarity that your eyes viewed and appreciated the flight. Your eyes are very efficient, and a perfect "camera" which modern and fully automatic camera inventors are trying to duplicate. The retina serves as the film that captures what the eyes see, and the brain interprets and appreciates what the picture from the eyes presented. The cranial nerves that we are about to describe, on the other hand, control the direction of the camera (eye), the aperture (pupil) and the lens adjustments for single clear focus.

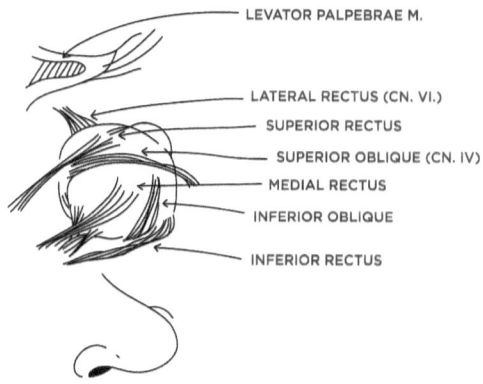

Figure 17. Muscles of the left eye looking lateral and upward. Note that all are supplied by CN III – Occulomotor Nerve except the Lateral rectus muscles which is supplied by CN VI – Abducens Nerve and Superior oblique muscles which is innervated by CN IV – Trochlear Nerve.

Cranial nerves III, IV and VI are traditionally discussed together as a functional group. This group is utilized by the brain to control the eye muscles, pupils, and lids with the purpose of maximizing and maintaining a single and sharp focus when looking at moving objects and fixed objects; when used for near vision (like when reading your favorite book) and for far vistas (like when looking at distant green mountains). The muscles that control eye movements are collectively called extraocular muscles or EOM's. CN III (Oculomotor Nerves) innervate most of the EOM's. The CN III supplies the following muscles and their corresponding functions: 1. The *levator palpebrae* muscles that move the upper lid upward; 2. The *medial rectus muscles* that pull the eyes inward toward the center; 3. The *inferior rectus muscles* that pull the eyes downward and rotates the eyes slightly lateral; 4. The *superior rectus muscles* that pull the eyes upward and rotates the eyes slightly medial; and 5. The *inferior oblique muscles* that rotate the eyes outward and upward (Fig. 17). In addition to supplying these muscles, the oculomotor nerves also carry with them the *parasympathetic nerves* that arise from the *Edinger-Westphal Nucleus*, innervating the pupillary constrictor muscles and the ciliary muscles. These are efferent arms of the pupillary reflex. The two remaining muscles are the *superior oblique muscles* that rotate the eyes inward and downward and receive innervation from the CN IV (Trochlear Nerves), and the *lateral recti muscles* that pull the eyes to the side and are innervated by the CN VI (Abducens Nerves). To help recall the innervations of the different extraocular muscles, let us remember that, CN III supply all the eye muscles except the *superior oblique and lateral recti muscles*.

How do we see far or near vision and moving objects? The actors in this marvelously fine-tuned functions are the oculomotor nerve *nuclei* that reside in the midbrain together with the trochlear nerve *nuclei*. The abducens nerve *nuclei* are in the lower pons. The main directors of the action are the Frontal Gaze Centers (FGC) on both sides of the Pre-frontal area (the area that follows the precentral gyrus) while the assistant directors are the Pontine Gaze Centers (PGC), located just near the abducens nerve nuclei on each side. PGC also refers to Paramedian Pontine Reticular Formation (PPRF), but for simplicity, we will use PGC. Other important actors that join the CN III nuclei in the midbrain are the parasympathetic nerves that constrict the pupils and adjust the lens for near vision [24,25].

When you focus your eyes directly at the beautiful pink roses in the garden, your eyes stay at the center (primary gaze). During this time, the left and right FGC, through the corresponding *opposite* command posts of the PGC, direct the muscles of the eyes to be tonically *equal*. The bright summer glare reaches the retina where some ganglion cells send axons to the parasympathetic nucleus of the midbrain. The parasympathetic neurons, through CNIII, then direct the pupils to constrict to about 4 mm on both sides, while the upper lids go down just enough to protect the eyes from the glare. Suddenly, a pretty butterfly joins the roses and gets your attention as it flies towards you on the *right side* to about four feet. In this story, while the occipital lobes and the limbic systems are enjoying the view, the FGC on both sides are busy balancing the movements of the eyes, and when your attention shifts to the butterfly that is flying towards the right side, the occipital lobes sense the movement and inform the *left FGC of the direction of the movement*. This time, the left FGC is now dominating the balance, sending commands to its assistant director, the opposite *right PGC* (Fig. 18). The *right PGC* then transmits two exquisite and well-orchestrated commands through its axonal baton. One command goes to the same side, to the *right* abducens nerve nucleus. The right abducens nerve that supplies the *right lateral rectus* pulls the *right eye* to the *right*. The other *PGC* command occurs via its axons that *cross and ascend to the opposite left oculomotor nerve nucleus.*

These crossing axons that ascend are called *Medial Longitudinal Fasciculus (MLF)*. The *left oculomotor nerve nucleus* that supplies the *left medial rectus moves the* left eye to the right. The result of the orchestrated command is a simultaneous and unified movement of both eyes to the right side. Both eyes are *conjugately looking at the right side,* where the butterfly is flying.

The image of the butterfly, as it flies nearer, enlarges, and some visual messages reach the lateral geniculate ganglia (LGG) then to the *Edinger-Westphal Nucleus* (EWN). Both EWN sends axons as *parasympathetic nerves* that join the oculomotor nerves. These *parasympathetic nerves* then connect with the neurons at the *Ciliary Ganglia*. The *parasympathetic ciliary neurons* carry impulses to the *ciliary muscles* and the *constricting muscles of the pupils*. Thus, the pupils constrict as the butterfly nears and at the same time causes the lens to *increase its biconcave shape,* allowing the size of the butterfly's image to remain the same as it reaches the retina.

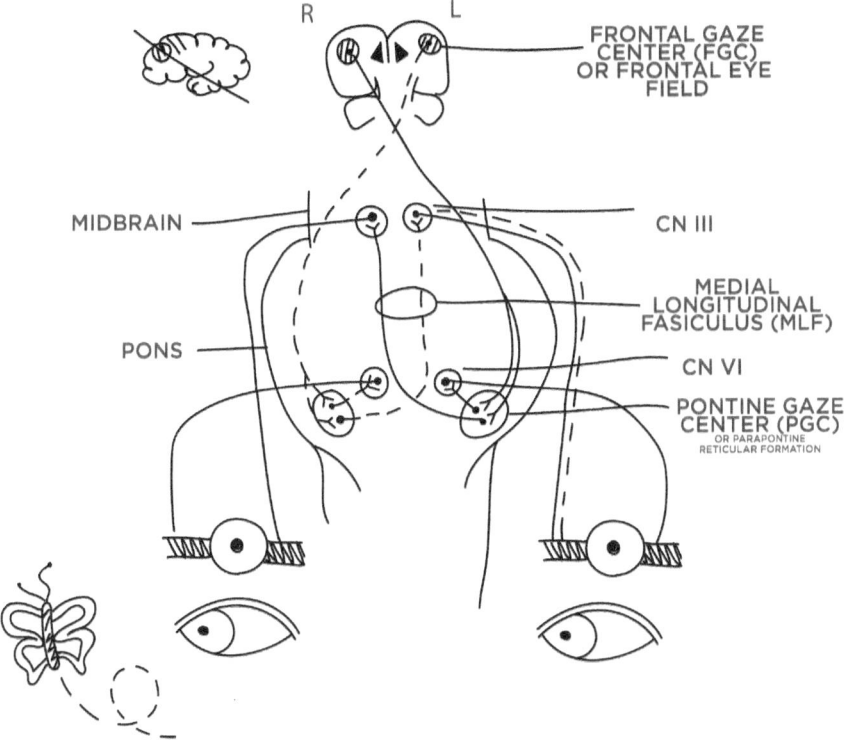

Figure 18. Horizontal gaze mechanism pathway. The left FGC senses the flight of the butterfly to the right. The left FGC dominates (dotted line) causing the eyes to move conjugately to the right, looking at the butterfly.

This process of *pupillary constriction* and *medial movement* of the eyes as the butterfly approaches nearer is a process of **accommodation**. The accommodation reflex is how the eyes can see clearly, near and distant images. The *levator palpebrae* muscles, which are supplied by the oculomotor nerves, *raise the upper lids to* allow the eyes to open some more. What has just been described is an enthralling flow of unconscious, fluid and finely coordinated movements of the muscles of the eyes that enable us to have a clear and single vision of our surroundings, a wonderful gift indeed. Now, let us analyze once again this experience from a functional anatomic point of view.

Please copy and draw or trace the Figure 18 as you are reading the *functional anatomy of horizontal gaze* mechanism. The tracing exercise will make you understand how the eyes can maintain a single and clear image while looking at a moving object like a flying butterfly. The location of the *right and left frontal gaze centers (FGC or Frontal Eye Field) is at the superior prefrontal gyrus on each side*. These are just in front of the motor strip or pyramidal gyrus or precentral gyrus. On primary gaze, the FGC commands are balanced at the center because the immobile flowers are in the middle of the visual field. When the butterfly flies to the right, the occipital lobe informs the FGC of the movement; this time the left FGC *recognizes this and now dominates the command*. The neurons at the left FGC will then send impulses through its axon, to the *opposite right pontine gaze* center *(PGC)* nuclei group in the lower pons. These activated neurons, in turn, send axonal impulses to the neighboring *right* abducens nerve nucleus which further send electrical waves to the *right lateral rectus muscle receptors* eliciting a muscle contraction, in effect *pulling the right eye to the right*. The other neurons at the activated *right PGC* send pulses through axons *that cross and ascend as medial longitudinal fasciculus (MLF)* to the *opposite side and terminate at the left* midbrain oculomotor nerve nucleus. The nucleus is then activated, and this time the impulses are propagated to the *left* medial rectus, causing the muscle to pull the *left eye to the right side*. Both eyes move to the right side in unison, looking at the butterfly and maintaining one clear focus. When two eyes move in unison, we say that the eyes are conjugately moving. In strokes that involve one side of the FGC, the opposite side or unaffected side dominate, resulting in a conjugate deviation of the eyes to the opposite side. For example, if there is a stroke involving the *right* FGC, the *left* FGC dominates, so the eyes are continuously positioned to the right side.

Because there is now absent influence or opposing right FGC, the eyes will remain in that position for a time. The eyes conjugately deviate *to the right side*. Because the lesion is on the right side, you may say that the eyes are *"looking at the side of the lesion"*.

On the other hand, if there are uncontrolled electrical discharges involving *the left FGC,* as in focal seizure or epilepsy, there will be an overwhelming dominance of the *left FGC* causing the eyes to deviate to the *right*. In this case, the eyes during the attack are conjugately deviated to the right side or, in this case, *"the eyes look away from the source of the seizures."* It is fascinating to see the effects of lesions that involve the horizontal gaze mechanism on eye movements. Crossed ascending pontine gaze axons, called the *medial longitudinal fasciculus* fibers are commonly affected by tiny strokes in elderly diabetics and multiple sclerosis in the young, causing bilateral medial rectus palsy or **internuclear ophthalmoplegia (INO).** In this case, both eyes deviate, "both are looking to the sides!" If the left PGC is involved, the supply to the left CN VI and the ascending and crossed MLF to the right CN III get affected causing both eyes to deviate to the right, or "away from the lesion." Pay attention to the laterality of the area, keep drawing it, and memorize (Do not worry if you forget ☺) the drawings to help you understand the different eye signs described above.

The pupillary control, as previously described, works in synchrony with the movements of the eyes in the process of accommodation. One will see in Fig. 13 that the ganglion cell axons (optic nerve) send electrical impulses to the Lateral Geniculate Ganglia (LGG). Some LGG neurons send axonal impulses to the pretectal neurons. This *retina-LGG-pretectal interconnection* serves as the *afferent arm* of the light reflex. *The pretectal neurons, on the other hand, send crossed and uncrossed axons to the Edinger-Westphal Nucleus (EWN) which consists of parasym*pathetic (PS) neurons. The EWN will then be the origin of the *PS nerves that merge with the oculomotor nerves* as they exit from the midbrain and become the *efferent arms of the light reflex*. The PS nerves reach the ciliary ganglion where they synapse with ciliary PS neurons and mix with ciliary sympathetic (SN) neurons which receive impulses from the Cervical Sympathetic Nerve plexus. Both PS and SN axons merge as short ciliary nerves. They innervate the *pupil constrictor* muscles and *pupil dilator* muscles respectively. They also innervate the ciliary muscles that control the biconcave shape of the lens. PS neurons *contract*

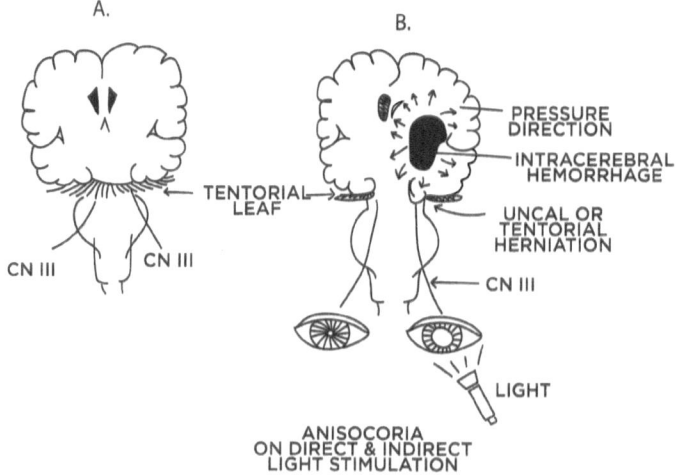

Figure 19. A. The tentorial edge around the brainstem where the uncus rests and below it is the exiting CN III – Occulomotor nerve. CN III carries on its top the Parasympathetic Nerve (PSN) that elicit pupillary constriction. B. Uncal herniation pressing on CN III disturbing the PSN, resulting to pupillary dilatation and anisocoria, allowing the Sympathetic Nerve to dominate.

the ciliary muscles which make the biconcave lens relax and increase the diameter, causing refraction of light that makes images smaller. The SN impulses *relax* the ciliary muscles, which in turn make the biconcave shape lens flat and refract objects to become bigger. PS nerve constricts the pupil while the SN nerve causes it to dilate (Mnemonics: COPS-constrict parasympathetic, and DAISY-dilate sympathetic). These two opposing autonomic nerves contribute to the efficient control of light to the retina through the process of accommodation.

One critical clinical condition that affects the PS nerve is related to *uncal herniation* from a large hemorrhage, infarct or severe edema of the brain. When both oculomotor nerves exit the midbrain, they run beneath the *tentorial leaf or edge,* where the tips of *both medial unci* (medial lobe of the temporal lobe) rest (Fig. 19 A). Both unci protrude a little and almost kissing the oculomotor nerve. It is because of this anatomic relation that pupillary dilatation in *uncal herniation* happens. The uncus can very well press on the oculomotor nerve, and the first manifestation is the *slowing down of the pupillary reaction or dilatation of the pupil* usually on the same side, causing **anisocoria** *(meaning, unequal diameters of the two pupils)* (Fig. 19 B). The risk of uncal herniation is one of the reasons why the pupillary reaction to light is considered a vital neurologic sign. *So what if there is uncal herniation? How important is it?* When the pressure in any part of the brain builds up, brain matter will seek to occupy areas with least resistance, and these are usually the spaces like the ventricular space, foramen magnum, and the quadrigeminal cistern (space where the brain stem passes through the tentorium). When one of the *unci herniates* and occupies the limited space of the quadrigeminal cistern, it will crowd the area and *push the brain stem, causing microscopic breaks of axons, blood vessels (shown as pathologic Duret hemorrhages in the brainstem), and other supporting structures of the brain.* The brain stem is considered the vital center where control of the cardiovascular system, respiration, and wakefulness reside. Displacing the brainstem may cause the patient to lapse into a coma or worse go into respiratory arrest or cardiovascular collapse and die. So, if a person has a *right-sided weakness and the left pupil dilates,* this may mean that there is intracranial pressure increase caused by a *lesion on the left side* of the brain. The increased intracranial pressure might cause the *uncus to herniate* and cause left pupillary dilatation or *anisocoria.* Anisocoria is an EMERGENCY!!

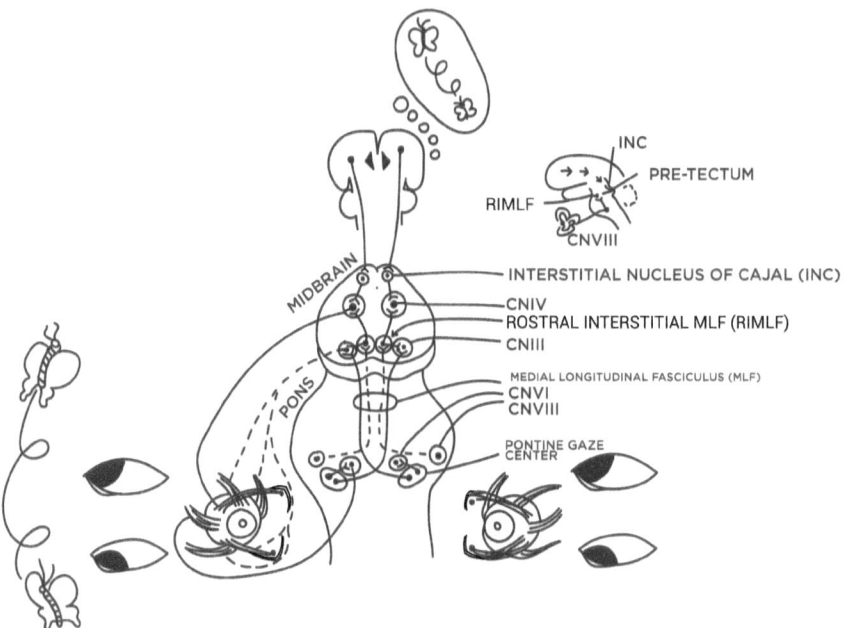

Figure 20. Vertical Gaze mechanism pathway. Cortical recognition of the flight direction of the butterfly is sent to pre-tectum, INC neurons which in turn send impulses to CN IV – Trochlear Nerve effecting appropriate eye movements. As this is happening, labyrinthine influences (dotted lines) are sent to the RIMLF further refining the eye movements in relation to head movements.

The upward or downward synchronous movements of the eyes allow the clear image of objects that are moving up and down. This important function is made possible through the **vertical gaze control mechanism** of the eyes. When the butterfly goes up, the vertical upward gaze accompanies the rotatory movement of the eye, movements that are *integrated by the rostral interstitial medial longitudinal fasciculus (RIMLF) and the interstitial nucleus of Cajal (INC)*. The RIMLF in both sides of the midbrain receive ascending *impulses from the vestibular system* through the MLF while the INC receives *inputs from the brain* through the pretectum (Fig. 20.). The semicircular canals provide inputs to CN VIII as they pick up movements of the head when following the flight of the butterfly. CN VIII then provide inputs to the RIMLF. The visual cortex and other brain centers interpret the position of the butterfly and send impulses also to the INC. This finely-tuned integration of systems will bring about appropriate movements of the eyes to provide a clear and single focus on the butterfly.

Tumors pressing on the midbrain like a pineal gland tumor or infarcts can cause the paralysis of the upward gaze, causing the eyes to deviate downwards -- looking like a sun setting on the horizon, the so-called "sunset sign." Pressures to the midbrain from above or below may sometimes cause irregular downward beats or "ocular bobbing." Case story:

A 32-year-old woman on her fifth month of pregnancy was discovered by the husband to be drowsy and difficult to awaken in bed. The night before, she complained to the husband about feeling dizzy. Both of them attributed the symptoms to the pregnancy. At the emergency room, when called and asked to put out her tongue, she opened her eyes and slightly opened her mouth but readily went back to sleep. Her right eye was also noted to be positioned downwards ("sunset sign") and deviated to the side while the left was at the center. On moving the head from side to side (Doll's head maneuver), the right eye remained in "sunset position" while the left was moving completely medially and laterally. On the brief opening of the eyes, the right eye showed a consistent partial weakness of the lid (ptosis), and on direct and indirect light reflex, the pupil on the right was bigger at four millimeters compared to two millimeters on the left eye (anisocoria) but were all briskly reactive. The left upper and lower extremities showed the mild weakness of 3-4/5 motor strength. CT Scan and MRI with angiography showed, a midbrain-pontine, small **cavernous hemangioma** (a form of an abnormal arterio-venous malformation) with hemorrhage. The multidisciplinary team decided to try conservative management. Doctors ordered complete bed rest, control of mild hypertension, close obstetrical and fetal monitoring. She slowly regained her consciousness, and the progress of pregnancy and fetal growth reached term. The caesarian section on the ninth month of gestation delivered a healthy baby boy. The mother slowly regained her neurological function except for persistent double vision when looking upward and to the right.

Clinical - anatomic Correlation:

The intracerebral hemorrhage most likely caused a mass effect on the oculomotor nerve nucleus on the right side to explain the ptosis and larger pupil on the right (anisocoria). The "sunset sign" of the eye on the right side was due to the disturbance of the right pretectum-INM-INC system. The left-sided weakness was due to the involvement of the right corticospinal tract (pyramidal or motor tract) at the midbrain before crossing at the medulla. What about the drowsiness? You will get to understand this in Chapter XI, Anatomy of Consciousness.

Many clinical conditions could disrupt the integration of the visual and extraocular muscle movements. One, however, must remember that the muscles of the eyes can be affected by diseases of the muscles, like **myopathies** or by diseases involving the **neuromuscular junction** (junction between nerves and muscles). **Thyrotoxic myopathy** is an example of acquired diseases affecting ocular muscles. **Myasthenia gravis** is the most common disease affecting the neuromuscular junction. These diseases can cause varying degrees of weakness or paralysis of the ocular muscles.

On the other hand, just like the peripheral nerves, the cranial nerves CN III, IV, and VI can be affected directly in its course through the cavernous sinus, by which inflammation in this area like **Tolosa - Hunt syndrome** or **cavernous sinus thrombosis** can cause varying degrees of weakness of the extraocular muscles. The abducens nerve (CN VI), being the longest cranial nerve, is vulnerable to various diseases or conditions. Increased intracranial pressure commonly affects the abducens nerve causing diplopia or double vision. In this case, CN VI has no localizing value. Diabetes when poorly controlled predisposes to atherosclerosis of the tiny vessels (**vasa nervorum**) that supply the nerves. Atherosclerotic obstruction decreases blood supply to the nerve to cause ischemia or infarcts. Diabetic vasa nervorum obstruction commonly affect CN VI to cause weakness of lateral recti muscles that manifests double vision or diplopia.

Neurological Examination:

First, instruct the patient to remove corrective glasses if he is wearing one. Place your index finger two feet in front of the patient's center of vision and tell the patient to focus on your finger. The position of the eyes in the center is the **primary gaze.** Tell the patient to inform you if he sees double. Keep the focus for about ten seconds while looking for deviation of the eyes. Then move the finger along the horizontal plane and let the patient follow the movements from extreme right to left while watching for weakness or extra efforts of the eye muscles to maintain a conjugate movement. Next, move your finger upwards and downwards at the center and on either side while watching for irregular activities or weakness of the eyes. Mildly weak muscles of the eyes can compensate and hardly noticeable. In this condition, we do the "cover-uncover test" to catch the compensating weakness. Cover one eye while you are doing the same horizontal maneuver, and while maintaining the gaze to one side suddenly uncover the eye and watch for drifts and compensated return to conjugate eye positions. Repeat the procedures until you are satisfied with the result. During vertical gaze examination, you must observe the movements of both upper lids; compare both and watch out for drooping eyelids. If you are suspecting fatigue of eye muscles due to myasthenia gravis, you can let the patient focus continuously upward for about a minute and look for signs of fatigue or appearance of diplopia or double vision. You may time the process to be able to quantify the duration of fatigability. To test for pupillary reaction, focus light directly at the pupil and check for size and speed of pupillary response. The procedure is the **direct light reflex test**. To do an **indirect light reflex test,** do the same maneuver, but this time observe the movement of the *opposite pupil*. The response should generally be equally brisk. Also, watch the pupillary activity on both sides as the patient is looking at the movement of the finger towards the nose. The maneuver is the **accommodation reflex test**. Both should constrict briskly when both eyes move towards the center.

Now, go to your window, watch and savor the many things immobile, mobile, near, and distant and be thankful of the efficient control of the ocular muscles to allow you to see the beauty of the world with clarity even while moving.

Chapter VI-D

Cranial Nerve V- Trigeminal Nerve
(Functions: Face Sensation and Mastication)

All of us have experienced toothaches in our lives. Imagine if one cannot perceive the aches. An infection of the tooth which is unfelt allows the undetected infection to progress to a dangerous abscess and life-threatening sepsis. When an ant lands on any part of our face, we will feel it crawling and can even differentiate it from flies or mosquitoes. The experience sends an alarm which triggers brushing it away before it bites! If we are unable to feel the crawling ants, we will also not feel and prevent their bites allowing multiple bites on the face. The sensory branch of the CN V (Trigeminal Nerve) transmit these protective pain and touch sensations.

We love to eat tender and juicy steak and taste the mix of flavors that go with it. Part of the enjoyment is biting, gnawing and experiencing the soft quality of the beef. If for some reason one is unable to make a bite and grind, the joy of eating becomes miserably frustrating. The motor branch of CN V (Trigeminal Nerve) supplies the muscles of mastication (jaw muscles) to allow chewing and make feeding a pleasant experience.

CN V (Trigeminal Nerve) has two functional components. The trigeminal nerve sensory afferent and the trigeminal nerve motor efferent. We shall discuss their functional anatomy separately.

Functional Anatomy of CN V Trigeminal Nerve Sensory Branches

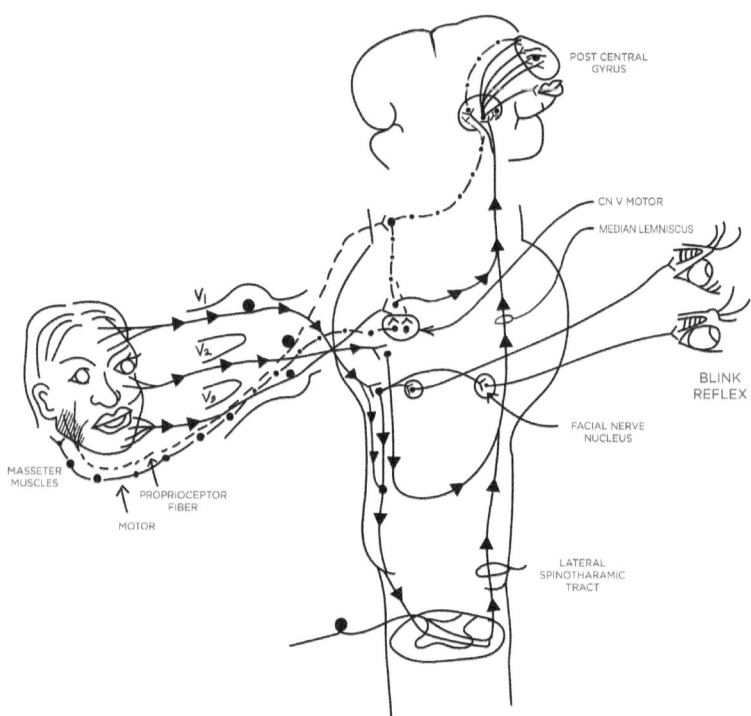

Figure 21. Cranial Nerve V – Three divisions of Trigeminal Nerve, V1, V2, V3. CN V-motor nucleus send efferent axons to masseter muscles (dotted lines). Proprioception afferent (broken line) fibers from the muscles. Sensory afferent nerve from half of the face (arrow), descending then ascending with the lateral spinothalamic fibers to the thalamic nucleus. Note synaptic connection with CN VII – Facial Nerve nucleus to effect a blink reflex when the cornea is stimulated.

Peripheral pain, temperature, and touch receptors are distributed diffusely in the face and other cranial structures like the sinuses, pharynx, nasal mucosa, and the base of the dura. *Proprioceptive receptors,* on the other hand, are distributed mostly in the *masseter muscles and extraocular muscles.* Just like the dorsal ganglia, the *pseudo-bipolar neurons of the receptors reside in the Trigeminal or Sphenopalatine or Gasserian Ganglia.* The sensory neurons in this station send axons to the trigeminal nerve sensory nuclei which are extensively distributed from the midbrain to the upper cervical spine (C3) in an organized and an orderly manner. The sensory receptors send impulses through the axons of the neurons at the Trigeminal Ganglia (TG), and these are bundled into *three divisions* that roughly *represent the corresponding cranial dermatomal distribution of the face (Fig. 21).* These are the *Ophthalmic Division (V1), Maxillary Division (V2), and Mandibular Division (V3).* Roughly the dermatomal areas of V1 are the forehead, the large part of the nose except the tip, the upper eyelid, the eyes, the brow, and the anterior ethmoidal sinuses. The V2 dermatomes, on the other hand, include the cheeks, the upper teeth, the tip and the alae of the nose, the maxillary sinuses, the palate, and part of the ears. The V3 dermatomes cover the area of the lower lip, the tongue, the lower jaw, the lower teeth, and part of the base of the dura. The neurons of the three ganglia divisions transmit impulses to the *second station at the brain stem.* The trigeminal nerve sensory mandibular division, particularly the *proprioceptive sensory fibers,* synapse with trigeminal nerve sensory nuclei at the midbrain level. Neurons in this area *(mesencephalic nucleus)* send synaptic connections to the trigeminal motor nerve nuclei. The neurons in this second station then send axons that *cross to the opposite side* to synapse with thalamic neurons at the third station. These thalamic neurons then send axons to its *destination* at the postcentral gyrus [26, 27].

The other sensory impulses, particularly for *pain or nociception and temperature, enter the second stations* at different levels in the pons, medulla, and C3. The *ophthalmic division second station* connects at the lowest level all the way to the posterior gray horn of the cervical spine (C3) then *cross to join the ascending spinothalamic fibers.* Axons of the neurons at the trigeminal nerve sensory nuclei or the second station *cross and* ascend to the third station of the thalamus, and then the neurons send axons to the *postcentral gyrus* and other areas of the brain. Sensory neurons at the second station in the brain stem *also send axons to different cranial nerve motor nuclei*. One of these is the Ophthalmic Division V1 that connects with the *motor neurons of the facial nerve (CN VII)*. This circuitry is the basis for the **corneal reflex**. The *cornea, when stimulated* with a wisp of cotton sends impulses through the *ophthalmic division* of the trigeminal ganglia. When pulses reach the ponto-medullary *second station for trigeminal nerve sensory nuclei*, some of the neurons transmit currents to both *right and left motor neurons of the facial nerve motor nuclei*. The facial nerve motor nuclei then send electrical potential to the *orbicularis muscles on both sides, causing a blink*. Remember this circuitry because corneal reflex is part of the examination of comatose patients. Testing its function gives us an idea about the status of the brain stem. In an unconscious patient, bilateral absence of corneal reflex may mean that the brain stem is severely affected and may spell poor prognosis, especially if other brainstem functions are abnormal. Unilateral lack of corneal reflex means either the trigeminal sensory nerve or facial motor nerves are affected in peripheral nerve diseases.

The neurophysiologic study called Blink Reflex Electromyography utilizes the reflex subserved by CN V and CN VII interconnections. The skin around the eyes, which is innervated by the CN V ophthalmic division, is stimulated, one side at a time. The procedure records the speed or latency of conduction of impulses from the stimulating electrode to the pick-up electrode of both eyelids that triggers a blink. The rate recorded and measured is from the CN V nerve to ipsilateral CN VII nucleus, and the first response is called the R1 wave. The conduction speed (latency) from the ipsilateral CN V nerve and contralateral CN VII nucleus and the second response is called the R2 wave. Diseases involving any parts of the trigeminal-facial reflex pathways will show absence or delays in the R1 and R2 latencies, physiologic abnormalities that imaging studies do not demonstrate.

Case Story:

Mrs. Martin, a 65-year-old widow, started complaining of pain involving the right lower jaw which she described as a toothache. According to her, it began as a small pinching pain over the right mandible which would occur occasionally, but within two months it became continuous but still tolerable. She consulted a dentist who prescribed pain medicines and requested for a panoramic X-ray of her teeth. Not finding any carious teeth or gum infection, the dentist advised her to continue taking pain medicines and placed her under observation. There was no satisfactory relief of the discomfort, and gradually the intensity of the pain became more severe that it disturbed her sleep. In distress, she said, "There were lightning-like, severe, stinging and unpredictable pains that jolted me...every attack made me cry in frustration!" These jolting pains happened when the surface of her face was touched or even when the air from the fan blew on her face such that she would always cover the right side of her face with a scarf. Unable to eat and sleep, she went back to the dentist who advised her to seek a neurologic consult.

Clinical - anatomic Correlation:

An agonizing disease called **Tic Duloreaux or Trigeminal Neuralgia** manifest as an *episodic, on and off, lightning-like, severe pain* that often has **trigger points** (this is an area nearby if touched can trigger the experience). Pain is experienced *along any or in a combination of the three divisions of the Trigeminal nerve*. In Mrs. Martin's excruciating pain, the V3 or mandibular branch of the trigeminal nerve is involved. Trigeminal neuralgia is usually *unilateral, has the same distribution, and is common among the elderlies*. The disconcerting experience is a form of neuropathic pain. **Neuropathic pain** is a painful manifestation of disease or injuries affecting the *nociceptive fibers or its central pathways*. Pain characteristically is felt along the sensory dermatomal distribution of the face and body. This understanding is essential because ordinary painkillers may not offer relief. Medicines for epilepsy are the same medicines found useful in managing neuropathic pain. Failure to recognize trigeminal neuralgia can sometimes lead to unnecessary teeth extractions when the pain happens along the distribution of the mandibular or maxillary divisions.

Neurological Examination:

With a wisp of cotton, touch the cornea (please see Fig. 53, p. 244) while the patient is looking up and away from the stimulus (this is a maneuver that prevents the patient from seeing the approaching wisp that could trigger anticipated blinking). The typical response is bilateral and brisk blinking. To test touch sensation, again using a light material like cotton, stroke the face lightly along the distribution of the three trigeminal nerve divisions. Ask the patient to compare how different one side from the other. The sensory examination responses of patients are a highly subjective test. The examination is repeated to observe for consistency of response. To examine pain sensation, use a pin to gently and lightly press on the skin along the same division of the trigeminal nerve. The patient should be able to detect the sharpness and should be felt similarly on the other side.

The corneal reflex test, with the Ophthalmic Division of CN V as the afferent arm and CN VII as the efferent arm, is important in assessing the function of the brain stem particularly in the examination of comatose patients. If the *brain stem is not functioning, it is incompatible* with life. The absence of corneal reflex on both sides denotes poor prognosis especially when accompanied by the following signs 1. Fixed dilated and unreactive pupils; 2. Absent doll's head maneuver; 3. The absence of eye movements on **caloric testing,** a test that stimulates the CN VIII vestibular organ with cold water through the eardrum; 4. The lack of spontaneous respiration, and zero motor movements in all extremities. All of these denote a poor prognosis. In some countries, a patient may be considered brain dead even if the heart is still beating (The heart has its generator of electricity to make it contract on its own,) allowing organ donation feasible. Countries have their *brain death criteria*.

Functional Anatomy of the Muscles of Mastication

How do chewing and biting work? The initiation of the motor movements of the muscles for mastication (i.e., Masseter Muscles) starts from the motor cortex or precentral gyrus. (Remember the homunculus and pyramidal tract?). The axons from the motor neurons merge with other axons at the internal capsule then descend anteriorly to the midbrain. The axons then *cross* to the opposite side before synapsing with the trigeminal nerve motor nuclei in the *midpons* at the second station. The trigeminal nerve motor nuclei then send axons through the sphenopalatine ganglion (does not synapse there) where different axonal branches arise to supply the muscles of mastication (Fig. 21).

Neurological Examination:

The muscles of mastication, which are supplied by the motor branch of the trigeminal nerve, can be tested by asking the patient to bite hard while touching the angle of the jaw to feel the bulk and tone of the jaw muscles. Another maneuver is to press the chin while the patient tries to open the mouth to assess the strength of the jaw muscles. Usually, the jaw should remain in the center, if the jaw deviates to one side, the muscles on that side are weak.

Clinical – anatomic Correlation:

In motor neuron disease where the trigeminal nerve motor nuclei may be involved, the bulk of the muscle atrophies or diminishes in volume; then eventually, in the advanced state of the disease, the jaw falls, and the patient will have difficulty chewing and will hold on to the jaw to keep it in place.

Chapter VI-E

Cranial Nerve VII- Facial Nerve
(Functions: Facial Muscles of Expression, Taste, Eye Closure, Lacrimation, Salivation, Sound Modulation)

Say cheeeeessseee! The typical command given by a photographer to a human subject to elicit a voluntary smile. When followed, simulates a happy expression of the face. Facial muscles are essential for *social expressions* of anger, gladness, surprise, sadness, disappointment, doubt, joy, sincerity, and many more. One can even fake the appearance. Actors are highly skilled in the art of expressing varied emotions by using their facial muscles. Appreciation of the taste of food can also be communicated through facial expressions like when it is sour or bitter. Tears that accompany the feelings of extreme joy; sadness; anger; or laughter complete the emotional expression. More importantly, tears protect the eyes by continuously providing lubrication to prevent drying of the cornea and providing antibodies to contain and control infections.

We mentioned in the previous chapter that masseter muscles are an integral structure in biting and chewing to appreciate the tenderness of the steak. Chewing and biting are also important to reduce the food size to a proportion that facilitates swallowing. The *salivary gland secretions* are also indispensable in the joy of eating because they soften the food and help make a bolus of the food for easy swallowing. Adding to the quality of appreciating the food is the gift of *taste*. The activities mentioned above are common needs in life and these are all due to the various functions of CN VII (Facial Nerve).

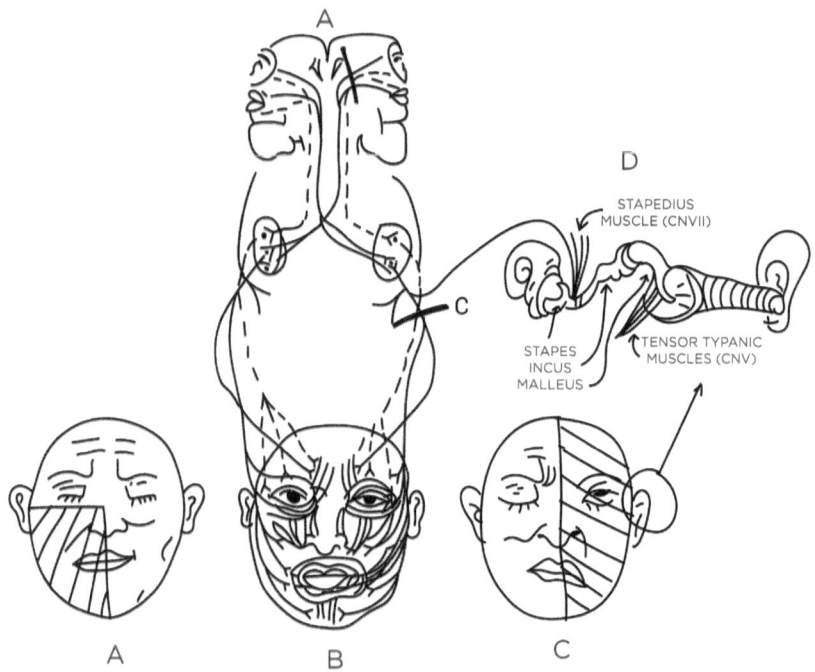

Figure 22. Cranial Nerve VII – Facial Nerve-Motor Component. D. Supply to stapedius muscle. B. Muscles of the face showing bilateral CNVII innervation of the upper half of the face (broken and solid lines) and unilateral innervation of the lower half of the face (solid lines). A. Lesions at the subcortical area (upper heavy line at *fig. B*) causing contralateral central facial palsy with sparing of the upper half of the face. C. Lesion involving the peripheral CN VII (lower heavy line at *fig. B*) causing Bell's Palsy.

There are three nuclei groups of CN VII (Facial Nerve):

1. The Motor Neurons of the Facial Nerve Nuclei (similar to the anterior horn cell of the spinal cord) is functionally divided into *upper motor groups* supplying the muscles of the upper half of the face, and the *lower motor groups* providing the muscles of the lower half of the face (Fig. 22).
2. The Nucleus Solitarious (NS) consists of neurons that receive taste sensations from the anterior two- thirds of the tongue and the upper palate via the geniculate ganglia. The axons from the taste buds are bundled together as short lingual nerves before joining the chorda tympani (as afferent nerve). There are a few sensory fibers from the auricular, periauricular, and external ear canals that send impulses via this nerve, too, but not shown in the figure (Fig. 23).
3. The Superior Salivatory Nuclei (SN) are composed of parasympathetic neurons that send axonal impulses to the pterygopalatine ganglia via geniculate ganglia (no synapse here) where neurons in turn pass the electrical wave to the lacrimal glands, the mucus glands of the nasopharynx, and the sinuses. Some of the axons of the superior salivatory nuclei reach the submandibular ganglia and sublingual ganglia whose neurons in turn supply the submandibular and sublingual glands respectively. The parasympathetic nerves to the salivary glands are bundled with other nerves as chorda tympani (Fig. 23).

There are *two components of the CN VII bundles on both sides*. These are *the* **facial nerve** and the special sensory nerve, the **nervus intermedius**. A large part of Cranial Nerve VII, the facial nerve, is dedicated to supplying the muscles of the face the so-called, *"muscles of facial expressions"* and the *stapedius muscles* of the middle ear. The smaller but equally important part of the bundle, the nervus intermedius, consist of the *afferent* nerves for special sensory function for taste and auricular discomfort and the *efferent* parasympathetic nerves for the salivary, lacrimal, and mucus glands.

The Facial Motor Nerve

As mentioned in Chapter III, the facial muscles, which include the muscles around the eyes (orbicularis oculi) and the lips (orbicularis oris), have their neural supply originating from the *precentral gyrus or motor cortex*, as shown in the *homunculus*. Descending axons from the pyramidal neurons, which will eventually supply the facial muscles, will pass through the internal capsule and the anterior part of the midbrain and then synapse with *two groups of facial nerve motor nuclei at the* second station. The *upper groups of motor neurons*, which supply the *muscles of the brow and the orbicularis oculi*, receive crossed and uncrossed *descending motor axons* (Fig. 22-B); therefore, the upper half of the face has *bilateral innervation*. The lower groups of motor neurons that supply the lower half of the face massively receive only crossed fibers from the corticospinal tract; therefore, the lower half of the face has unilateral innervation. The axons from the second station motor facial neurons at the lower third of the pons go around the nucleus of CN VI (abducens nerve) before they exit as facial nerves. The *facial nerves* therefore *bundle both the axons from the upper group and lower group of neurons* [28].

Case Story:

Mr. Hudson, a 54-year-old corn farmer, while tending to his animals, suddenly developed weakness of the left upper and lower extremities and fell. Upon seeing the father fall, the son frantically rushed beside him and noticed the slurred speech that cannot be understood. The son drove Mr. Hudson quickly to the emergency room where the duty-doctor noted his left face sagging; however, he was able to blink and wrinkle both brows and forehead. He was able to close both his eyes tightly. He understood all questions and was able to express himself despite the slurring verbally. His tongue slightly deviated to the left upon protrusion. The other cranial nerves were normal. The motor strength of his left upper extremity was 1/5 while that of the left lower extremity was 3/5. There was no sensory deficit. There was a Babinski sign on the left. An MRI revealed an early small infarct at the right internal capsule.

Clinical – anatomic Correlation:

A lesion *above* the facial nerve nucleus such as an infarct at the level of the internal capsule, which Mr. Hudson had, results in a weakness of the *opposite face, but only in the lower half of the face muscles because of the bilateral innervation of the upper half of the face* (Figs. 22-A & B). The corticospinal tract involvement at the internal capsule spared the ability of the brow to move and the eye to close. Neurologists refer to the lesion above the nucleus as *supratentorial in location*, with the tentorium as the anatomic boundary separating the brain from the brainstem. If the affectation is the peripheral nerve of CN VII, which carries the motor nerves to both upper and lower parts of the facial muscles, the result is paralysis of the entire side of the face. A common site of inflammatory injury to the facial nerve is at the stylomastoid foramen, a tight canal where the nerve exits from the skull to supply the facial muscles. The manifestation is often referred to as *Bell's palsy*. Charles Bell described the syndrome in around 1829, for which he was given credit, when he detailed the motor and sensory anatomy of the CN VII and described manifestations of lesions involving the peripheral facial nerve [29]. The left brow fails to wrinkle on frowning and the left eye does not close completely. Failure to close the left eye completely exposes the cornea to foreign body or flow of air. The result is a stinging irritation in the left eye, frequent blinking and lacrimation. Also, the left side of the lips does not participate in pouting and upon smiling, the left side sags or is paralyzed (Figs. 22-B & C). The understanding of this concept is of the essence because patients who develop Bell's palsy are often worried that they might have a stroke. Reassuring them that the lesion involves the peripheral nerve of CN VII, not the brain, and therefore is not a stroke, provides immeasurable relief from anxiety. Also, expensive hospitalization and diagnostic workup are avoided. Informing patients that recovery from facial deformity attributed to Bell's palsy is complete in about 85%, is also very reassuring.

The *facial nerve egresses from the brain* at the ponto-medullary junction and *enters the internal acoustic canal and*, together with the *nervus intermedius, enters* the *facial canal* at *the mandibular area and exits at the stylomastoid foramen*. The nerve passes through the *Geniculate ganglia* where the stapedius nerve takes off (Fig. 22-D). The stapedius nerve supplies the stapedius muscle that provides a tone to the stapes and serves to regulate sound wave vibration. When a loud noise occurs, the muscle contracts and decreases the movements of the stapes and effectively dampens the transmission of sound waves to the cochlea (**stapedius reflex**). This reflex protects the ears from the destructive effects of deafening sound to a certain extent. This stapedius nerve can be involved in diseases or injuries to the internal acoustic canal, a canal which lies on top of the middle ear. When a poorly controlled middle ear infection extends and involves the internal acoustic canal, the facial nerve at this level can be affected and can produce a syndrome of Bell's palsy with hyperacusis, loss of taste at the anterior 2/3 of the tongue, and loss of lacrimation on the side of the area affected. Paralysis of the stapedius muscle can result in loss of control of the stapes and would clinically manifest as **hyperacusis** or exaggeration of sounds commonly perceived at usual intensity. It is for this reason that a history of ear infection should always be sought, and the external canal examined by otoscope.

The motor nuclei of both facial nerves receive synaptic connections from trigeminal nerve ophthalmic division sensory nuclei at the level of the pons and medulla. The link will complete the corneal reflex with the trigeminal nerve-ophthalmic divisions as the afferent arm and the facial nerves as the efferent arm. The motor nuclei of the facial nerves also receive synaptic connections from the neighboring acoustic nuclei of CN VIII (Vestibulo-acoustic nerves) to complete the *stapedius reflex* to loud noise which protects the hearing apparatus from damage.

The Nervus Intermedius

The Nervus Intermedius is the smaller division of CN VII that carry both afferent and efferent nerves. They accompany the facial nerves as they enter the internal acoustic canal (IAC). The *efferent* nerves are axons from the parasympathetic nucleus of the Salivatory Nucleus (SN). These axons pass through the IAC, facial canal, and geniculate ganglia (do not make synaptic connections here) and join the *greater petrosal nerves*. These nerves synapse with the neurons at the pterygopalatine ganglia. The post ganglionic neurons of the *pterygopalatine ganglia* supply the lacrimal, nasopharynx, sinus, and mucus glands. Some of the neurons extend their axons through the *chorda tympani nerves* to

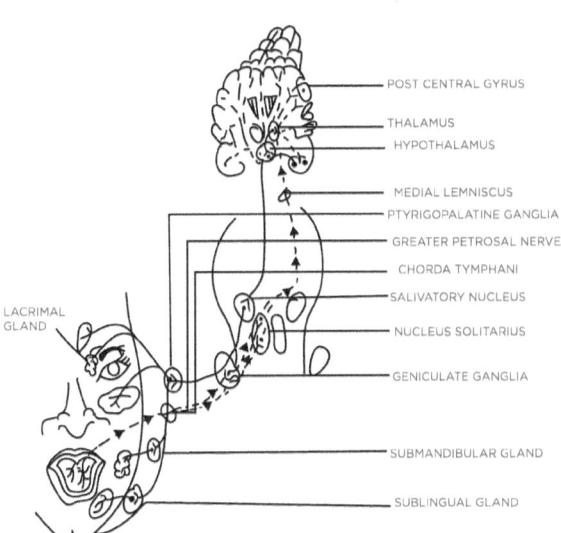

Figure 23. Cranial Nerve VII – Facial Nerve for Taste and Parasympathetic nerve to Glands. Taste fibers (arrows) to the Nucleus Solitarious then ascending at the opposite side towards the thalamus then to the cortex. Hypothalamic fibers (solid lines) descending to the Salivatory Nucleus then to the salivary and lacrimal glands through respective ganglia.

innervate the *submandibular* and *sublingual ganglia* (Fig. 23). These postganglionic neurons supply corresponding glands.

Transmission of taste sensation is one of the essential functions of CN VII (Facial Nerve). There are five basic taste sensations- *sweet, salty, sour, bitter,* and *umami* (amino acid taste sensation). Taste receptors are distributed diffusely in the tongue, soft palate, and even the larynx. These five sensations have specific *taste bud receptor channels or proteins* that allow transduction or transformation of chemical reactions into electrical depolarization that release adenosine triphosphate (ATP) into the receptors of the afferent axons. The receptors from the anterior 2/3 of the tongue, soft palate, and a part of the larynx transmit these electrical impulses through the *chorda tympani, greater petrosal nerves and synapse with the neurons at the geniculate ganglia (GG)*. The neurons from the GG, the first station, transmit impulses through the *nervus intermedius* and synapse with the second station neurons of the Nucleus Solitarius (NS) at the lower pons and upper medulla. The NS neuronal axons, in turn, cross and join the *medial lemniscus* as it ascends the brain stem to reach the third station at the thalamus. The thalamic neurons will distribute the taste impulses to the middle part of the postcentral gyrus (tongue and lips of homunculus) where sensation for taste is integrated with the hypothalamus, amygdala, and insula to provide the emotional and behavioral components of the taste perception. The integration with other cortical centers is how one appreciates the taste and flavors of food. The posterior 1/3 of the tongue transmit taste sensation through CN IX (Glossopharyngeal Nerve) which we will discuss later.

Salivatory secretion is also a necessary function of CN VII. How does sight of food trigger salivation? How does the green mango elicit more salivary secretion than the ripe mango? When chewing, saliva helps in the masticatory process to transform food into an ingestible consistency. Salivary flow is mostly a nerve-mediated reflex. The afferent arm comes mainly from two sources. The first consists of the *cortical sources* (conditioned reflex) which are descending impulses from the various cortical locations triggered by *sight of food, the smell of food, and thought of food*. This descending impulse will synapse with the superior Salivatory Nucleus (SN). The second source of afferent arm consists of the *taste and mastication impulses* (unconditioned reflex) transmitted through the nervous Intermedius, the glossopharyngeal nerve, and the vagus nerve for taste, and the trigeminal motor nerves for mastication. When these afferent impulses reach the brainstem, synaptic connection with the different levels of the SN occur. The neurons at the SN are mainly parasympathetic neurons that send efferent axons through the nervus intermedius and eventually to the greater petrosal nerve and chorda tympani to stimulate perioral, mucosal, submandibular, and sublingual gland secretions. The parotid glands likewise receive efferent impulses through the glossopharyngeal nerves. The sympathetic nerve has a limited role in the salivary or gustatory function, but it does increase blood flow to the acini of the salivary gland, thereby increasing the volume of the saliva.

> *Thine tears floweth.*
> *Is it for joy or sorrow?*
> *Or hath the dust of summer blown*
> *a sting on thine eyes that burrows*
> *or to stir my senses, to strike my heart?*
> *It is more powerful than arrow.*
> -- a. san luis

The *lacrimal gland* secretes a salty fluid that bathes the external eyes to protect it. Tears are protective to the cornea and conjunctiva. Basal tears are secreted continuously to wash these structures. Reflex tears, on the other hand, are responses to injuries or potential injury to the cornea and conjunctiva. Foreign bodies like dust that land on the cornea can trigger pain and reflex tears. Its afferent arm is the ophthalmic branch of the trigeminal nerve which sends synaptic innervation to the salivatory nuclei of the facial nerves, a group of parasympathetic neurons whose efferent axons eventually innervate the lacrimal gland through the greater petrosal nerve. Emotional tears, on the other hand, are cortical and hypothalamic descending influences on the SN that trigger tears after a hearty laugh or a sad milieu or cry because of pain. Tears are indeed powerful emotional participants in the expression of feelings.

Neurological Examination:

To test the facial motor function or the muscles of expression, let the patient show his/her teeth or make a grin. Observe the symmetry of the facial folds during the movements and sustained facial contraction. Then, to examine the orbicularis oculi muscles, make the patient close the eyes forcibly against your fingers' effort to open them. Mild weakness can be detected this way. Then let the patient wrinkle the forehead, as in anger, to test the frontalis muscles. Bell's palsy consists of the failure of the upper lid to close; upper and lower facial weakness; and other manifestations depending on the severity of the paralysis and the part of the facial nerve involved. One eye is continuously open so conjunctival irritation triggers increased lacrimation and frequent blinking of the opposite eye. Drooling of saliva on the weak side can be observed due to the weakness of the orbicularis oris or muscles of the lips.

If the lesion is above the chorda tympani, taste sensation on the same side of the anterior 2/3 of the tongue will disappear. For taste sensation evaluation, the patient is instructed to keep the tongue protruded. Then apply on one side of the anterior two-third a cotton swab soaked in either sugar water and the sour lemon juice. The patient signals that taste is perceived then points at appropriate multiple taste descriptors like bitter, sour, salty, sweet, none. If the facial nerve at the internal acoustic canal or petrous bone area is affected, the stapedius muscle will weaken resulting in **hyperacusis**, a magnified perception of hearing on the same side. In hearing intensity test, the patient compares the sound of a tuning fork from each side of the ears. One can use cellophane crumpling as the stimuli. The ear the patient describes consistently as stronger than the other is the afflicted side. The examiner, serving as the control, does the same maneuver to himself and compare the result with the experience of the subject.

Chapter VI-F

Cranial Nerve VIII-Vestibulocochlear Nerve

(Functions: Hearing and Balance)

Bronx, New York. At ten o'clock in the evening while sitting by the window of an apartment, you notice the place is still very much awake. You hear the different sounds of motor engines, the clanking of garbage covers, shouts of people, wailing of the ambulance siren and the sound of horns with different notes. They are near and distant, yet amid all these noises, you notice a distinct, exquisite and sweet music of a violin resonating in the air. How can you identify the different and distinct sounds and yet be able to filter them and appreciate the notes of the violin?

How come when one has a stuffy congested nose, the hearing seems to be decreased or distant?

Try bending your head and body and do complete turns ten times then try to walk in a straight line. Are you able to walk straight and what is your feeling? Dizzy? Every day, you bend, turn your heads, and make forward and backward movements, turning while the hands are holding on to something yet most of the time you do not fall or trip. Did you ever ask yourself why you can do this?

Cranial Nerve VIII (Vestibulo-Acoustic Nerve) consists of two different components, these are the **Cochlear Nerves** that transmit stimuli from the eardrums that trigger discriminative hearing and the **Vestibular Nerves** that transmit stimuli from the vestibular apparatus (semicircular canals and utricles and saccules) that provides delicate balance in all our activities.

The Cochlear Nerve.

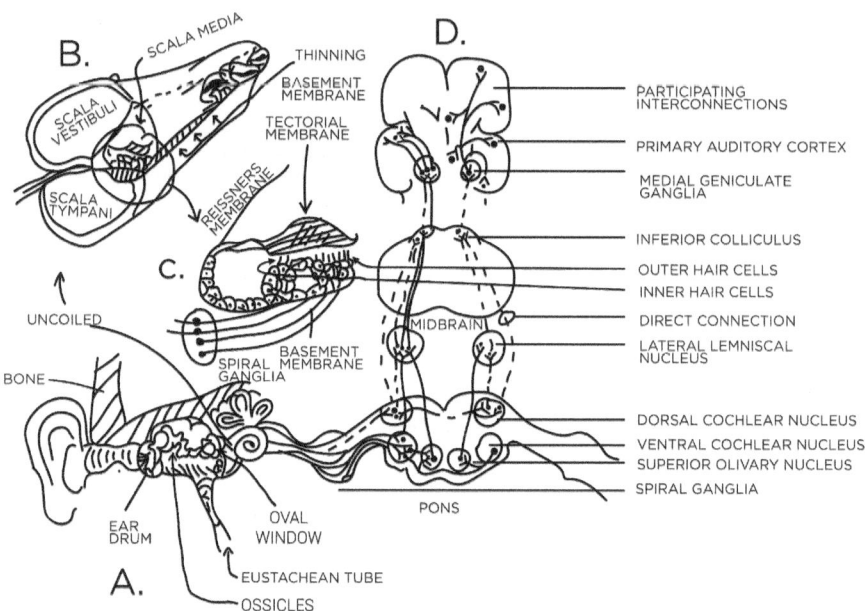

Figure 24. Cranial Nerve VIII – Auditory or Cochlear Division. A. 3 ossicles in the middle ear transmitting sound waves to oval window of the cochlea. B. Cochlea uncoiled showing 3 tubes or scala filled with different fluids allowing transmission of sound waves that cause differential displacement of the basement membrane, which is thicker but shorter at the base and thinner but longer at the apex. C. Hair cell's stereocilia displaced against the stiff Tectorial membrane. Electrical impulses from stereocilia are transmitted to the spiral ganglia then to the various nuclei group in the pons. D. Central connections from Pons, Inferior colliculus, Medial geniculate ganglia to Primary auditory cortex.

In the midst of neighborhood noise, a beautifully distinct sound of a violin calls one's attention. The pinna of both ears caught many of the sound waves that get amplified in the external ear canals. The sounds then vibrate the eardrums and get transmitted to the bony ossicles found inside air-filled middle ears whose only opening is through the auditory tubes or Eustachian tubes that are connected to the nasopharynx (Fig. 24 A). The ossicles consist of the *malleus, incus,* and *stapes*. When a loud bang suddenly happens, the stapedius muscles which is innervated by the CN VII (not seen in the illustration) pull the stapes away from the oval windows while the tympanic tensor muscles which are innervated by CN V, pull the malleus. These muscular contractions cause tension to the tympanic membranes, in effect dampening impending transmission of sounds and preventing damage to the inner hair cells of the cochlea (***Cochlear Reflex***). Nasal congestion can close one Eustachian tube creating increased pressure in the middle ear space and in effect dampening ossicular transmission of tympanic vibration. That is why, when one has severe nasal congestion, at times hearing seems "distant" or decreased in the affected ear.

Sounds with high amplitude and low force energy are transmitted in the air and transformed mechanically as vibrations by the ossicle system and are changed to low amplitude but high energy force. The ossicles transmit the vibrations to the oval windows of the cochlea. The vibration induced by the stapes through the oval window is strong enough to create pressure waves in the perilymph of the *Scala Vestibuli* which in turn create similar waveforms in the endolymph of the *Scala Media*. The waveforms created is identical because there is no resistance from the vestibular membrane. The wave displacements allow the transfer of the pressure waves to the *Scala Tympani* then to the round windows (Fig. 24 C). The waveforms at the Scala Media displace the Basilar Membrane in varying degrees, depending on the frequencies of the sound waves. The radial fibers that make up the basilar membranes are the shortest and stiffest at the base and longest and malleable at the apex, creating critical differences of displacements. When the pressure wave moves from the bottom to the top, the high-frequency sound gets to displace the basilar membrane earlier than the low-frequency sounds (>20 Hz) as they near the zenith. This critical differential displacement separates the various frequencies of noise we hear around us, allows localizing where the sound comes from, and even eliminates the extremes and their time differences [30,31,32]. The characteristic of the basilar membrane explains why the sound of the violin is heard as distant with distinct frequency against the other nearby sounds and noise. But how can we identify notes or different noises? The *Organ of Corti* contains: 1. Stiff but minutely mobile tectorial membrane (TM); 2. Outer hair cells (OHC) which are located underneath the head of the TM and are more in numbers compared to the inner hair cells (IHC); 3. IHC is situated at the base of the TM and is fewer in numbers; 4. Dendritic branches of the spiral ganglia neurons; 5. Afferent nerves from the IHC and efferent nerves to the OHC; and 6. Other supporting structures (Fig. 24 D). The OHC serves as the amplifier or modifier of pressure waves. When the basilar membrane is displaced, the OHC moves upward, allowing displacement of its cilia against the TM. The cilia, acting as a switch, trigger entry of potassium (K^+) to the cilia, eliciting depolarization and shortening of the cell body – *electro-mechanical transduction*. The OHC's shortening and lengthening mechanism gets reflected the basal membrane and allowing feedback vibration to the organ of Corti – *reverse transduction*. The efferent impulses from the brain also influence the OHC contractility. The electro-mechanical and feedback transduction and efferent impulses from the brain can enhance and modulate cochlear sensitivity and selectivity to sound frequencies. These perhaps permit fine-tuning and identification of notes and noises. How are the pressure waves transmitted to the brain? The IHC is the primary transmitter of cochlear outputs to the brain. Displacement of basal membrane raises the IHC and the cilia against the TM, triggering a cascade of K^+ entry to the cell, the opening of channels to calcium (Ca) and releasing glutamate transmitter to the afferent dendrites of the neurons of the spiral ganglia (*first station*). At this point, the journey of the transduced sound waves gets out of the cochlea.

The *spiral ganglia neurons*, bundled as cochlear nerve, join the vestibular nerve upon entering the internal acoustic canal (Fig. 24 B). The facial nerves also pass through the same acoustic canal. After exiting the canal, the vestibulocochlear nerves enter at the ponto-medullary junction and synapse with the neurons of the *Dorsal Cochlear Nuclei* (DCN). The DCN is located at the lower pons and the *Ventral Cochlear Nuclei* (VCN) at the medulla (*Second station*). The VCN contains five *cell types* with *distinct morphologic and physiologic features* that discriminate *stimulus onset, offset, and frequency modulation* (refining further the distinction of noise and the tune and rhythm of the violin). The *VCN* sends crossed and uncrossed fibers to the following areas: *Superior Olivary Nuclei (SON), Lateral Lemniscus Nuclei (LLEN), and Inferior Colliculi (IC).*

The crossings of fibers allow differential recognition of one side from the other for localization and rhythm and allow bilateral perception even if there is a lesion on one side. The neurons of SON send ascending fibers to LLEN and IC. The neurons of DCN, on the other hand, send axons across with few synaptic connections with LLEN neurons and most direct link with IC neurons, which is the *third station*. The *DCN* direct connection with the IC neurons is considered a *fast-acting system*, which is operant in *the startle response* to sudden loud noise. The longer processing time due to the interconnections in the brain stem may explain some sound processing for discrimination. When impulses reach the third station at the IC, they synapse with specialized neurons in this area. The IC neurons then send pulses to the *fourth station* at the Medial Geniculate Ganglia (MGG) where their neurons subsequently send electrical waves to the *Primary Auditory Cortex* which is responsible for the characterization of sound sensation as pitch and rhythm. The *secondary auditory cortex and cortical interconnections allow hearing perceptions* that will distinguish sounds like speech, music or noise. The audio transmission at this point does not only discriminate the sound of violin from the noise but also colors it as a beautiful, distinct, and clear music and even relates it to familiar tunes in the past.

Case Story:

Mr. JC, a 43-year-old bank manager, had a cough, high-grade fever, and headache for three days. Just before admission, the wife noted that he was still asleep at noon on a Monday workday. In the emergency room, his neck was rigid on flexion; he was drowsy and had to be prodded several times to give verbal responses which were garbled and incomprehensible. An immediate CT scan of the brain showed normal findings. A lumbar tap was done to analyze the cerebrospinal fluid (CSF). The CSF showed the abnormal presence of too many white blood cells, highly suggestive of acute bacterial meningitis. Appropriate antibiotics were immediately started to treat the infection. After 36 hours, his fever disappeared, and the headache became tolerable. On the fourth day in the hospital, after breakfast, he became agitated because he could not hear anything at all; he lost his hearing. Deafness on one side or both sides can happen as a dreadful complication of pyogenic meningitis. The small penetrating vessels to the ponto-medullary areas supplying the nucleus of CN VIII or the exit cochlear nerve can be infiltrated by inflammatory cells (arteritis) causing sensory-neural deafness.

Clinical - anatomic Correlation:

Deafness or *decreased hearing* and *tinnitus* are common symptoms linked with the cochlear neural apparatus and its connections. Diseases can directly or indirectly affect the ear canal, the bones or ossicles of the middle ear, the cochlea, the auditory nerve (part of CN VIII), and the cochlear nerve nucleus at the ponto-medullary junction and cause deafness. The ear canal can be blocked by a foreign body, a mass or cerumen and can cause failure of sound waves reaching the eardrum. The negative pressure created by a congested nasal mucosa that is obstructing the Eustachian tube can dampen sound vibration transmitted by the three ossicles of the middle ear. Middle ear infections (otitis media) is also a common cause of deafness in developing countries. The cochlea and its organ of Corti can be affected by viral diseases such as mumps, blockage of its blood supply caused by stroke or inflammatory cells, degeneration of the cells of the organ of Corti, due to toxic medicines (ototoxicity), or noise pollution. The vasa nervorum, which are the tiny blood vessels supplying the cochlear nerve, can be blocked by inflammatory cells from meningitis like what happened to the case of Mr. JC. The Schwann cells that produce myelin to wrap around the cochlear nerve can turn into a tumor (schwannoma) and strangulate the nerve to cause gradual deafness. The CN VIII nucleus and their ascending fibers at the ponto-medullary junction can be directly disturbed by obstructing or rupturing the blood vessels supplying this part of the brainstem. The central station at the superior gyrus of the temporal lobe when affected by a stroke, manifests not as deafness, because the patient can hear, but cannot identify sounds. The disturbance is called **auditory agnosia**, the inability to discriminate and interpret the sensation of sound. Electrical discharges from seizures involving the superior temporal lobe produced positive manifestations in forms of *auditory hallucination* or *seizures and possible associated episodic aura* of an annoying ringing of the ears.

Clinical Examination:

Clinically, there are two types of hearing problems: abnormal transmission of sound through the ear *(conduction deafness)* and failure to transmit auditory electrical signals (*sensory-neural deafness*). The initial test consists of comparing the hearing perception on each side of the ears by using the ticking sound of the watch (circa 1970) or by snapping or rubbing of the fingers. **Rinne's test** is done with the vibrating tuning fork applied at the mastoid area and as soon as the sound disappears, the tuning fork is immediately placed 1-2 cm away from the ear of the same side. If the vibration sound is no longer heard (bone conduction greater than air conduction) there is conduction deafness. If the sound persisted (air conduction is longer than bone conduction), the ear is normal. However, if the air conduction is shorter compared to the examiner's hearing, this may indicate sensory-neural deafness on the same side. **Weber's test** is done by placing the tuning fork in the middle of the forehead and if the vibrating sounds are heard equally on both sides, the ear is normal. If the sound is heard only on one side, there might be conduction deafness on the same side or sensory neural deafness on the opposite side. The use of *Audiometers* can quantify the loss, but this requires cooperation from the patient. *Auditory Evoked Potentials* can measure the speed of travel of the stimulating click sounds from the source to the inferior colliculus and the central station of the temporal lobe. The right and left sides of the ears are tested and compared and established laboratory norms of conduction speed (latency) based on the different wave forms are determined. Asking the patient to identify the sound of a coin that drops on the floor, shaking off a bunch of keys, or the ringing of a bell will test for *auditory agnosia* and will test the ability to lateralize sound.

The Vestibular Nerve.

Watching the U.S. Open Men's Singles Championship between Novak Djokovic and Rafael Nadal is indeed an exciting treat and is also an enthralling display of vestibular mechanisms in action. Did you notice how Nadal was able to focus on the fast-moving ball at 120 miles per second while at the same time running very fast towards the ball and hitting it back with a powerful topspin at almost 100 miles per second to the opposite side away from Novak? And Novak, with similar intense focus on the ball, ran mightily to reach for the ball with his racket and whacked the ball back towards Nadal! The ball moving swiftly back and forth, players fiercely in graceful abundance, ran, stopped, swung, and hit the ball until one succumbed to human limitations. Isn't it amazing how each player, while running, suddenly stopped for a split second and hit the ball full swing without losing balance? The vestibular apparatus, the semicircular canal, the utricle and saccule finely coordinated with the visual cortex, frontal gaze center, brain stem nuclear group, cerebellum, spinal cord, and extraocular muscles are all very much operant in this sport. Too complex? It is but let us try to understand it.

Let us rewind the story but this time focusing only on the normal vestibular functions. When Nadal saw the ball going to the left, he suddenly turned his head and body to the left. The *vestibule-ocular reflex (VOR)* allowed him to see *one single ball* while in motion. The sudden acceleration and deceleration of movements triggered the *vestibule-spinal reflex (VSR)* that allowed body and arm to move in coordination to maintain balance and posture, while the *vestibule-collic reflex (VCR)* allowed the head-body balance despite the head movement. The motion is not only vestibular in action because most of the described responses had the strong and active participation of the *sense of proprioception and visual perception* about body and space orientation. (Sounds fancy and complicated, too? Yes, it is, but you do not need to memorize. Just know that there is a complex integration of different body systems for such movements.)

The vestibular apparatus consists of two main parts: the three *Semicircular Canals (SCC)* and the *Utricle and Saccule* (Fig. 25 A). The SCC is like the circa 1970 tires where you have the outer tube, representing the bony part of the SCC, and inside it is the inner tube representing the membranous membrane of the SCC. Let us cut the three tires and sew the cut-edges together at their ends -- with one positioned vertical, another one horizontal and one at a 45° angle. All the arches point to the external side. Now we have three elongated and close set of tubes on each side of the ears. The *perilymph* of the SCC is similar to a fluid that fills the space between the exterior and interior tube, while the *endolymph* of the SCC is like a fluid that fills the interior tube. Now we have two tubes with different fluids inside. The perilymph resembles CSF with a high Na: K ratio, while the endolymph resembles plasma with a high K: Na ratio. Located at the end where the inner tubes fuse is the *ampulla* which contains the diaphragmatic membrane or cupula that moves in reaction to endolymphatic pressure.

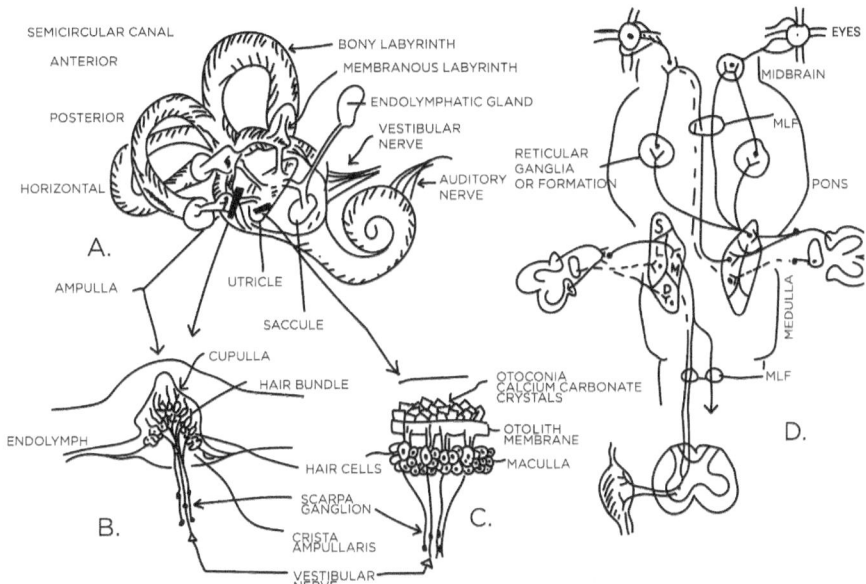

Figure 25. Cranial Nerve VIII – Semicircular Canal or Labyrinthine Organ Division. A. Parts of semicircular canal (labyrinthine apparatus) B. Cupula inside each ampulla C. Otoconia inside utricle. D. Ponto-medullary labyrinthine nuclear groups interconnections and eye muscle connections.

Within the copula is connective tissue crista ampullaris where hair cells rest and move from side to side in unison with the copula. (Fig. 25 B). Head angulation changes trigger fluid movement inside which causes the walls to move together with the hair cells. The movement of the crista ampullaris causes the hair cells to move back and forth, inducing depolarization that is transmitted as electrical impulses. Movement of hair cells away from the membrane causes excitation while movement of hair cells toward the membrane elicits inhibition. The three SCC on one side is an exact duplicate of the other side, with their positions perpendicular to each other and covers the same direction as a pair. The effect of this relationship is a balanced and coordinated "push-and-pull effect" that covers all angles of movement. An example of such movement is a forward movement causing the Right, North-East (NE) and Left, South-West (SW) plain of the labyrinth to move and strike the hair cells of the ampulla, causing them to sway in different directions, with the SW causing excitation and the NE causing an opposite inhibition.

The *Utricle* and the *Saccule* have endolymph as well but the equivalent of the copula of the SCC is the *otoconia* which have more mass and made-up of calcium carbonate; as such it is sensitive to gravitational force and linear acceleration that is transmitted to the *otolithic membranes* (Fig. 25 C). To cover the different dimensions of head movement, the *Saccule lies vertically* while the *Utricle lies horizontally* when in an erect posture. Movement of the otolithic membrane displaces *the hair cells in the macula*. The hair cells get depolarized and send transduced electrical impulses to the *bipolar neurons of Scarpas Ganglion*. The neurons extend fibers as vestibular nerve through the internal acoustic meatus together with the facial nerve and cochlear nerve. It enters at the ponto-medullary junction where some axons synapse with four groups of vestibular neurons while some go directly to the cerebellum (Fig. 25 D). The SCC hair cells respond to angular and velocity motion while the *Saccule and Utricle* to linear and acceleration motion [33,34,35]. So, when Nadal saw the ball to the left and turned his head to the left, the angular movement of the SCC could have been triggered and the sudden acceleration of the head movement triggered the Utricle and Saccule. The result was a vision of one ball, position change of extremities to balance, and toning of the neck to keep head-body orientation.

The cerebellum has a great influence in balancing the impulses coming out and going into the vestibular apparatus. The vestibular neuronal complex serves as the primary processor of vestibular input and implements direct, fast connections between incoming afferent information and motor output neurons. The *cerebellum is the adaptive processor*; it monitors vestibular performance and readjusts central vestibular processing if necessary. Vestibular sensory input integrates with incoming somatosensory and visual sensory data. The Vestibular nucleus consists of the *superior, lateral, medial, and descending nuclei* group on each side (Fig. 25D). *Superior and medial neurons* relay impulses to the cranial nerve nuclei that control the eye muscles to participate in the *Vestibulo Oculomotor Reflex (VOR)*. The *medial group* is also involved in *Vestibulo Spinal Reflex (VSR)* and coordinates eye and head movements that occur together. The *lateral vestibular nucleus is primarily engaged in VSR*. The cerebellar projections to the vestibular nuclear complex have inhibitory influence that refines vestibular activities. The cerebellar flocculus adjusts and maintains the *gain of the VOR*. The nodulus of the cerebellum changes the *duration of VOR responses* and is also involved with the processing of otolith input. Anterior superior vermis affects the VSR and when impacted by a stroke cause profound gait ataxia with truncal instability.

We have just described the intricate participation of the cerebellum in processing vestibular afferent impulses and how its efferent output influences motor functions. The overall effects are unconscious adjustments of the eyes to have one single moving vision and constant refined muscle activities that participate in balance and controlled movements. Nadal and Djokovic, tennis greats, run back and forth, maintaining a single image while running and doing complex activities including creating a strategy on how to whack the ball to an intended target...cognitive cortical participation!! The runs, the sudden stops, the swings of the arms, the twisting of the body, the deceleration, the balance and the timing are all integrated into the vestibule-cerebellar system of these great players. Amazing isn't it?

Case Story:

Mrs. Rossi, a 40-year-old teacher shouted in distress and panic upon waking in the morning. She was seen immobile, flat in bed, with eyes closed, and holding the edge of the bed. "I feel like I am falling and turning," she nervously shouted. After a while she vomited thrice and was nauseated with every movement. She remained immobile in bed, begging to be brought immediately to the hospital, but the husband and son were unable to do so because every effort to move her caused more anxious attacks of subjective vertigo (as opposed to objective vertigo where the surroundings are felt to be the ones turning or moving). Mustering enough courage, Mrs. Rossi tolerated the experience so that she could be brought to the car and rushed to the nearest emergency room.

In the emergency room, her heart rate was 96/minute, she had a blood pressure of 139/90 and her respiration was 20/min. The doctor did a quick neurological assessment, then alleviated the anxiety of the patient by reassuring her that aside from the dizziness, the rest of the brain was functioning well. She was greatly relieved after being informed that it was not a stroke. She was administered Metoclopramide for the dizziness. The doctor described the presence of horizontal nystagmus with the fast component to the left. There was no motor and sensory deficit and there were no other cranial nerve abnormalities. Upon lateral flexion of the head, the doctor was able to reproduce the nystagmus and the symptoms consistently on the left lateral flexion of the head. The doctor wrote a diagnosis of Benign Paroxysmal Postural Vertigo (BPPV) or Acute Vestibular Neuritis. The disease is also called Benign Postural Vertigo of Barany, named after the man who first described the problem in 1921.

Clinical – anatomic Correlation:

The sense of imbalance or dizziness (general feeling of imbalance) or **vertigo** (the illusion of swaying or movements most common in rotatory objective or subjective experience) are the most common symptoms afflicting the vestibulo-cerebellar and central system. When there is a sense of imbalance, the functions of one side of the *vestibular apparatus*, the *vestibular-cerebellar connections* and the *cerebellar incoming* *and outgoing connections* should always be pictured in mind to help us determine the possible location of the problem. The most common disease-causing vertigo is **Benign Paroxysmal Positional Vertigo (BPPV) or Acute Benign Positional Vertigo** which is usually not associated with deafness. The vertigo is acutely severe and exacerbated by head movement and this is then followed by gradual recovery in a week or a month. **Meniere's disease** is due to obstruction of the flow of the endolymph, causing increased pressure manifested as sudden severe vertigo (patients may fall during the experience), tinnitus and hearing loss due to the involvement of the hair cells of the organ of Corti in the cochlea. Paroxysms of vertiginous attacks could be due to episodes of "puncture-drainage-relief", and "sealing-increased pressure-recurrence of vertigo" mechanisms. When acute vertigo accompanies deafness, a stroke due to obstruction of the labyrinthine artery which is a branch of the posterior inferior cerebellar artery should be suspected.

The brain of Mrs. Rossi received the abnormal or unbalanced signals from the vestibule-cerebellar system and in turn interpreted and expressed them as dizziness, mainly vertigo, an illusion of turning and sense of imbalance that she anxiously experienced. The abnormal impulses reached the brain through the vestibulo-cerebellar and thalamocortical connections. Comparative anatomic studies have shown that ascending vestibulo-cerebellar and median geniculate fibers synapse with the neurons at the *ventroposterior intermedius* (VPI) *thalamus*. The thalamic neurons in turn project to the *parieto-insular vestibular cortex (PIVC) and the postcentral gyrus at about the face area of the homunculus*. This pathway allows conscious decisions to accelerate, to decelerate, to stop or to take a balanced position. This pathway also can explain anxiety reaction and unnecessary worries that may magnify the experience of imbalance or vertigo. The other important reason is that, this cortical pathway is stimulated by various head positional maneuvers to facilitate adaptation to the lack of balance that will pave to earlier tolerance and recovery, a rehabilitation strategy.

Neurological Examination:

The three semicircular canals are positioned strategically with each other to cover all possible angular movements of the eyes, while the utricle and saccule sense linear acceleration/deceleration activities of the eyes and head. The cells inside these structures that detect the movements are the *hair cells*. Typically, when the eyes focus to the front and there is no head movement there is *symmetric tonic activity* stimulating the vestibular system. While moving, there is a constant interplay of *increasing* activity of one side with a corresponding *decrease* of action on the opposite side, depending on the direction of movement. The result is a perception of that movement and fine reflex activity that results in a clear vision and similar operations of relevant parts of the head and body. This reflex action a vestibule-ocular reflex (VOR) where the cortical stimulation actively opposes the direction of the eyes. The opposing movement results in physiologic fast, fine, and jerky movements of the eyes opposite to the course of the eyes, This is called jerking "*nystagmus.*" The constant eye movement and corresponding opposition to it can sometimes appear clearer when one peers through the window of a running train and looks at the passing series of electric posts. The many milliseconds of efforts to fix the vision of each electric posts create jerky nystagmus, commonly described as "optokinetic nystagmus."

When you let the gentle gaze at and follow your finger as it moves laterally and then vertically, you might be able to elicit nystagmus physiologically. If there is an imbalance due to disease or injury to one side of the vestibular apparatus or the nerve, especially if it involves the horizontal canal, *horizontal nystagmus* could be elicited away from the locale of the lesion. If the superior and posterior semicircular canals are affected, a rotatory type of nystagmus will show due to the participation of the horizontal canal in the movement. *Rotatory nystagmus* can be *due to peripheral or central* pathologies. When *vertical nystagmus* appears during the maneuver, it usually indicates a brain stem lesion. The bilateral vestibular disease has no differentiating impulses to the brain, so there is either a little vertigo and nystagmus or none at all. Slow growing tumor, like vestibular neurilemmoma may not cause vertigo or nystagmus because the brain has enough time to adapt to the imbalance.

The caloric test is a procedure that stimulates specific gravity changes in the endolymph by irrigating the external ear (after checking the absence of obstruction or perforation of the eardrum) with contrasting temperatures of cold and warm water. The temperature either increases or lowers the specific gravity by convection. With warm water and the patient in a prone position, the specific gravity goes down allowing the endolymph to move upward towards the cristae, triggering excitation of the nerve. The vestibular nerve transmits the stimulus to the opposite pontine gaze center in the brain stem, where the extraocular muscle favors turning of the eyes *away from the source* of the stimulus, but the vertiginous experience and the *nystagmus are towards the stimulus*. The caloric test is a very helpful test because it provides objective evaluation and is not dependent on the cooperation of the patient. It is also indispensable in assessing the integrity of the brainstem, in differentiating brainstem or cortical cause of decreased sensorium, and in distinguishing true coma versus catatonia (a psychiatric problem). This test however elicits so much discomfort to conscious patients. This test is now rarely used in awake patients. Ice caloric test is still a standard test in the evaluation of comatose patients and in assessing brain death.

Chapter VI-G

Cranial Nerve IX- Glossopharyngeal Nerve

(Functions: Taste, Salivation, Baroreflex, Swallowing, Ear & Palatal Sensation)

Memorial Day is barbecue picnic day all over America. You salivated after smelling the scent of strawberry-wine marinated barbecue, so you got a large serving. While savoring the taste of the tender meat and the sour-salty special sauce that goes with it, you suddenly realized that the last bus service is about to leave, so you made a big bite, swallowed vigorously, almost choked on the food and followed it with soda. The barbecue party is a very familiar scenario without realizing how fine-tuned our scent- the salivation-taste-chewing-swallowing cycle of feeding is. Do you know how much CN IX Glossopharyngeal Nerve contributed to this story?

The pleasant scent of barbecue is transduced into electrical stimulus, through *CN I (Olfactory Nerve)*, that eventually reaches the medial or inner temporal structures and the hypothalamus. The *hypothalamic neurons* then send *descending* impulses to the *Inferior Salivatory Nuclei* (shared superior salivatory nucleus with parasympathetic nuclei of CN VII). The salivatory nuclei neurons then send axonal fibers, as part of the *glossopharyngeal nerve*, through the jugular foramen. These particular *parasympathetic nerves* follow a circuitous route as they enter the skull joining the *tympanic nerves,* then join the lesser petrosal nerves again as they *exit the foramen ovale* where they synapse with the neurons at the *Otic Ganglia*.

Glossopharyngeal Nerve-Parasympathetic Nerve to the Parotid Gland

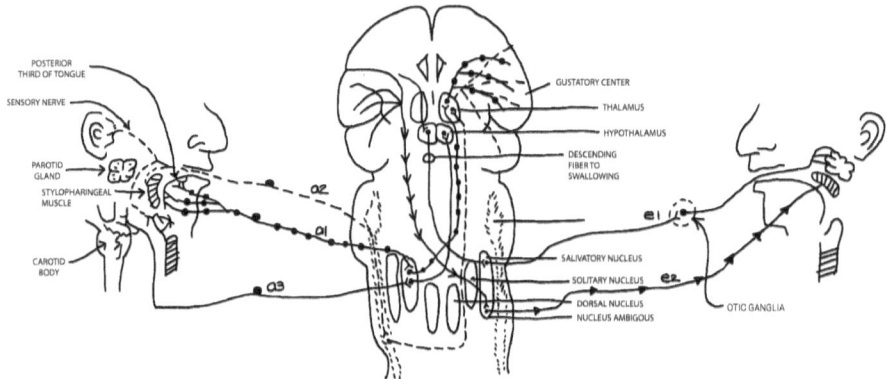

Figure 26. Cranial Nerve IX – Glossopharyngeal Nerve. Efferent nerves, from Nucleus Ambiguus, supply the parotid and mucus glands (e1) and stylopharengeal muscle that participates in swallowing (e2). Afferent nerves, a1 from posterior third of tongue for taste (dotted line); a2 from somatic sensation of external ear, posterior tongue and upper pharynx (broken line); and a3 from baroreceptors and chemoreceptors of the carotid body (solid line).

The otic ganglia neurons or postsynaptic parasympathetic neurons of CN IX send axons that pass through the left and right mandibular divisions of the CN V (Note: CNV has no parasympathetic function) to innervate the *parotid glands and tongue mucus glands, causing salivation* (Fig. 26-e1). Because the parasympathetic nuclei of CN VII share the Salivatory Nucleus, the *submandibular and sublingual* nerves get stimulated, too, through the same pathway. These glands also contribute significantly to the salivation [36].

Glossopharyngeal Nerve's Role in Swallowing

Upon seeing the last bus, the brain triggers the voluntary need to feed fast. The act of eating is a cognitive-emotional trigger that reaches the *pre-central motor gyrus* neurons which in turn send descending impulses to the *Nucleus Ambiguus (NA)*. The neurons from this station will send impulses to the *stylopharyngeal muscles (the only muscles supplied by the glossopharyngeal nerves)* which, together with the other muscles of the pharynx and larynx (supplied by vagus nerves and cranial part of the accessory nerves), propel *food down to the esophagus* (Fig. 26-e2). The primary afferent sensory fibers of the pharynx (pharyngeal plexus) come from the bipolar neurons at the *inferior GG* which sends impulses to the inferior part of *Nucleus Solitarius* (Fig. 26-a1) and *spinal nucleus of the trigeminal nerve*, thus facilitating the *efferent chewing mechanism of the mandibular muscles* [37]. Now you know that rushing ones eating call into action delicate integration of swallowing tools to prevent choking. What do you think will happen if one of these cranial nerves get affected by diseases? You are right. The delicate and efficient swallowing mechanism gets impaired predisposing one to choking or for saliva and food to be misdirected to the lungs causing *aspiration pneumonia*.

Glossopharyngeal Nerve for Taste

Taste sensation from the anterior two-thirds of the tongue is transmitted by CN VII as described in the Facial Nerve chapter. Taste sensation from the posterior third *of the tongue is transmitted via the glossopharyngeal nerve*, particularly the taste sensations for *bitter and sour* (Fig. 26-a1). The CN X (Vagus Nerves) transmit the transduced taste sensations at the base of the tongue and around the tongue. To recap, the taste sensation in the entire mouth is innervated by *cranial nerves VII, IX, and X*. When the taste-specific buds in the posterior third of the tongue transform or transduce the *tastants* (chemicals with taste characteristics) into electrical impulses, the depolarization is transmitted centrally to synapse first with the neurons at the *inferior glossopharyngeal ganglia (GG)*. The axons of the inferior GG neurons join the other glossopharyngeal nerve fibers and enter the jugular foramen, then synapse with the *caudal or inferior parts of the Nucleus Solitarius (NS) whose neurons are also shared by the facial and vagus nerves*. The neurons here, in turn, ascend and project to the *ventroposterior medial nucleus* of the thalamus. The thalamic neurons then project to the *primary gustatory cortex* which is in the area of the inferior parietal postcentral gyrus, and from here to the *secondary projection areas* which will provide cognition, emotion, and color to the experience of taste. In our case, a particularly discriminating "barbecue" taste.

Pain, temperature, and touch sensation of CN IX

Sensory receptors from the *skin of the external ear*, the *internal surface of the tympanic membrane, the walls of the upper pharynx, and the posterior one-third of the tongue* send impulses to the neurons of the *superior and inferior glossopharyngeal ganglia* (Fig. 26-a2). The neurons here in turn send axons through the jugular foramen to the *medulla* where the *axon descends* to synapse with the spinal trigeminal nucleus neurons. The trigeminal nucleus neurons send ascending impulses to the opposite Ventroposteromedial thalamic nucleus (VPM). The thalamic neurons then send pulses to the postcentral sensory gyrus and other areas of the brain that decipher the sensations into a meaningful experience.

Clinical Story:

One wintry morning, while Mr. McLee, a 76-year-old farmer, was feeding his sheep inside the barn, he noted that all of a sudden he was exerting more effort to carry the pail of warm water and was veering and trudging to the left. He decided to sit down and yelled for help but his voice was hardly audible. Alarmed and besieged by confusion, he mustered enough control of a near panic emotion, and with a rod on his right hand, pummeled the side of the emptied bucket. The noise succeeded in getting the attention of his wife, Jane, at the other end of the barn. Rushing fast and concerned, she saw him slumped at the side of the post, coughing while struggling to stand and to talk.

The emergency room physician noted that Mr. McLee could talk but his speech was slurred and was interrupted regularly by paroxysms of coughing. He was able to relate what happened to him though with much effort to be understood. The doctor noted that when Mr. McLee raised both arms, the left hand drifted and moved clumsily. The left side of the face and right side of the body had decreased sensation to pain and touch (**crossed deficits**). Both pupils were briskly reactive but the size of the left was smaller than that of the right (**anisocoria**). There was mild rotatory nystagmus when looking to the left. On stroking the right upper palate, there was a gag but when done on the left, there was none. He was diagnosed to have a *left lateral medullary syndrome* caused by a stroke. Worried and concerned, the ER physician immediately referred the patient to the stroke service which ordered MRI procedure and started appropriate medical treatment protocol.

Clinical – anatomic Correlation:

The different tracts and cranial nerve nuclei can be affected readily at the medulla because the structure is small in diameter. The branches of the posterior inferior cerebellar artery (PICA) supplied the small medulla. In Mr. McLee's case, the right-sided sensory deficit of the body and the *left* facial sensory deficit meant that the spinothalamic fibers, that carry the crossed sensory fibers from the spinal cord, and the uncrossed trigeminal sensory fibers on the left side of the medulla are affected. Involvement of the inferior cerebellar peduncle tract explains the struggle to carry the pale, veering to the left, clumsiness of the left hand, and the rotatory nystagmus. The smaller size of the pupil and mild ptosis on the left are due to the affectation of the left descending sympathetic tract that arises from the hypothalamus down to the spinal cord. The *Muller's muscle* that raises the lid, together with levator palpebrae muscles (innervated by CN III), is supplied by the sympathetic nerve. Involvement of the left Nucleus Ambiguus of both CN IX and CN X explains the slurring, the difficulty of swallowing the saliva, absent gag on the left side, and resulting paroxysmal coughing. The problem of swallowing and the inability to "sense" the presence of materials in the throat allow saliva to passively flow to the larynx, triggering protective frequent or paroxysmal coughing. Without this protective mechanism of coughing, aspiration of saliva and other materials can lead to aspiration pneumonia.

The procedure, gag reflex test, is touching the upper pharynx elicited a gag which is a motor reaction. The *afferent arm is the glossopharyngeal nerve sensory component* while the *efferent limb of the reflex,* which is the motor component, is carried out by *the vagus nerve.*

What Mr. McLee had was an infarct involving the **lateral medullary syndrome** which was initially described by Gaspard Vieusseux in 1810 and Adolf Wallenberg in 1895. These two scientists, reported series of cases with neuropathologic correlation involving this part of the medulla due to obstruction of the posterior inferior cerebellar artery (PICA) [38].

The ER physician became worried and concerned because, aside from the deficits described previously, there was a risk of involving other medullary fibers and nuclei that control vital functions such as the cardiovascular and respiratory centers and wakefulness systems. The ER physician is aware that the brainstem, particularly the medulla, is a critical structure of the CNS requiring very close monitoring for any signs of deterioration.

Both the CN glossopharyngeal nerves and CN vagus nerves mediate the Carotid Sinus and Carotid Body Reflex. The Carotid Sinuses at the base of both Internal Carotid and Common Carotid Artery bifurcations have baroreceptors embedded in their walls. The stretch effect of arterial blood pressure activates the baroreceptors. These receptors are sensitive to pressure changes like the rises in systole and drops in diastole. The *chemoreceptors,* on the other hand, are embedded near the baroreceptors and are sensitive to changes in low pH, pO2, and high pCO2 levels. The receptors' transduced electrical discharges are transmitted to the neurons at the *inferior glossopharyngeal ganglion* which then sends axons that join the other glossopharyngeal nerves through the jugular foramen (Fig. 26-a3). The vagus nerves, on the other hand, transmit transduced impulses from the *baroreceptors of the Aortic Arch* and the *chemoreceptors of the Carotid Sinus.* Upon entering the medulla, the axons from both glossopharyngeal and vagus nerves descend to synapse with the *Inferior Nucleus Tractus Solitarious (NTS)*. The NTS neurons send axons to various *reticular formations at the medulla and to the hypothalamus* to mediate cardiovascular and respiratory reflex responses to changes in blood pressure and pH, pO2, and pCO2. The *glossopharyngeal nerve impulses are inhibitory* and will be discussed with the vagus nerve in the next chapter. Now you know that the medulla is a host to the cardiovascular control, making it a vital part of the brainstem.

Chapter VI-H

Cranial Nerve X- Vagal Nerve
(Functions: Taste, Salivation, Carotid Sinus Reflex, Hering-Breuer, Visceral Organ Control, Swallowing, Phonation, External Canal Sensation)

Running for the first time at the famous New York Marathon takes a lot of long, patient and disciplined preparation. In one of your training, after running 10 miles, you noticed that your heart was palpitating at 110 per minute and your blood pressure was going up to 160/100. Are you going to worry? Will the heart rate and blood pressure recover? Your respiration also is heavy and fast, will you worry about this too?

The vagus nerve contains afferent axons of receptors or ganglionic neurons from various parts of the body structures and organs. An example of this is the afferent sensation for taste from the epiglottis and base of the tongue. The vagus nerve a participant, together with CN VII and CN IX, in the transmission of taste to the brain. It also contains efferent axons from the brain stem-medullary nucleus to supply various parts of the body. An example of this is the efferent parasympathetic supply to the pharyngeal mucosal and gastrointestinal glands and its participation in the swallowing and breathing synchrony. It also contains afferent and efferent autonomic fibers or axons participating in cardiovascular and respiratory reflexes.

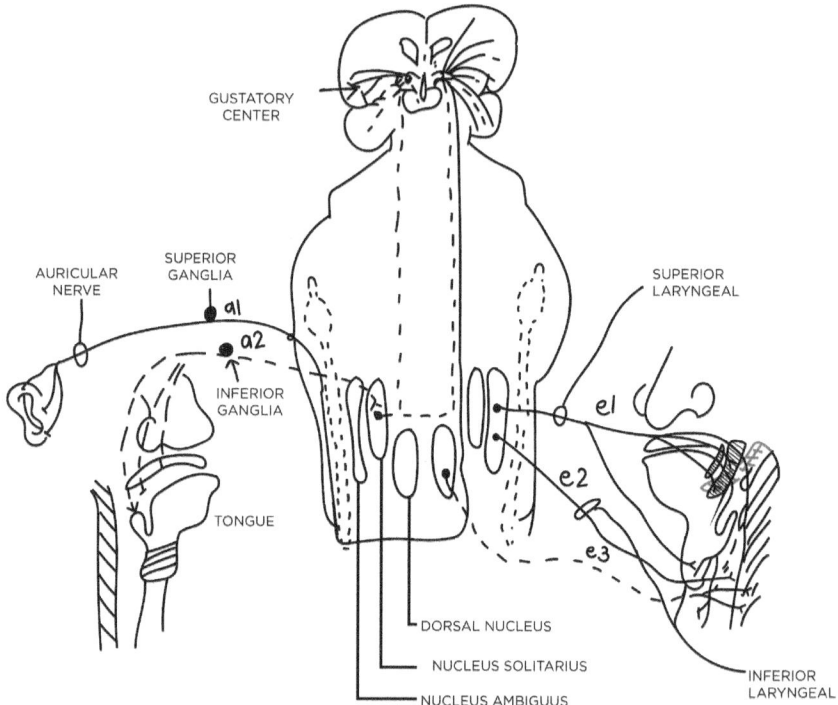

Figure 27. Cranial Nerve X – Vagus Nerve. Afferent nerve from pinna and external canal of the ear joining the CNV sensory fibers, descending and crossing, to ascend and terminate at the thalamus (a1). Taste sensation around the mucosa and base of the tongue and epiglottis to Nucleus Solitarius (a2). Efferent nerve from Nucleus Ambiguus (e1) to mucosal glands of the pharynx and glottis and cricothyroid muscles; (e2) to larynx and vocal cord; and (e3) paraympathetic pharyngeal nerve to the pharyngeal muscles.

CN X Vagus Nerve-afferent fibers

A vagal afferent nerve carries nociceptive and touch sensation fibers from the ear in its route to the brainstem to join the other medial lemniscus sensory fibers. When you inadvertently push the cotton bud while cleaning the ear canal, the pain felt is transmitted through a branch of the vagus nerve. *Receptors from the external canals and ears* send impulses, through the **auricular nerves**, to the neurons of the **superior ganglia**. The superior ganglia neurons then send afferent fibers to the *medulla*. Upon entering the medulla, the superior ganglia fibers *descend* and synapse with the *trigeminal spinal nuclei of the lower medulla*. The neurons subsequently send crossing fibers through the *medial lemniscus* to the *thalamus*. The thalamic neurons send axons to the primary sensory area at the *postcentral gyrus* (Fig. 27-a1).

Taste perception is transmitted mainly by afferent nerves of CN VII (anterior 2/3 of the tongue) and CN IX (posterior 1/3 of the tongue). *The surrounding structures* like the mucosa, around the tongue, taste buds at the base of the tongue, and epiglottis have taste receptors also that transduce and transmit impulses through CN X vagus nerve. One can imagine an expert wine taster "rolling" the wine all over the mouth, using much of the vagal nerve function in the transmission of delicate impulses from the taste buds before spitting it out. He then grades the aroma, texture, fullness, sweetness, bitterness and many other taste details. The impulses are transmitted to the *inferior ganglia* and from there to *the medulla* where axons *descend* and synapse at the *inferior Nucleus Tractus Solitarius (NTS), the second station (Fig. 27-a2)*. The neurons then send bilateral impulses to the third station at the *thalamus whose neurons, in turn, forward the electrical waves* to the *Gustatory Center* at the *inferior postcentral gyrus*. It is at the gustatory center where the discriminatory details of the taste of the wine eventually result to a grade.

CN X. Vagus Nerve-efferent Arm

The parasympathetic neurons from the medullary Salivatory Nucleus send impulses to the Parotid Gland via Glossopharyngeal nerve, while the surrounding secretory mucosal glands of the pharynx are supplied by the Vagus nerve to add to the salivary secretion of the oral cavity.

The efferent arm of the vagus nerve carries with it different branches to many areas of the mouth, neck, chest, and the abdominal structures. The vagus nerve gives off two branches, the superior laryngeal nerve and the inferior laryngeal nerve also called recurrent laryngeal nerve (Fig.

27). The superior laryngeal nerve gives off two branches (Fig. 27-e1). These are the internal laryngeal nerve which innervates the pharyngeal mucosa above the glottis and the external laryngeal nerve which controls the inferior cricothyroid muscles that keep the larynx open for breathing. These are important for swallowing-breathing synchrony.

The inferior laryngeal nerve or recurrent laryngeal nerve (Fig. 27- e2) is predisposed to injury from thyroid or mediastinum located surgeries, as well as tumors in the area, because of its proximity to these neck structures. This nerve is essential for phonation, and injury to this nerve causes hoarseness or loss of voice. When a patient presents to you exerting much effort in speaking with a hoarse and airy voice and is later found to have one vocal cord paralyzed, doing a CT Scan or MRI of the mediastinum is essential because tumors in this location can readily press on the recurrent laryngeal nerve.

The parasympathetic neurons at the Dorsal Nucleus provide the pharyngeal nerve (Fig. 27 – e3) that innervates the pharyngeal muscles for its autonomic or involuntary portion of swallowing.

The afferent and efferent limbs of the vagus nerves mediate the Carotid Sinus and the Hering-Breuer Reflexes (HBR). *Baroreceptors from* the aortic arch and *chemoreceptors* from the carotid sinus send impulses through CN X to the *inferior ganglion neurons* (Fig. 28 – a1) *and then to the inferior medullary Nucleus Solitarius (NS), the second station,* which is considered the *integrational hub of the reflex*. The glossopharyngeal nerve together with the vagal nerve also sends impulses to the NS (this was mentioned in Chapter IV-F). Neurons of NS transmit depolarizing waves to the *parasympathetic neurons of Nucleus Ambiguus (NA)* and the *Dorsal Motor Nucleus (DM)*. The neurons here send axons as the parasympathetic *efferent arm* of the reflex, *also mediated* by the vagus nerve (Fig. 28 – e1). The efferent vagus nerves descend to form cardiac, esophageal, and pulmonary plexuses. The cardiac plexus innervates the heart muscles and the sinus nodes. The parasympathetic vagal nerve transmitter is acetylcholine which *decreases heart rate*. During exercise, like jogging, a sympathetic drive happens to cause the blood pressure and heart rate to go up because of the oxygen demand. When blood pressure increases bring about stretching of the walls and these are detected by baroreceptors. The baroreceptors then react by sending inhibitory impulses to the brain through the same glossopharyngeal and vagus nerves.

CN X. Vagus Nerve Autonomic Reflex arms

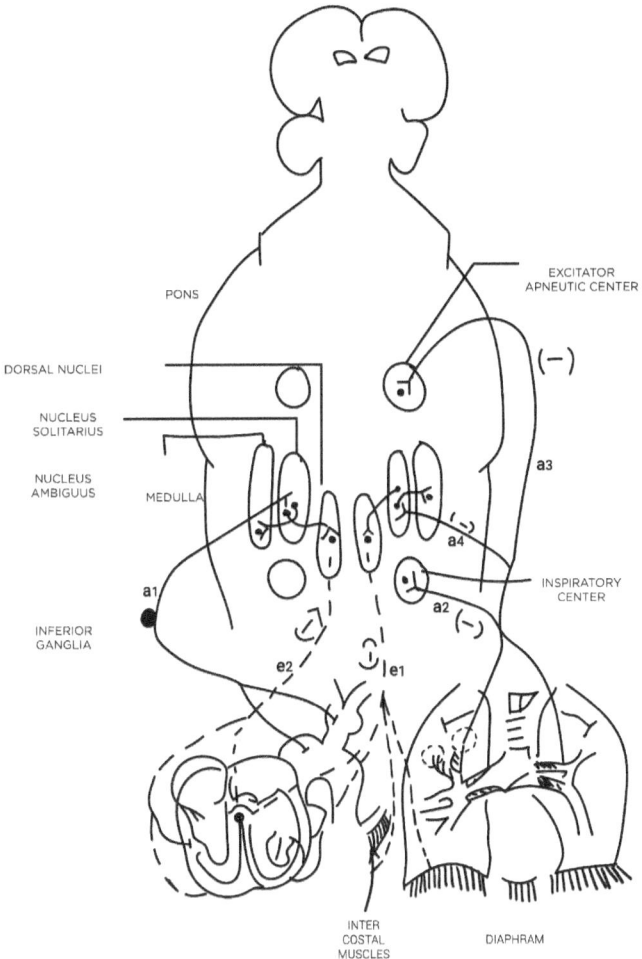

Figure 28. Cranial Nerve X – Vagus Nerve Autonomic Reflex Arms. Inhibitory afferent nerve (a1) from baroreceptors and chemoreceptors of the Carotid Sinus and Aortic Arch to the Nucleus Solitarius (NS). Inhibitory efferent nerve (e2) from Dorsal Nuclei (DN) to sinus nodes and walls of the heart; and intercostal and diaphragm muscles. Hering-Brewer Reflex, afferent inhibitory nerve from stretch receptors of bronchiolar and alveolar smooth muscles to Inspiratory Center (a2), Excitatory Apneutic center (a3), and to NS (a4) that in turn send impulses to DN and Nucleus Ambiguus (NA). DN neurons send vagal efferent (e1) to the heart and muscles of respiration.

The result is containment of the blood pressure and heart rate not to go beyond limits and also to allow fast recovery. This relationship enables this reflex to rapidly adjust the blood pressure to normal levels in different situations. When there is an increased sympathetic drive and increased blood demand in contracting muscles during running, rapid heart rate happens to meet the oxygen demand of the muscles. When the running stops, then the inhibitory effect of the *vagus and glossopharyngeal nerves* will slow down the heart rate and result to lower blood pressure.

In the *Hering-Breuer Inflation reflex (HBIR)*, the stretch receptors of the bronchiolar and alveolar smooth muscles are stimulated during inhalation, sending inhibitory afferent impulses, via the vagus nerve, to the *inspiratory center (IC) of the medulla* (Fig. 28 – a2), *apneutic center (AC) of the pons* (Fig. 28- a3) and *Nucleus Solitarius (NS, Fig. 28-a4)*. Direct inhibition of the IC and the AC which is excitatory to the IC, allows arrest of inspiration to favor expiration [39,40,41]. Neurons from NS send synaptic impulses to Nucleus Ambiguus and Dorsal Motor (DM) nucleus. The net effect of these connections prevent the parasympathetic neurons from inhibiting the heart, thereby causing increased heart rate and prevention of the alveoli from overexpansion by inhibiting inspiration. This reflex is operant in lower animals and during infancy. In adults, the threshold for the afferent impulses to commence is high such that it is only called upon when there is an increase in the tidal volume as experienced in vigorous exercise. In adults, the peripheral chemoreceptor from the carotid artery and inspiratory centers in the brainstem which are more responsive to changes in carbon dioxide (CO_2) levels, pH and very low oxygen (O_2) take over the HBIR. In adults the threshold for the HBIR is high oxygen demand in running exercise where the tidal volume increases causing more stretching of the bronchial and alveolar stretch, thus more frequent inspiratory-expiratory cycle (panting) and increased heart rate (tachycardia). Knowledge of the neural control mechanism of respiration is critical in understanding the different settings of the mechanical ventilators when respiratory support is urgently needed. This past decade, treatment of intractable seizures, pain, cardiac arrhythmia, depression, and other clinical conditions include vagal nerve stimulation (VNS). Stimulation of vagal nerve can cause decrease in heart and respiratory rates but at a certain threshold. Subthreshold stimuli are used in VNS treatment interventions [42].

The parasympathetic nerves coming from Nucleus Ambiguus and Dorsal Motor Nucleus of the medulla, via the vagus nerve, give off thoracic, cardiac, and gastro-intestinal branches that, in turn, form cardiac, pulmonary, esophageal, and gastric plexuses. The *parasympathetic vagal branches supply all the organs except the adrenal glands. These plexuses mediate Gastro-esophageal peristalsis.*

Case Story:

Mr. JP Perez, a 56 year- old electrical engineer, suddenly and briefly complained of dizziness while having coffee at 8 AM. He fell and mumbled briefly. Friends immediately rushed him to a nearby hospital where he was found to respond only to painful stimulus by hyperextension of the head and all extremities (decerebrate posturing). The ice caloric test showed normal ocular muscle responses. Respiration was deep and fast at 36/min. Heart rate increased at 110/minute. Reflexes were hyperactive in all extremities. There was bilateral Babinski. On CT Scan, there was a huge right cerebellar hemorrhage that was estimated at 50 ccs or more. Mr. Perez was intubated and connected to a respirator; however, after about three hours the blood pressure dropped to 30 palpatory and the respiration became shallow and irregular at 30/min. He subsequently died six hours after the initiation of inotropic agents. Post-mortem autopsy showed cerebellar tonsillar herniation that was pressing on the medulla.

Clinical – anatomic Correlation:

Clinicians give the brain stem much "respect" or concern because of the following reasons:

a) All the nerves that enter and leave the brain pass through it. If affected in its entirety, quadriplegia and sensory deficits of the entire body can result.
b) The Reticular Activating System (islands of gray neurons scattered in the brainstem up to the hypothalamus) that participates actively in wakefulness reside here. Its affectation can cause coma or varied forms of sensorial changes.

c) Control of the respiration, heart, and blood pressure also reside here. If these vital functions are affected arrhythmias, hypotension and cardiopulmonary arrest can result.
d) The neural control of the eyes, swallowing, balance, and taste are in the brainstem. Their affectation can cause much discomfort such as double vision, dysphagia, dizziness, imbalance and loss of taste. The dysphagia puts patients at risk of developing aspiration pneumonia.

The implication of lesions in the brainstem is not only on the possible poor quality of life outcome but also on the risk of death. Early recognition of signs and symptoms of brainstem involvement is a must so appropriate life-saving measures can be instituted immediately. The medulla, in particular, hosts the vital centers. When the cerebellum herniates through the foramen magnum (tonsillar herniation) and presses on the medulla, the blood pressure may drop, and the respiration becomes irregular and shallow. The cerebellar herniation caused the demise of Mr. Perez. Early recognition of cerebellar hemorrhage and immediate surgical evacuation, if indicated, can prevent death and may allow full recovery. It is therefore essential to immediately initiate a referral to neurosurgery when the diagnosis is cerebellar hemorrhage or infarct. Family participation should be pursued in the decision as much as possible.

Chapter VI-I

Cranial Nerve XI- Accessory Nerve
(Swallowing and Head Movement)

While watching the US Open Tennis championship match between Novak and Rafael, you kept on turning your head from left to right and then right to the left, following the balls as they crossed from one court to the other. Then you raised your hand in triumph every time your favored player made a point. Just imagine if you could not make all these moves, would the joy of watching the game be the same?

The Accessory Nerve is an efferent nerve and it originates from two sources. One source is from the Nucleus Ambiguus where it joins the Vagal Nerve at its lower part in supplying the motor muscles of the soft palate and the larynx as it participates in the act of swallowing (Fig. 29 – e1). The other source arises from the lateral horn of the upper cervical gray matter at C2 to C5, supplying the trapezius and sternocleidomastoid muscles that allow head rotation and raising of the shoulder and arm (Fig. 29 – e2). Some investigators do not include the Accessory Nerve coming from the Nucleus Ambiguus because the nerve arising from this lower part of the medulla joins the vagus nerve in supplying the muscles of swallowing. The lateral horn of the gray matter in the upper cervical cord is the source of the spinal cord portion of the Accessory Nerve – the Spinal Accessory Nerve. [43].

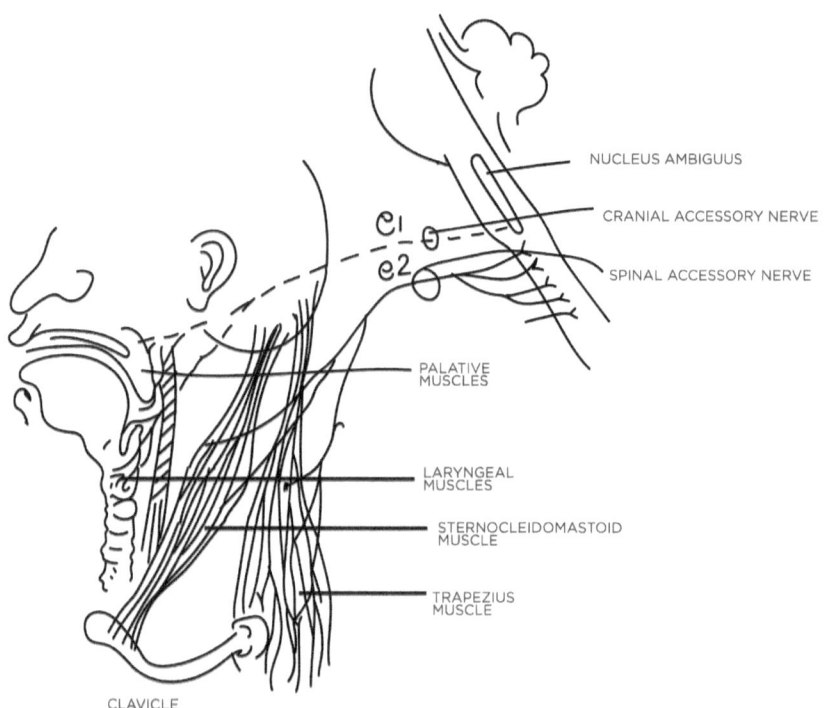

Figure 29. Cranial Nerve XI – Accessory Nerve. Efferent nerve (e1) from Nucleus Ambiguus to the soft palate and pharynx and (e2) from upper cervical motor neurons to the muscles of the neck.

Clinical Story:

Mr. Chan, a 62-year-old Chinese businessman, felt what he described as the stiffness of the left neck which he would often massage. He attributed the neck stiffness to his work which required long hours in front of the computer. He later noted that his head would periodically turn to the right and found it difficult to control. After about a year, the head-turning became more frequent, longer and exaggerated to a point where it was bothering his work at the computer and this time causing slight pain at the back of the nape. He said, "No matter what I do, I could not control the turning of my head; but according to my wife she did not see this during my sleep."

Physical examination and neurological examination were all normal except for the involuntary tonic (continuous) contraction of the left sternocleidomastoid muscle with the associated turning of the head to the right. Mr. Chan was diagnosed to have *sporadic spasmodic torticollis or cervical dystonia*. The cause and mechanism of this bothersome and distressing illness are still poorly understood. The pathologic disturbance is believed to be at the basal ganglia and classified as a **movement disorder**.

Clinical – anatomic Correlation:

The cortical homunculus has neck and shoulder representations which approximate the group of neurons that initiate neck muscle movements. The basal ganglia and the cerebellum participate actively in the more delicate control of actions which subsequent chapters shall elaborate. The more delicate control of muscle movements is mostly coming from the integration of the cortical motor cortex, basal ganglia, and the cerebellum. An example of this interaction is the control of head movements through the sternocleidomastoid muscles which are supplied by the accessory nerve. When any disease process disrupts the integrating influence of the basal ganglia on muscle movements, different movement-related manifestations may result.

An example of this is **spasmodic torticollis or neck dystonia** which is a sustained involuntary contraction of the sternocleidomastoid muscles, causing the head to turn to the opposite side. The spontaneous movement is present only during waking time.

In some cases, the other muscles may develop similarly sustained contraction causing generalized dystonia. Other diseases that involve these muscle groups are neck injuries that affect the peripheral nerve of the CN XI particularly those involving the anterior triangle of the neck, causing an inability to turn and straighten the head. A degenerative disease of the motor neurons (motor neuron disease or amyotrophic lateral sclerosis) will manifest as weakness, atrophy, and fasciculation of the trapezius and sternocleidomastoid muscles that may cause "head drop," the inability to raise or maintain the posture of the head.

Chapter VI-J

Cranial Nerve XII- Hypoglossal Nerve
(Functions: Swallowing and Sound Formation/Phonation)

When you put out your tongue to catch and taste the falling snow, the strength of its muscles will allow you to do this and keep it out for a time and at the center and even move it left and right. Licking ice cream is fun too when the tongue is strong. You can even make the "yodel sound" when its strength intact. The tongue participates in the joy of eating by bringing the food towards the esophagus through a reflex mechanism. Try talking without moving your tongue. Can you express the words clearly and make the sounds audible?

The tongue has a homunculus representation at the precentral gyrus at the mouth area. Motor neurons for the tongue send axons to merge with the other motor axons of the corticospinal tract at the internal capsule (Fig. 30 - A). Then it continues downwards, and just before reaching the hypoglossal nucleus, the axon decussates and synapses with the opposite hypoglossal nucleus at the medulla. Clinically, understanding this crossing to the opposite side is important. If there is a lesion on the right and above the brainstem (bold line), the tongue weakness is seen on the left side (Fig. 30-B). The corticospinal tract crossing means that when the tongue muscles push the tongue forward, the normal right side will overcome the weak left side, causing the tongue to deviate to the left away from the lesion. The nucleus at the medulla, in turn, sends impulses to the tongue muscles, allowing the tongue to protrude and move backward to guide food or saliva to the back of the oral cavity in preparation for swallowing.

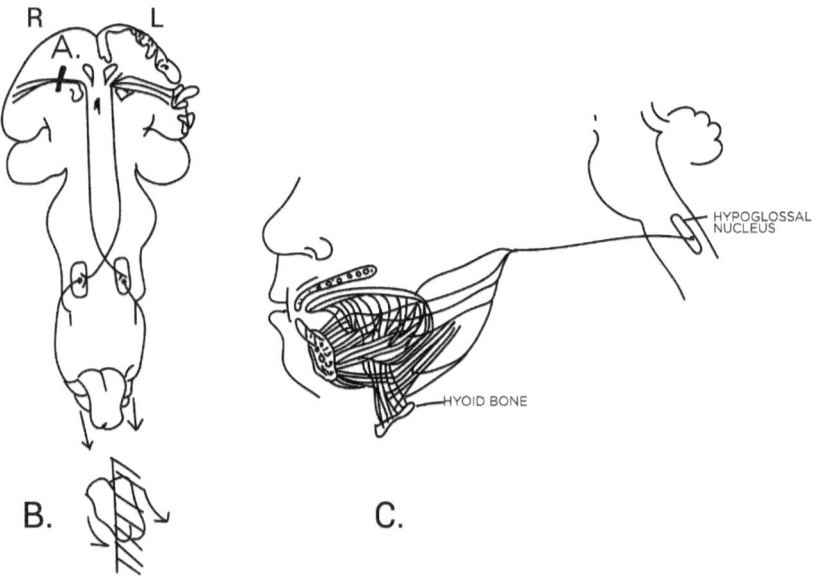

Figure 30. Cranial Nerve XII – Hypoglossal Nerve. A. Motor neurons for the tongue at the homunculus send axons to the opposite hypoglossal nucleus at the medulla. Right sided lesion shown as bold line. B. Tongue when protruded deviates toward the left side. C. Hypoglossal motor neurons innervate the tongue muscles.

If one side of the nucleus is involved, the same side of the tongue will become weak together with fasciculation and atrophy. The genioglossus muscles at the base of the tongue recently were shown to have bilateral innervation. The bilateral innervation could perhaps explain why one expects the tongue weakness after a stroke to recover spontaneously [44]. The tongue also participates in sound formation and phonation. When one side of the tongue gets weak, slurred speech happens, and if there is too much weakness, phonation or speech can hardly be understood. Drooling at the weak side maybe be seen because of the difficulty in handling saliva. Traumatic intubation, over inflation of endotracheal tube balloon or overstretching of the neck during intubation can injure the hypoglossal nerve occasionally. This predisposition to injury is because the nerve passes laterally to the base of the tongue on its way to innervating the muscles [45]. Most recently, the hypoglossal neurons were shown to have weaker electrical discharges during REM sleep. This finding explains the posterior displacement of the tongue during deep REM sleep and may explain the snoring and upper airway obstructive sleep apnea. Stimulation of the hypoglossal nerve causes the tongue to move forward and relieve the airway from obstruction. Hypoglossal nerve stimulation is now an option in the management of upper airway obstruction sleep [46,47,48].

Case Story:

A hard working chef, Mr. Doble worked early morning till dark, happy with the fact that he could mix the best Spanish dishes that satisfied each customer. His small, dainty restaurant was always full and one of the most popular in the city. He, however, had a secret that no one knew, and that was he had an irregularly irregular heartbeat called **atrial fibrillation**. One spring morning, while baking bread, he was surprised to drop the tin pan and could hardly move his left hand. He immediately sat in an armchair nearby just in time, for his left leg was starting to give way as well. He yelled with much effort, "....ngggiiiiittttooo!!!" He was alarmed to notice that he could not say Juanito's name with clarity. Juanito who was just across the table saw the sudden change on Mr. Doble. He tried to make him stand but the

200-pound weight was just too heavy for him to carry and he could not understand the garbled things he was saying. He called 911.

The ER physician noted that Mr. Doble when asked, could understand and follow everything. His slurred verbal responses were hardly understandable. It took a lot of effort for him to raise his left arm for a few seconds when told to do so. He could not lift the left leg as well but was able to flex it briefly. There was no subjective or objective sensory deficit of any kind. All the functions of the cranial nerves were normal except the deviation of the tongue to the left when asked to put it out. The deep tendon reflexes on the left side were hyperactive when compared to the right and there was a Babinski sign on the left. The MRI showed a new and small lacunar infarct involving the right internal capsule. After treatment and rehabilitation he was able to recover fully and went back to his love of cooking, but this time with preventive medicines, well-controlled diet, the lower weight of 170 pounds, and an additional assistant.

Clinical – anatomic Correlation:

The internal capsule is where the axons from the motor neurons of the pre-central gyrus (corticospinal tract) merge and bundled before they go down to the brain stem and cross to the opposite side at the level of the medulla. Because of the merging, an infarct on the right internal capsule can cause paralysis of the left side of the body. Notice that sensory symptoms and signs are absent. The absence is because only the motor fibers were affected by a small lesion, causing a pure motor weakness (a pure sensory deficit can happen too if it involves the thalamus). The small lesion is called a **lacune**, a small cavity. The tongue deviated toward the left side because the fibers from the opposite homunculus that innervates the left are where the infarct is. The tongue muscles can push forward, and if the left muscles are weak, then the deviation is to the left. Lacunar infarcts produce pure motor or pure sensory deficits, and the prognosis is fortunately good that a full recovery is possible as in the case of Mr. Doble. Even if the functional recovery is favorable, it is essential to know that this is considered a risk factor for another stroke—a stern warning not to push your luck! Mr. Doble heeded the advice.

Neurological Examination:

Listening to the sound produced by the patient while talking and letting the patient imitate the phonation of, "lalalalalala" or "mememememe" or "Mississipi-Mississipi," one may uncover a characteristic slurring in the pyramidal tract or hypoglossal nerve involvement. The pyramidal tract was affected in Mr. Doble's case. Sometimes a nasal twang can be heard indicating an upper palate weakness due to vagus nerve involvement. A sudden irregular and poorly controlled loud voice when talking is an explosive speech due to cerebellar pathology. In basal ganglia diseases where there are involuntary tongue movements, there is a lot of effort exerted in phonation. The patient is instructed to protrude the tongue to know which side is weaker. If this is not obvious, letting the patient push the tongue against the inner cheek, with the examiner's hand over the cheek, will help estimate the degree of weakness when compared to the other side.

Motor denervation from motor neuron disease may show fasciculation and atrophy upon examination of the tongue at rest or when slightly protruded.

Chapter VII

The Spinal Cord and Peripheral Nerves
(Functions: Sensation, Motor Strength, Reflexes, Autonomics)

Imagine a bee buzzing toward you!! When one's forearm is in danger of being stung by a bee, an immediate reaction is flexion of the forearm to avoid the bee followed immediately by the opposite arm driving away or swatting the insect with one's palm. Simultaneously, maintaining balance and vision. Even the legs get coordinated to move away from the insect and to run. While this is happening, the body balances and the eyes coordinate with the neck muscles to maintain focused vision on the bee and possibly its other companions while maintaining a posture of flight or fight. You will also notice the heart rate and the respiratory rate going up. How can these highly complex movements be coordinated smoothly, instantaneously, and with swift precision? It is incredible to know that most of these complex activities find expression through the spinal cord and peripheral nerves.

There are four topics covered in this chapter, the sensory functions, the motor functions, the reflexes, and the autonomic nervous system. Covering these four functions emphasize the need to evaluate the status of these four systems in the neurological examination.

The Topography of the Spinal Cord

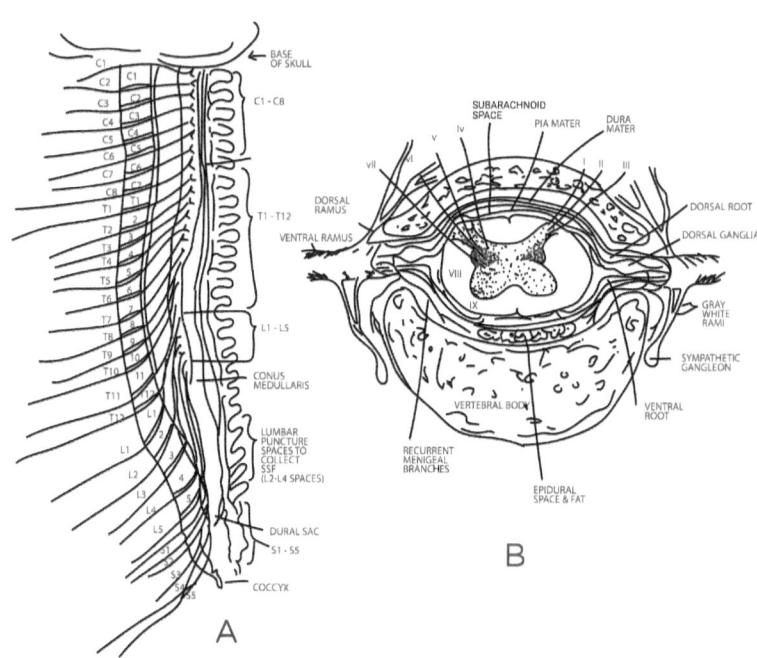

Figure 31. A. Spinal vertebrae, spinal cord, spinal nerves and anatomic divisions. Note end of spinal cord (conus medullaris) at T12-L1 level. C8 nerve exits below the T7 vertebrae. B. Cross-section of spine and parts. Note dorsal ganglia just going out of neural foramen. Gray mater of spinal cord grouped into I to X lamina.

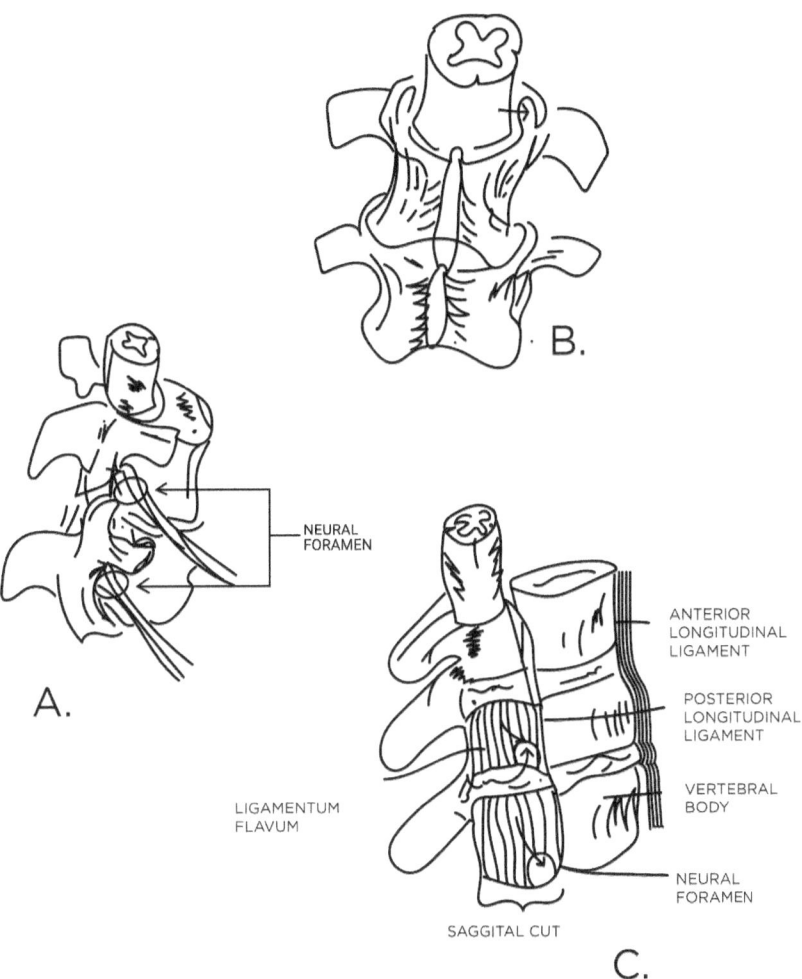

Figure 32. A. Lateral view of 2 spinal vertebrae. B. Posterior view of 2 spinal vertebrae. C. Saggital section of spinal veretebrae and components. Arrows shows exit directions of nerve roots to neural foramen.

The Backbones

The spine or the backbones or the spinal column or vertebral column is a fundamental structure that houses the spinal cord, its coverings (the pia-arachnoid and dura), its rootlets that enter and exit the cord and partly the neural foramen, and the *dorsal ganglia* (Fig. 31-B). It consists of bony vertebrae arranged one on top of the other in a column and had five anatomic divisions: the seven cervical vertebrae, the twelve thoracic vertebrae, the five lumbar vertebrae, the five sacral vertebrae, and the vestigial coccyx (Fig. 31-A).

The vertebral column is dynamically able to move backward, forward, laterally, and rotatory but to a limited degree. These movements are made possible by the facet joints and the compressible discs (Fig. 32). These joints may sometimes weaken and cause displacement of one vertebra over the other (**listhesis**), and this movement can very well press on the exiting or entering nerves to cause symptoms. Like any joints, degenerative osteophytes can grow between facet joints and press on the nerve roots. Discs may herniate and if it gets directed to one side can compress the nerves at the neural foramen, where nociceptive nerves enter, to cause pain. If the disc herniation is large enough, this may press the spinal cord and cause weakness and sensory symptoms like numbness or pain. Diseases or injuries to the dynamic and anatomic functions of the spinal column can very well cause symptoms involving the spinal cord and nerves.

The Spinal cord

The spinal cord is divided into four functional segments based on which spinal neural foramen of the spinal vertebra the nerves exit (Fig. 31-A). These functional segments are: **Cervical (C)1-8** cord segments (C1 to C7 nerves egress at the top of the vertebra while the rest, C8 to S5, exit under their corresponding vertebra), **Thoracic (T) 1-12** segments, **Lumbar (L) 1-5 segments,** and **Sacral (S) 1-5 segments**. The spinal cord usually ends at the L1-L2 level in adults, and this is also where the cauda equina begins, also called *filum terminale,* or *conus medullaris*. The cauda equina consists of lumbar and sacral nerves that still have to exit caudally at their corresponding neural foramen

[49]. These anatomic boundaries have great clinical importance. Space where the lumbar and sacral nerves "float" provide adequate space for CSF dynamic studies (this is continuous with the CSF circulation) and CSF fluid diagnostic analysis. During lumbar tap procedures, needles are inserted between L3-L4 vertebrae because there is minimal risk of injuring the spinal cord in this area. If a patient complains of radiating pain on the right lower limb with weakness, the usual consideration is a root compression on the right L4-L5 or L5 –S1 levels; but one cannot entirely rule out the possibility that the problem might be involving the same roots but at the level of the conus medullaris at L1-L2. The manifestations caused by pathology at this level is called **conus medullaris syndrome.** Remember that the spinal cord ends at about the L1-L2 level in adults. Therefore when requesting an MRI, be sure to include L1 spine in the view.

The spinal cord has paired content, i.e., the left side has similar anatomic and functional structures as on the right side (Fig. 31-B). The butterfly-shaped gray matter occupies the inner central portion of the spinal cord. The gray matter is divided into a) *posterior horn*, b) *intermediate zone* (seen only at T1 to L2 segments *for autonomic neurons*) and c) *large anterior horn* is where the anterior motor neurons are.

The gray matter consists of scattered groups of neurons subdivided into *ten (10) functional neuronal group*s labeled as Lamina I to IX from the posterior to the anterior of the spinal cord, with lamina X being the area around the central spinal canal (Fig. 31-B). *Lamina I-VI* are generally *recipients of sensory*-related functions and where interneurons exert their modulating effects. *Lamina VII,* which is found only from T1-L2 segments, is where sympathetic autonomic nervous function emanates while *Lamina VIII to IX* has *motor-related functions.*

The white matter is the outer part of the spinal cord that consists of *ascending and descending myelinated and unmyelinated axons --* collectively called **tracts or funiculae.** The names of the tracts of the white matter are according to their cord positions (eg., lateral, medial, anterior, posterior, and combination, eg. anterolateral), and according to where the initiating impulses begin and terminate (e.g., *lateral corticospinal tract,* from the precentral cortex to various levels of the cord or *lateral spinothalamic tract,* from the spinal cord to the thalamus).

Descending Fibers of the Spinal Cord

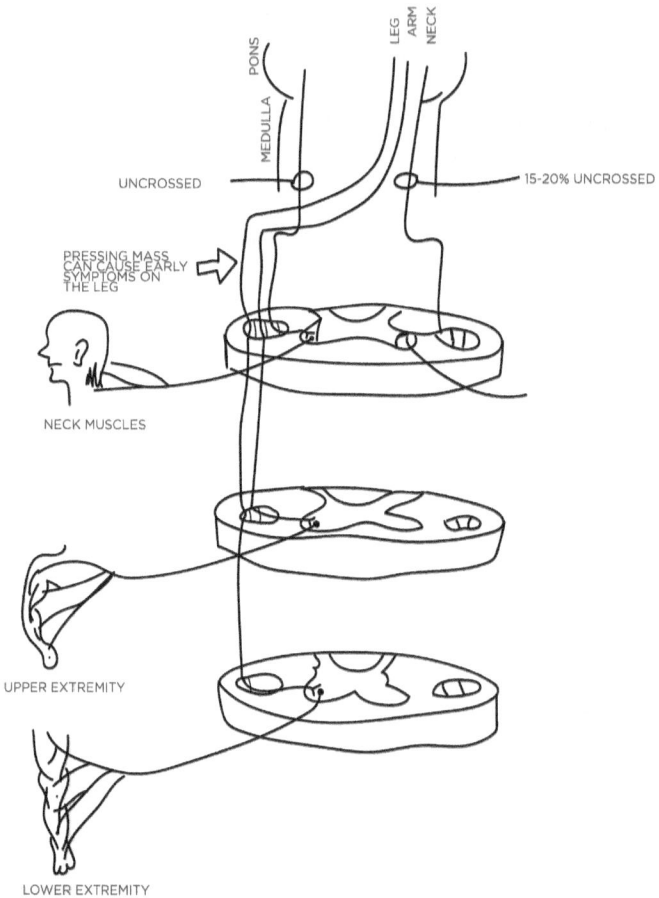

Figure 33. Descending cortico-spinal fibers and topographical arrangement. More medial fibers exit early and supply the upper portions of the body and most lateral fibers exit last and supply the legs.

There are many *descending fibers* in the spinal cord and the most clinically known is the- corticospinal or pyramidal tract. Ninety-five percent of these long and thickly myelinated descending fibers cross at the lower medulla. The *cortical pyramidal tract n*eurons (Brodmann area 4) and some contributions from premotor gyrus, postcentral gyrus, and parietal lobe is the origin of the corticospinal tract. The corticospinal tract descends in the spinal cord as **Lateral Cortico Spinal Tract (CST)** and is topographically arranged in such a way that the medial side connects first with upper parts of the body, while the most lateral side links with the lower extremities (Fig. 33 and Table I-A). Most of the CST that cross the pyramid at the level of the medulla synapse with the alpha motor neurons at Lamina IX and the interneurons at Lamina IV to VIII. The *five percent* uncrossed CST descends as *Anterior CST* destined to innervate mostly the cervical Lamina VII bilaterally, and they *modulate the motor neurons innervating the neck and upper extremities*. The Anterior CST participates in maintaining *neck tone and posture.*

Case Story:

Mrs. Jones, a 45-year-old sales manager of a boutique, is a health buff. When she woke up one summer morning, she experienced piercing and lightning-like pain just below her right armpit while she was jogging. The discomfort caused her to stop and rest. The pain stopped so she went back home and attributed it to muscle sprain. That night, she could not sleep because the pain recurred, but this time on both armpit areas. She consulted an ER doctor who prescribed pain medicines which afforded moderate relief and sound sleep. The following morning, the pain was again gone. The next week, a nagging mild and tolerable pain in the same area would occasionally recur but did not bother her. Mrs. Jones and her husband decided to spend a week in a Long Island beach with their two children. While they were on the way, she started feeling numbness on the right leg. While frolicking in the beach, the left leg was beginning to become numb, too. She decided to skip the bonfire and went to sleep instead, hoping that the numbness would disappear. When she woke up to prepare breakfast she felt the numbness progressing to involve the inguinal and buttocks on both sides. She immediately consulted at a nearby hospital where she underwent MRI of the lumbosacral spine. The result was normal, so the doctor decided to order for the MRI of the thoracic spine. The imaging study turned out to be normal as well.

The family cut short their vacation so that they could bring her to a specialist who believed that the numbness was related to the pain she was experiencing and that the MRI was read as normal because the problem most likely was higher at the cervical level of the spinal cord. A repeat MRI, this time at the level of the cervical spine, was done. The MRI showed a tumor delicately located at the back of the spinal cord at the C7-T1 level.

Clinical – anatomic Correlation:

The topography or body map of the pyramidal tract is such that the axons that supply *the upper extremities are medially located* and are the first to synapse with the anterior horn. The axons that innervate the *lower extremities remain in the lateral position at the cervical level* as shown in Fig. 33. This topographic arrangement explains why *a cervical compressive pathology to the spinal cord can sometimes cause numbness or weakness or both at the distant lower leg first instead of the upper extremities.* It is for this reason that every time there is paraparesis (weakness of both lower extremities) or paresthesia (numbness), *one should always ask the patient if there are pains* and other sensory disturbances at the neck and or subtle weakness of the upper extremities because the *pathology might be at the cervical level,* just like what Mrs. Jones had. The MRI is expensive. MRI of the lumbosacral and thoracic spine was the wrong site. Clinically, the lesion was in the cervical spine, which should have been the target of MRI instead. It is also a wise practice that if a lumbosacral MRI is negative for somebody with leg weakness or numbness and a spinal cord lesion is suspected; one should consider doing a cervical MRI.

Table I. Descending fibers, origins, terminations and functions

A. Cortical Descending Fibers

Descending Fiber	Origin	Termination	Function
Lateral CST	Precentral gyrus	Lamina VII-IX	Initiation of Motor function
Lateral CST	Premotor	Lamina IV-VII	Motor modulation
Lateral CST	PostCentral	Posterior horn cells	Motor modulation
Lateral CST	Parietal area	Posterior horn cells	Motor modulation
Anterior CST	Parietal area	Cervical Motor horn cells	Modulate arm and neck muscles
Anterolateral CST	Parietal area	Posterior and intermediate horn	Modulation head, neck, posture muscles

B. Brainstem descending fibers

Tecto spinal tract	Superior colliculus	Cervical Lamina VI-VIII	Reflex head movements as response to visual stimuli
Rubro spinal tract	Red nucleus	Lamina V-VII	Flexion of extremities
Vestibulo-spinal tract	Lateral vestibular n. or Dieter's nucleus	Cervical and lumbar Lamina VII-IX	Facilitates spinal reflex to maintain neck muscle tone and posture
Reticulospinal tract	Pontine & medullary tegmenti	Complex connections	Reflex excitation of axial (mostly) and limb muscles.
Medial longitudinal faciculi	Different neurons of the brain stem	Upper cervical neurons	Regulates head position.

Other Descending Fibers of the Spinal Cord

There are other important descending fibers that are enumerated in Table I-A and B. These tables show the different descending fibers, their origin, their termination, and functions. These *descending fibers, in general, are modulators* to afferent sensory inputs and *coordinators* to the eventual muscle tone or movements. The other descending brainstem neuronal fibers are *coordinators of tone, reflexes, visio-spatial function, and opposing muscles*. These fibers are responsible for the different actions and reactions made after a bee sting. The summation of the motor functions plus synaptic connections from the *superior colliculi- spinal linkages* (for visio-spatial motor coordination) allows the victim of a bee sting to focus on the prey while allowing neck tone and head balance. The *red nucleus- spinal connection* which (facilitates flexor and extension coordination of muscles) allows the affected arm to move in conjunction with the defensive movement of the opposite forearm to swat or drive away the insect. The vestibulospinal tracts modulate cervical posture, and the *reticulospinal tracts* (axial and limb coordination) allows the stance of fight or flight readiness. The varied functions described above provide a general idea of how important these other descending fibers are. You do not have to memorize these interconnections. Just understand that all actions described above can happen every millisecond in our daily activities, and they are finely tuned and critically coordinated and made possible through these intricate interconnections in our brain and spinal cord. What is fascinating is that we are unaware of these coordinated movements and reactions.

The spinal cord motor neurons send axons and contribute to the formation of the peripheral nerve. The motor neuron axons exit as *ventral (anterior) roots or rami*. The *first branches are small dorsal rami* that supply the *paraspinal muscles* (muscles in between the spinal vertebrae} that contribute to the stability of the spine. The ventral rami will proceed and join the sensory nerves as a bundled peripheral nerve. The motor neurons from the spinal cord segments contribute to the peripheral nerves that would correspondingly innervate groups of muscles. **Myotomal distribution** refers to the group of muscles with their corresponding spinal cord innervations. C 1-3 segments supply the neck muscles; C3-5 makes up the phrenic nerve that supplies the diaphragm; C4-T1 contributes to movements of the upper extremities, and the entire T12 sections provide the trunk and abdominal muscles; L1- S5 supply the lower extremities and related muscles. Note that peripheral nerves that supply the musculature contain contributions from two or more spinal cord segments. When one points a finger to an interesting object, C5-T1 spinal cord segments contribute to the act because these levels contribute to the radial nerve that mainly supplies the extensor muscles of the pointing finger.

Ascending Fibers of the Spinal Cord

The ascending fibers contribute much to the reaction of the body to the bee sting in the forearm. After a tiny break of the skin and the venom from the stinger introduced to the body, the transformation of chemical reactions into electrical impulses at the bare nerve endings happen. The neurons then transmit these nociceptive impulses at the dorsal ganglia to the posterior gray of the spinal cord. The nociceptive axons synapsing with posterior gray horn nociceptive neurons located in I, III, and IV Lamina of the spinal cord (see Fig. 7-A). As mentioned in Chapter IV, descending influences from brainstem raphe nucleus, periaqueductal gray and reticular formation synapse with interneurons at Lamina II to modulate nociceptive transmission. Posterior gray neurons, at 1-2 levels higher, transmit nociceptive sensations to the opposite side by crossing anteriorly to the spinal canal. The crossed axons then ascend as the **lateral spinothalamic tract.**

Being able to guide the left hand that would swat the bee requires precise orientation to space and exquisite control of muscle tone. These need intact proprioceptive sensation for the swatting extremity. The receptors for this function are the Golgi tendon organs that detect muscle tone. The target of the swatting palm, on the other side, is the location of the sting at the forearm, and the recognition of the area is mediated by nociceptive sensation through the bare ending receptors. Large myelinated IIb and A alpha fibers transmit tone and position sensations to the dorsal root ganglia. From the dorsal root ganglia, the impulses subsequently reach the spinal cord where the axons are bundled together as *fascicles (gracilis coming from the leg and cuneatus from the upper extremities)*. The fasciculus gracilis and cuneatus ascend at the posterior column without crossing (see Fig. 7-B). These would then synapse with the *gracilis and cuneatus nucleus* at the brainstem medulla (note that the 2nd order neuron is NOT in the spinal cord but the medulla). The axons from these medullary nuclei will then cross to the other side as ascending medial lemniscus which will transmit impulses to the ventroposterolateral (VPL) thalamic nucleus. The thalamic neurons will then project these impulses to the post-central gyrus and other areas of the cortex.

Table II shows other ascending fibers, origins, terminations, and functions. Clinical assessment of the actions of two anatomic structure in the table is possible. These are the *lateral spinothalamic* tract that mediates pain, temperature and touch, and the *posterior column* that transmits position, vibration, tone and discriminatory touch sensation. This table also shows that *non-conscious proprioception* occurs through the posterior column as *collateral fibers terminating at lamina VII (not all fibers ascend thru gracilis and cuneatus posterior column)*. The neurons from this lamina, in turn, send axons to the cerebellum giving us an insight of how proprioception contribute to balance. Aside from connection through lamina VII, there are also ascending and descending interconnections within the spinal cord that influences muscle tone.

The autonomic nervous system (ANS) is a vital part of the central nervous system that regulates involuntary or non-conscious functions of the heart, blood vessels, lungs, glands, gastrointestinal tract, bladder, sex organs, and pupils. *Smooth muscles* provide functions *to these organs*. Most of these structures are controlled by the ANS that innervate smooth muscles as distinguished from corticospinal tract and motor nerves that supply *skeletal muscles*. The ANS sympathetic neurons that reside in the intermediate gray horn (lamina VII) of the spinal cord send axons that join the sensory and motor peripheral nerves. There is therefore always a possibility that diseases that affect the sensory and motor nerves can involve the autonomic nervous system. In clinical situations where there is a need to investigate the sensory level and the myotomal distribution determined, the inclusion of the evaluation of the autonomic functions is imperative. The two functionally opposing autonomic nerves are the Parasympathetic (PSNS) and Sympathetic Nervous System (SNS).

Other ascending fibers of the spinal cord

Table II. Ascending Fibers of the Spinal Cord. Origin, Nerves, Tracts, Terminals, Functions

Origin	Nerve type	Tracts	2nd terminal	3rd terminal	Destination	Functions
Muscle spindles, golgi tendon	A alpha, Ia	Dorsal Column, gracilis (leg), cuneatus (arm)	Medulla, Nucleus gracilis and cuneatus	Contraleteral VPL, Thalamus	PostCentral gyrus, Brodman 1-3	Proprioception, Position sense
Pascinian Corpuscle	same	same	same	same	same	Vibration
Meissners Corpuscle	same	same	same	same	same	Discriminatory Touch
Bare Nerve Endings	a-delta, c fibers	Lateral Spino-Thalamic tract	Lamina I-VI	Contralateral VPL Thalamus	Primary & Secondary sensory cortex	Pain, Temperature, Crude touch
	same	Anterior Spino Thalamic tract	Lamina VII	Periaqueductal gray, intralaminar thalamic n.		Light touch
	same	Spinoreticular fibers		Reticular- medial thalamic formation	Diffuse cortical areas	Arousal, motivational, Attention, Affective reaction to pain
Receptors of dorsal column	Alpha, Ia	Spinocerebellar tract	Collateral From gracilis tract to Lamina VII (C8-L2)	Ipsilateral, vermis of the anterior cerebellar lobe, thru inferior peduncle		Nonconscious sensation of muscle position and tone of leg

Autonomic Nervous System of the Spinal Cord

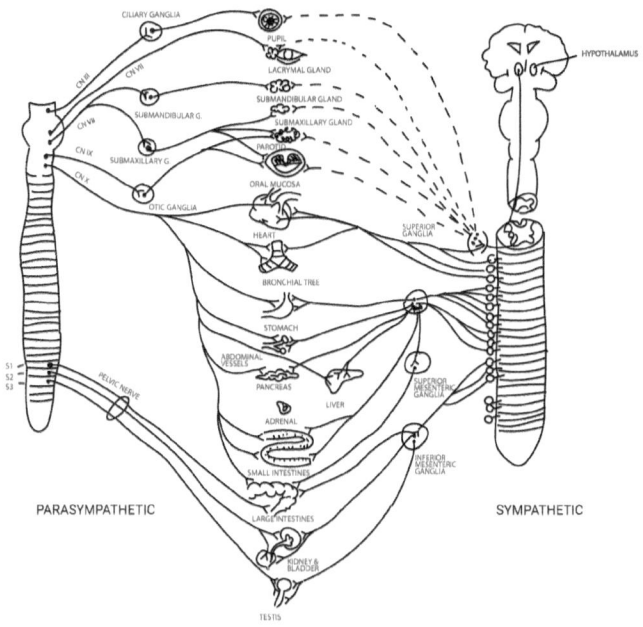

Figure 34. Autonomic Nervous System and innervated structures. A. Parasympathetic Nervous System exit mostly through the brainstem and Spinal S1-S3. Note extensive supply by the Vagus nerve. B. Sympathetic Nervous System exit mainly at T2 to L3 spinal levels.

In general, the PSNS blocks or slows down while the SNS excites or speeds up. *The PSNS* afferent and efferent systems are mostly located in the brainstem particularly CN III, VII, IX, X, while the rest are at the intermediate gray of S2-S4 segments of the cord (Fig. 34 – A). The *SNS*, on the other hand, are stationed at the intermediate gray of T1 to L2 segments of the spinal cord (Fig. 34 - B). The SNS neurons at the intermediate gray are also called *preganglionic neurons,* and they receive *descending sympathetic* axons from the neurons of the cortex (particularly the limbic structures), hypothalamus, and brainstem. The axons of the sympathetic neurons from the intermediate gray exit the spinal cord to join the motor fibers for a short distance, then synapse with the *post-ganglionic sympathetic neurons* in the paravertebral sympathetic ganglia. This understanding is essential because diseases involving different levels of the cord or peripheral nerve distribution can cause autonomic abnormalities as well. The most common manifestations are a loss of bladder and bowel control and failure of erection. This knowledge emphasizes the need to do a rectal examination to determine if there is laxity of the rectal sphincter and to palpate the suprapubis for bladder retention.

Case Story:

Jockey Martinez, 30 years old, has been riding racehorses since he was 10 years old, and after turning professional at the early age of 18, he has since won more than ten major awards in big horse racing events. In one of the practice-runs against four horses, while running inside the pack, his horse tripped hurling Mr. Martinez over the safety fence of the oval. Witnesses said Mr. Martinez turned over more than three times upon hitting the ground and then remained immobile. When the aides reached his side, he was found conscious but could not move his four extremities and could not feel anything below the shoulder. He was immediately immobilized with a neck brace and body brace and gently laid in a stretcher without bending any parts of the spine. Upon reaching the emergency room, MRI of the cervical spine showed a cervical vertebral fracture of C3 and forward displacement of C3 anteriorly with spinal cord compression from the intraspinal hematoma. He was intubated immediately and placed on respiratory support. He had indwelling catheter insertion and immediate surgical evacuation of the hematoma and stabilization of C3 to C5 spine at the operating room. His anal sphincter was lax with no contraction. He was paralyzed on all extremities and could not feel from the shoulder down. He survived the surgery and underwent extensive rehabilitation.

A year since the tragic accident, Mr. Martinez was moving around on an electric wheelchair specially designed for him using the two digits of the right hand to navigate. He could already make a hearty laugh and was able to talk using a voice aide. The suprapubic catheter remained hidden and was on laxatives for his bowel movements. His only complaint was the disturbing on and off lightning-like and pricking pain on the left shoulder that radiated to the entire hand, and when the left palm was touched, he described it to be hypersensitive. The skin on his left arm was cold, dry and scaly and the nails were also dry and pale. A doctor told him that the pain was neuropathic pain. He has acclimatized to the fact that he has no erection. He no longer has sexual desires.

Clinical – anatomic Correlation.

The quadriplegia and sensory loss was due to the traumatic injury to the spinal cord brought about by the fracture of the C3 vertebrae. The descending sympathetic tract was similarly injured to explain the loss of bladder and bowel control.

Reflex sympathetic dystrophy (RSD) or complex regional pain syndrome (CRPS) is a form of neuropathic pain associated with trophic autonomic nerve changes like warmth, swelling and redness in the early stage of the disease, and cold, dry skin, hair loss and dry nails in the late stage. CRPS is usually felt near or around the musculoskeletal injuries or nerve injuries. The pain can have a component of **hyperalgesia** (pain felt disproportionate to the pain stimulus, like a pinprick) or an element of **allodynia** (pain experienced after a non-painful stimulus, like touch). The neuropathic pain of Mr. Martinez is most likely CRPS with allodynia.

The link of the central nervous system (CNS) with the body is the peripheral nervous system (PNS). It carries impulses from the spinal cord to different recipients of the body parts (motor and autonomic nerves) and at the same time carries impulses from the body parts toward the spinal cord and eventually to the brain (sensory nerves). The PNS has three parts, these are (Fig. 35):

1) the *roots* and
2) the *dorsal ganglia* which are still in the protection of the vertebrae and the dura (though the dorsal ganglia are partly outside the confines of the spine and dura);

   Clinical – anatomic Correlation: There are diseases specifically affecting the roots (Acute Guillain-Barre Disease or Chronic Polyradiculitis) or the dorsal ganglia (dorsal ganglionitis, Herpes Zoster Infection). Tapping the Cerebrospinal Fluid (CSF) that bathes these structures provides a specimen for various diagnostic tests. The neural physiology can be tested by Nerve Conduction Velocity (NCV) Studies while Electromyography (EMG) tests the muscles that peripheral nerves innervate. These two tests, EMG's-NCV's, are studied together to arrive at possible diagnosis.

3) the *plexuses*, which are the merging of nerve roots from several segments of the cord. Examples are brachial, axillary and lumbosacral plexuses;

   Clinical – anatomic Correlation: Brachial plexitis (inflammation of the brachial plexus) or brachial-axillary nerve injuries in babies due to pulling of the upper extremities during difficult deliveries are examples of diseases that may affect the plexuses.

4) the *peripheral nerves* are bundles of the efferent motor and autonomic fibers from the different segments of the cord supplying the skeletal and smooth muscles respectively, and afferent sensory fibers which receive impulses from varied receptors located in different parts of the body;

   Clinical – anatomic Correlation: Peripheral nerves can be injured, causing weakness of muscles that they innervate and produce some characteristic forms of dysfunctions with certain examination maneuvers. The median nerve is a bundled peripheral nerve with efferent contributions from C6 to T1 segments of the spinal cord

The Topography of Peripheral Nervous System

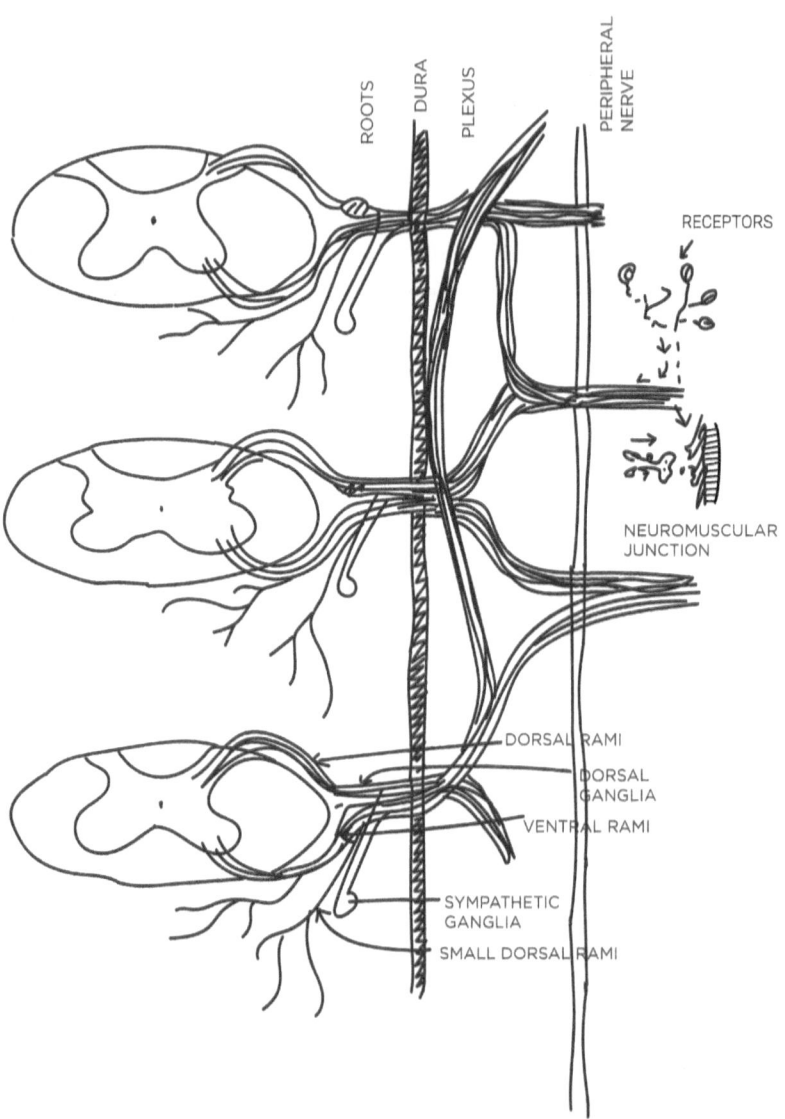

Figure 35. Division of Peripheral Nervous System into roots, plexuses and peripheral nerves.

and afferent receptors from the palmar surface of the thumb, index and middle fingers. The muscles supplied are the flexors of the first three fingers and the thenar muscles. Injury to the nerve, as in *Carpal Tunnel Syndrome*, results in numbness or *pain in its afferent distribution* and *loss of grip or, worse, loss of thumb function* also called *"ape hand."*

Table III. Differences between ulnar and median nerve injury.

Ulnar nerve	Median nerve
Deficit is primarily in 4th and 5th fingers	Deficit is primarily in 2nd and 3rd fingers.
Deficit is most prominent at rest and when the patient is asked to extend his fingers.	Deficit is most prominent when the patient is asked to make a fist.
Often accompanied by inability to abduct or adduct the 2nd, 3rd, 4th, and 5th finger.	Often accompanied by difficulty opposing the thumb.
Often accompanied by apparent atrophy of the first dorsal interosseous muscle of the hand	Often accompanied by wasting of muscles of the thenar eminence
Deficit described as "claw hand" when at rest or when fingers are hyperextended, "Benedictine hand"	Deficit described as "ape hand" due to inability to use the thumb on grip or "Benedictine hand" on flexion of the fingers.

When told to make a grip, the fingers supplied by the median nerve fail to flex resulting in a hand posture called, *"pope's hand or benediction hand"* which looks like the hand of a priest when blessing, also called *"shooting hand,"* (Fig. 36-A, see also Table III.). Injury to the ulnar nerve causes extensor muscle weakness of the 4th and 5th fingers and partly the 3rd finger resulting in the so-called, "claw hand" in a resting position. Only the 1st and 2nd fingers that respond to hand extension while the others remain flexed, resulting in the "benediction hand", too (Fig. 36-B & Table III). The radial nerve innervates much of the extensor muscles of the hands. Injury to the radial nerve results in "wrist drop." (Fig. 36-C).

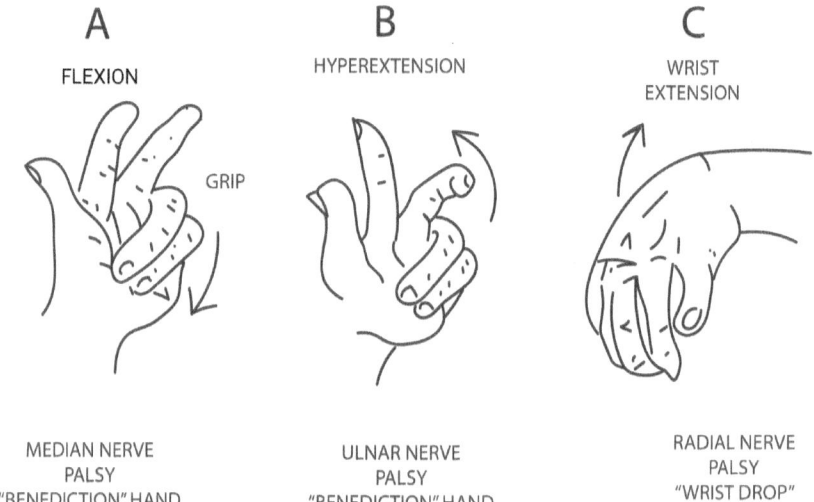

Figure 36. Characterestic hand features associated with nerve injuries of the upper extremity. A. Median nerve injury on gripping results to "benedectine hand sign." B. Ulnar nerve injury results to similar "benedictine hand sign" but elicited on hyperextension of the fingers. C. Radial nerve injury causes wrist drop.

5) the *neuromuscular junction* where the efferent motor nerve ends as *pre-synaptic terminal* and where neuro-transmitters are released to interact with the *post-synaptic receptors of the muscle fibers. The binding of neurotransmitters with receptors trigger a K and Na shift in the muscles allowing continuation of electrical transmission that will eventually trigger muscle contraction.*

Clinical – anatomic Correlation: Specific diseases may involve the terminal of the efferent nerves (presynaptic) as in *Botulinum toxicity or Lambert-Eaton Disease,* or at the muscular receptors (postsynaptic) as in *Myasthenia Gravis.*

Case Story:

Mrs. Fox, a 60-year-old avid golfer who played every weekend and holidays, had just finished the 18th hole for par to her delight at about noon. On the way to the locker, she noted numbness on both plantar surfaces of the feet but did not mind this. While having dinner that night, the numb sensation was alarmingly noted to have reached below the knees. The numbness started to worry her, so she made an appointment with her family doctor. When she woke up the following morning, she frantically shouted for help to her son, "Please help me. I cannot move my legs!" Confused and in panic, she cried, "I am paralyzed, oh my God!" The son asked if she could feel her legs, she said that she could feel the legs. The son, also worried, reassuringly said, "That is good because that means the nerves are still working!" She rushed her immediately to the emergency room.

She was found to have subjective symmetric numbness below the knees. The upper extremities are normal at (5/5) while both lower extremities are paralyzed (0/5). The rectal sphincters were normal. Deep tendon reflexes were absent in all upper and lower joints. Babinski sign was not present. She was admitted to the ICU to observe for any progression. The initial consideration was Guillain-Barre, so she was infused with Immune globulin. That afternoon, the weakness progressed to involve the upper extremities and the respiratory muscles, necessitating intubation and respiratory support. After ten days, she became stronger which allowed removing her from the respirator. She began oral feeding and underwent rehabilitation. She was discharged wheelchair-borne on the third week after demonstrating that she was able to feed herself. She began to recover her muscle strength gradually, and by the sixth month she was again striking golf balls in the driving range and honing her game. Another month later, she was back in the fairways enjoying the game, and one time she excitingly told her doctor that she had a hole-in-one! What remained from her illness was a tolerable tingling sensation in the legs.

Clinical-anatomic Correlation

In diseases involving the roots of the peripheral nerve or the so-called radiculopathies (radicle- roots), as in Guillain-Barre Syndrome (GBS), an acute polyradiculopathy is characterized by a *slight* sensory manifestation, *dominant* symmetric motor weakness, and *sparing* of the bladder and bowel functions (an autonomic nervous system function). The most prominent characteristic is the *absence* of deep tendon reflexes.

What is striking in Mrs. Fox's case was the fast or acute appearance of symmetric sensory and motor symptoms. There are other causes of muscle weakness. Muscle diseases, like hypokalemic paralysis or thyrotoxic myopathy or neuromuscular junction diseases like myasthenia gravis, also show symmetric weakness; but there are no sensory manifestations, and often the reflexes are present. An acute spinal cord disease like transverse myelitis or traumatic cord injury, as in the case of Jockey Martinez, similarly can cause symmetric weakness with an equal degree of sensory deficit. A clear dermatomal level and myotomal distribution can be demonstrated as well as autonomic nervous system affectation, like bladder and bowel paralysis. The deep tendon reflexes below the lesion will show a hyperactive reaction.

In summary, we have briefly described the parts of the peripheral nerve in general terms and have given examples of how diseases affect the different structures. We gave an example, too, of how the roots can be disturbed by an illness that manifests as Guillain-Barre syndrome and briefly considered some cases which may mimic the disease, and also described their differences. We will now split the peripheral nerve into their bare functional components and detail some of their characteristics, which is a way of reinforcing the understanding of the peripheral nerves.

The Motor Component of the Peripheral Nerves.

The anterior horn cells carry modified and modulated impulses from higher parts of the brain and bring them to action through different muscle groups that function as tone stabilizers, rotators, flexors or extensors. The overlapping innervations and multiple muscle groups acting in harmony allow smooth and precise coordinated movements. The nerve type that transmits rapid impulses are the thickly myelinated A alpha nerves (Table II). The quick transmissions allow immediate muscular reaction as a protective mechanism or swift, appropriate actions necessary in our daily activities.

Reflexes are involuntary and reproducible physiologic reactions to various stimuli on receptors that send impulses, through afferent nerves, to target neurons. These target neurons, in turn, send efferent nerves to innervate skeletal or smooth muscles completing the *reflex arc*. A typical example is the deep tendon reflex (DTR, also called myotatic or stretch reflex) which is used clinically to evaluate the functions of the different spinal cord levels and the peripheral nerve innervations. There are other reflexes previously described involving the cranial nerves, like the pupillary light and accommodation reflexes described in Chapter IV-C. Stimulating the cornea (CN V-ophthalmic branch afferent) with a wisp of cotton and causing a blink response of both eyes (CN VII efferent) as described in Chapter IV-D is a corneal reflex procedure. Understanding the mechanism of the DTRs is essential for correct interpretation of reflexes elicited by the neurologic hammer.

Muscle spindles are seen within the muscles and contain *intrafusal fibers* with annulo-spiral sensory receptors of stretch and motor fibers that contract within the muscles. They primarily detect muscle stretch. When you tap the tendon of the knees with a neurologic hammer, the vibration stimulates the *intrafusal* sensory receptors transmitting the impulses through *afferent Ia and II nerves* (Fig. 37 A – a1). The nerves branch at the gray matter to synapse and excite the anterior motor neurons whose alpha fibers innervate the quadriceps extensor muscles (Fig. 37 – e1); at the same time the other branches innervate the *inhibitory interneurons* which send impulses to the motor neurons that supply *the antagonistic flexor muscles,* causing them to relax (Fig. 37 – e3). The result is a brief jerky extension of the leg or a kick. Upon stimulation of the anterior motor neurons, the *gamma motor neurons* around them

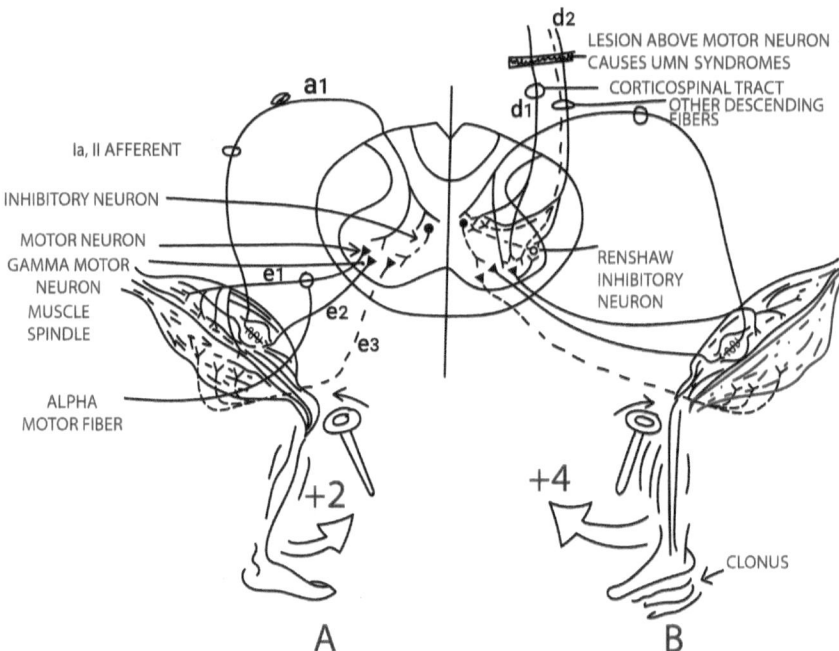

Figure 37. Knee jerk reflex. A. Reflex arc, afferent arm (a1) from the muscle spindles to the motor neuron and inhibitory interneurons and efferent arms (e1) to the quadricept extensor muscles, (e2) to muscle spindles and to opposing flexor muscles (e3). Note normal reflex of +2. B. Descending influence to the anterior and inhibitory neurons, (d1) corticospinal tract and brainstem descending influences (d2). Lesion involving the descending fibers (bold line) eliciting hyperflexia +4 and presence of clonus.

are also stimulated, causing the activation of *gamma fibers* that innervate the motor ends of the *intrafusal muscles*. The intrafusal muscles contract, *setting the tone for another contraction when a reflex stimulus is initiated (Fig. 37 – e2)*. The pathways explain the mechanism of monosynaptic or stretch reflex or DTR [50]. Readiness of muscles to contract, set by the spindles and the muscular contraction, and relaxation of opposing muscles, provide a mechanism of maintaining *muscle tones*.

Tables I and II show various descending and ascending tracts that serve to modify and regulate the activities of the motor neurons and muscle spindle sensory perceptions at the spinal level. The corticospinal tracts can modify the reflex by synaptic connection to motor neurons and interneurons (Fig. 37 – d1). Descending brainstem inhibitory influences likewise affect stretch reflex activities (Fig. 37 – d2). Diseases above a lesion in any of the spinal cord levels remove these inhibitory influences (Fig. 37 – bold line), resulting in a hyperactive reflex response on examination (upper motor neuron sign). If the peripheral nerve is affected or injured, the axons of the anterior horn cells fail to transmit impulses to the muscles resulting in diminished or absent reflexes (lower motor neuron signs) [51]. We tend to limit our association of reflexes to the DTR and pupillary light reaction, unmindful of the fact that in our daily lives, reflexes allow us to maintain muscle tone necessary for balance, posture, and all our motor activities that are working 24 hours a day!

The Concept of Upper Motor and Lower Motor Neuron Signs

When there is *upper motor neuron (UMN)* signs the manifestations are a *weakness, hyperreflexia, the presence of Babinski sign, and spasticity*, while the *lower motor neuron (LMN)* signs are a *weakness, hyporeflexia, flaccidity, atrophy, and late appearance of fasciculations and fibrillation*. To understand this concept, one should consider the level of the spinal cord *lesion* and the *spinal level being tested*. If the test is on a spinal level *below* the spinal cord lesion, the manifestations are upper motor neuron signs. UMN signs because the corticospinal tract and the *descending influences are "stopped"* by diseases above the spinal cord level being tested, causing the release of inhibitory effect to the gamma and motor neurons. If *the examination is involving precisely the level where the lesion is, then* the manifestations are lower motor neuron. LMN because the disease disturbed the reflex arc participants.

Neurological Examination:

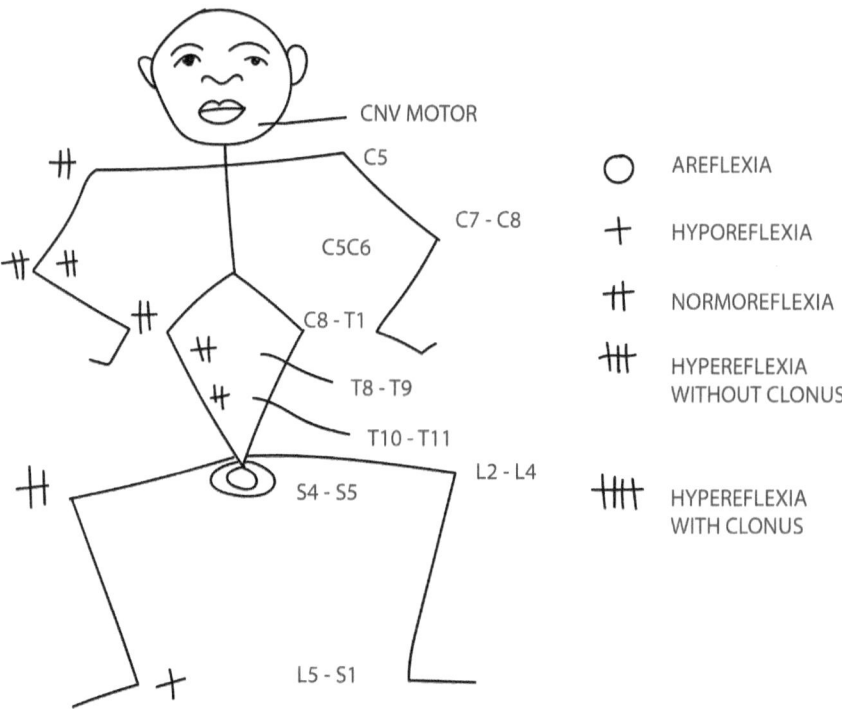

Figure 38. Popular cartoon to show where deep tendon reflexes and corresponding spinal levels are tested. Degree of responses measured from 0 to +4.

The reflex response to tapping by a neurological hammer is usually graded 0 to +4 with grade +2 as normal, a grade of +3 is hyperreflexia, and a grade of +4 is hyperreflexia with clonus.

Different types of examination of reflexes are deep tendon reflexes, abdominal reflexes, cremasteric reflex, Hoffman's reflex, Clonus and Babinski sign. Figure 38 shows a human cartoon showing the various joints used for deep tendon reflex examination and their corresponding spinal levels. Reflexes are graded as, (0) for absence of reflex; (+) for hyporeflexia; (++) for normal; (+++ to ++++) for hyperreflexia. For other areas, only their presence or absence are noted because responses may be difficult to elicit. Examples of these areas are the ankle, palmo-mental, cremasteric, and abdominal reflexes. Gentle tapping of the joints that are in their readiness position is the ideal way of doing the examination. Avoiding the factor of weight bearing and conscious control can produce a reliable result. The maneuver is done by carrying the arm or having the leg rested in the floor or bed. Examining while asking questions is one trick to remove conscious control of reflex movements.

Abdominal reflex is done by stroking gently and medially the abdominal skin by quadrants. The standard response is a quick abdominal muscle contraction. Cremasteric reflex test, on the other hand, is done by gently stroking the upper and inner thigh of males. The typical response is that the scrotum rises then goes back to original position. Do this examination only when deemed necessary and with consent from patients or legal relatives.

The motor examination begins by observing the patient move, walk, reach out, and stand from a sitting position, sitting from lying, tiptoeing and reaching out for something. Patients with Parkinson's disease (PD) often complain of weakness when there is none on motor examination. On observation, PD patients may have the limitation of arm swing, slow movements, and hesitancy or shuffling movements of the legs on initiating the act of walking. Patients with ataxia may also complain of weakness when the real problem could be an imbalance due to vestibular or cerebellar diseases. Pay attention also to the posture during walking. In PD, the patient often walks in stooping posture. Patients with true weakness or paresis on one side will show a limp on the affected side or dragging of the affected foot.

Examine all the big joint flexors and extensors against the resistance of your hand. The maneuvers may fail to demonstrate the very mild weakness of the legs because of the compensation by strong quadriceps muscles, but when told to squat or stand up without the support of the hand, the defect can be manifested as a struggle to get up. For mild tibialis anterior weakness, letting the patient walk on toes or soles may unmask the lag or limp in the affected leg. Muscle groups or myotomes showed to be weak have specific neural innervations.

The segments of the spinal cord have corresponding sensory and motor areas of innervation. These are mapped as sensory dermatomal (Please refer back to Chapter III) and motor myotomal distributions. Most overlap the innervation of the areas except for few areas of the extremities, like the dorsum of the feet which is largely innervated by L5. The following ways examine the myotomal distribution:

C3,4, and five supply the diaphragm (the large muscle between the chest and the belly that we use to breath). Let the patient take deep breaths; observe and feel the upward and downward movements of the diaphragm. Look for symmetry. When there is paralysis on one side, the affected side fails to follow the movement of the opposite side, and most likely this is related to phrenic nerve (C3-C5 innervate injury at the side of the weakness.

The test to estimate the strength of the patient's muscle groups, press or pull against the function of these muscles with the assumption that the muscle strength of the examiner is 5/5 which is normal. In this traditional measure, the denominator represents the normal strength of 5 while the numerator changes in grade relative to the denominator. To simplify the examination, we use the functions of the muscle or group of muscles for flexion and extension because their innervations roughly represent the different spinal cord levels or peripheral nerve innervations (Fig. 39).

Extension of the arm on the side tests the deltoids which are supplied by C5 while flexing the elbow tests the biceps which have a C5-6 innervation. Extending the elbow tests the triceps which has a C6-7 innervation. Flexing of the fourth finger by pressing against the thumb tests the small flexor muscles which are largely innervated by C8-T1 (median nerve. Extension of the hand tests the forearm external extensor muscles which are innervated by C6-7 (radial nerve). At the lower extremities, an extension of the hip tests the gluteal muscles that are innervated by L4-L5 (gluteal nerve) while flexing of the hip tests the iliopsoas muscles which is innervated by L2-3 (femoral nerve) tests.

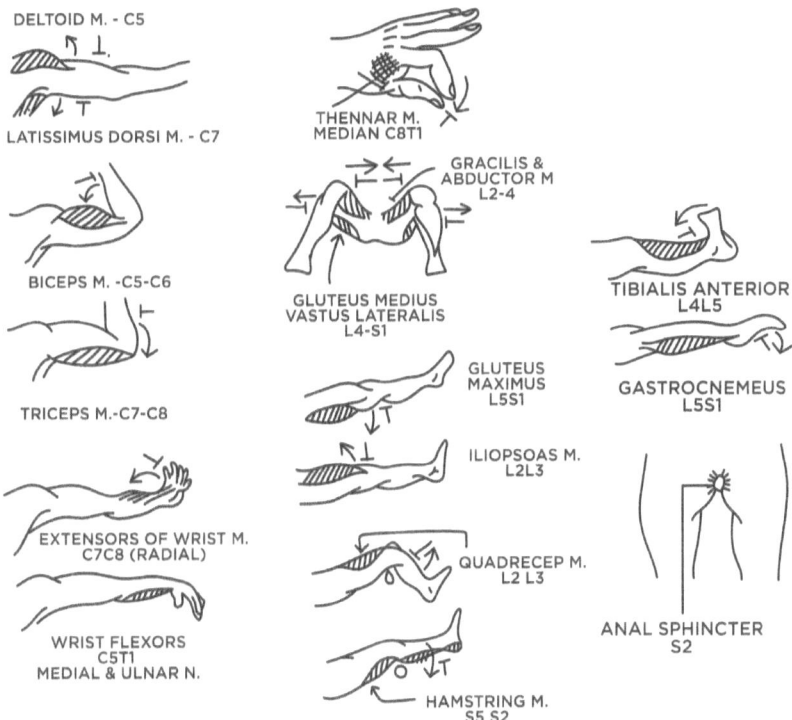

Figure 39. Myotomes and spinal level innervations. Directions of force movements (arrows) to test tones and strengths.

Knee extension tests the quadriceps muscles which are innervated by L3-4 and flexion of knees are largely due to contractions of the hamstring with L5-S1 (sciatic nerve) innervation. Flexion of the foot through the anterior tibialis muscles have L4-5 (peroneal nerve) innervations while the extension of foot tests the gastrocnemius muscles which are innervated by S1. Toe extension tests the extensor halluces longus which is innervated by L5.

Case Story:

Mrs. Hoesct, a pretty 32-year-old dance teacher and a mother of two was diagnosed to have multiple sclerosis (MS) two years ago when she complained of blurring of vision, dizziness, numbness from the shoulder and below, and slight weakness of both legs. MRI showed MS plaques at the left side of the optic chiasma, on both periventricular areas, at the right ponto-cerebellar peduncle and in both lateral and posterior columns of C5 down to C8 cervical cord. The symptoms disappeared gradually after one month of treatment which allowed her to continue her passion for teaching dancing. She kept taking her medicines. A follow-up examination showed the persistence of bilateral hypoactive (+) brachioradialis (C5-C6) reflexes, while knee-jerk reflexes (L2-4) were hyperactive (+3). There was also Babinski sign on both feet.

Clinical - anatomic Correlation:

If MS plaques involve the spinal cord at C5 – C8, signs *below* this level will demonstrate upper motor neuron signs like hyperreflexia on knee-jerk reflexes (L2-L4) and bilateral Babinski sign. Brachioradialis reflexes at C5 - C6, where the MS plaques are located, will show lower motor neuron signs like hypoactive reflexes. Treatment modified the appearance of the other manifestations in the upper and lower extremities.

The Sensory Component of the Peripheral Nerves.

The basis for the distribution of sensory receptors in the body is on its functional necessities, like Golgi tendons in muscles for tone and position, Pacinian corpuscles in the skin for vibratory sensation and bare ending receptors in many parts of the body for pain and touch sensation (Table II). The bodies of the neurons transmitting the sensory impulses from the periphery lie in the dorsal ganglia. Remember that the dorsal ganglia are exclusively a house of sensory neurons. The action potential is transmitted from the dorsal ganglia to the posterior part of the cord toward the neurons in the posterior gray horn for pain, touch, and temperature sensations. The axons of the dorsal ganglia neurons that will transmit discriminatory sensory impulses pass through the posterior column where it will be named fasciculus gracilis (coming from the legs) and fasciculus cuneatus (coming from the arms). These long axons continue to ascend until they synapse with nucleus gracilis and cuneatus at the medulla. These dorsal ganglia neurons that provided this long tract carry sensory impulses for vibration, proprioception, and other discriminatory sensations.

We have emphasized that each level of the cord has sensory innervations mapped in the dermatomal distribution. To help localize the disease process, evaluate progression or improvement of the disease use the dermatomal map. When determining the location of the disease, it is also essential to assess motor and autonomic nerve status. For motor function, we use myotomal levels. For autonomic nerve affectation, observe the distribution of changes in the skin temperature, texture, sweat, color, including rectal sphincter tone and bladder fullness after voiding.

Neurological Examination

Practical instruments can be used, including one's fingers. One can use a wisp of cotton for light touch, art painting brush that gives better control for gross touch test. When using a pin, punch it through a stick applicator for better and consistent light application. A cloth cutter's liner that rolls for faster procedure and mapping of pain are practical. Tuning fork at 260 cps, to test posterior column pathways, is applied to bony areas of the dermatome tests for vibration. For temperature, application of small test tube with cold or warm water along the dermatomal distribution and identifying them is a test seldom used because it follows the same pain distribution. Neurological hammer is a favorite tool to test for deep tendon reflexes. A two-point compass to determine the ability to identify the two points when applied almost simultaneously and a certain distance. With the eyes closed or covered, assure the patient that there will be no harmful stimuli. All instruments for sensory examination are tested in normal areas first to allow patients to familiarize with the sensation. They are instructed to describe what is felt when the device is applied and to compare if the feeling in the corresponding area is the same, lesser in degree or felt more. Procedures are repeated to determine consistency in this highly subjective examination.

Only patients who can cooperate undergo detailed sensory examination. Gross sensory examination for patients' with disturbed consciousness or with cognitive problems is limited often to graded pain stimuli. When there is a need to examine the anal and perineal areas (S4-5 level), seek written permission from patients or legal surrogates after explaining to the patient and family the importance of the procedure. During the conduct of examining the S4-5 sensory innervation, a member of the clinic staff should be present to serve and provide reassurance to the patient or family. Do the evaluation in collaboration with the patient. The patient's experience should guide the focus of the examination. Begin with touch sensation; the stroke of the wisp of cotton or brush is done in regional distribution, always comparing both sides and repeated for consistency, always to find out if there is a difference or not and, if there is, the degree of variation. Pain stimulation by using pinprick is applied lightly for the superficial sensation of the skin. When there is a decreased sensation, *hypoaesthesia* is the term used, while the sensory loss is *anesthesia*. Watch out for exaggerated pain sensation in mild painful stimuli, this is called *hyperaesthesia* but if the pain experienced with a standard stimulus, it is called *allodynia*. Frequent practice and doing this repeatedly to patients will shorten the examination time. One may skip temperature examination because it follows the same pain pathway and termination, but for some patients who have a phobia or anticipated anxiety with the prick stimuli, this would be a more acceptable examination.

Vibratory test, position sense test, and test for two-point discrimination evaluate the posterior column. During the trials, patients are blindfolded to avoid anticipated and guessing responses. Start by letting the patient experience and feel the vibration of the tuning fork applied over the bony protuberances of the body. Then let the patient compare the degree of vibration felt between corresponding dermatomal areas of the body. The position-sense examination is done with the patient seated and comfortable. At first, the flexion and extension test is done on large joints like the wrist for instructional purposes. Next is to do the maneuver in digital joints of the hands and feet. In two-point discrimination tests, apply simultaneously two pointed calipers at 2-5 mm distance from each point. Then ask the patient to determine if there were one or two points applied. The shortest length that the patient can feel the two points when applied simultaneously is usually 2-13mm. Compare the test on both sides and corresponding areas of the body. In general, the maneuver uses the tip of the fingers or toes. Where there is a failure to feel the two points, most likely is the dermatomal level that the posterior columns innervate.

Letting the patient identify the written number on the palm, the shapes of coins and other small objects, and the textures of different materials laid on the hand are tests for the secondary or discriminatory sensation that evaluates the function of the postcentral gyrus.

Make and draw the dermatomal distribution of the sensory disturbances.

The Autonomic Nervous System

The Autonomic Nervous System (ANS) is a complex integration of various structures of the central nervous system that is purely involuntary. It is responsible for maintaining homeostasis in the body in response to external and internal stimuli. This function is made possible by two main components that oppose each other but in a coordinated and automatic way. These two components are the Sympathetic Nervous System (SNS) and the Parasympathetic Nervous System (PSNS). One can say that the general function of the SNS is "fight or flight," while the PSNS is "rest and digest" and "feed and breed." In general, the sympathetic system dominate during the intense and heightened reaction to an external or internal threat to the body. The parasympathetic nerve takes control when a person is at rest and in a relaxed state. As an example, when one sees a swarm of bees, the entire body responds to the experience through the SNS that automatically increases the heart and respiratory rates, dilates the pupils, causes piloerection, and the body is set in an alert and ready-to-run state. When the bees are gone, the PSNS starts to dominate. This time, the heart rate decelerates, blood pressure goes down, respiration slows, piloerection disappears, and pupils go back to their usual size. Usually, the laughter of relief follows!! Whew, that was close!!

Anatomy of the Autonomic Nervous System

The ANS has central nervous system components (CNS) and peripheral nervous system (PNS) components that integrate to modify and regulate impulses that are eventually transmitted to the body as shown in Figure 34. The CNS-ANS participants are divided into cortical, brainstem, and spinal cord groups. The PNS-ANS participants consist of three sympathetic ganglia, cranial and peripheral nerves, and neural plexus at the walls of the innervated organs.

Cortical and subcortical structures participating in the ANS functions are the insula, medial prefrontal regions, amygdala, stria terminalis, thalamus, and hypothalamus, and they receive interconnecting impulses from brainstem structures, thalamus, olfactory bulb, optic nerve, and other cortical areas. These structures, in turn, send pulses to the brainstem nuclear groups and the intermediate gray horn of the spinal cord. The cortex provides the *cognitive, emotional, and behavioral autonomic reactions* [52].

Brainstem centers of the ANS include the periaqueductal gray, parabrachial pons, nucleus tractus solitarius, nucleus ambiguus, salivatory nucleus, dorsomedial nucleus, and intermediate reticular zone of the medulla. Chapters VI-C on CN III, Chapter VI-E on CN VII, Chapter VI-G CN IX, and Chapter VI on CN X describe cranial nerve ANS connections involving the brainstem. These neurons receive afferent inputs from the cortex, and the spinal cord and some have interconnections within the brainstem. The efferent autonomic outputs from the brainstem are basically parasympathetic.

Preganglionic neurons and postganglionic neurons transmit the autonomic impulses at the cranial and peripheral nerves. **Preganglionic neurons** refer to a group of neurons that send efferent axons to another group of neurons, named **post-ganglionic neurons**. Outside the brain stem or spinal cord are these post-ganglionic neurons that relay impulses to the "target" organs. *An exception where preganglionic neurons have no postganglionic connection is the direct sympathetic preganglionic connection to the medulla of the adrenal glands which respond by releasing noradrenalin and epinephrine directly to the bloodstream.*

Parasympathetic Nervous System (PSNS)

The preganglionic efferent *parasympathetic neurons* (PSNS) of the cranial nerves are in the brainstem. The neurons send impulses outside the brainstem to many postganglionic neurons of several ganglia, and in turn, the neurons innervate smooth muscles to elicit specific functions. The autonomic nervous system of the cranial nerves has been described in the earlier chapters on cranial nerves. Some of the neuroanatomic and functional PSNS examples are as follows:

- CN III preganglia is at the Edinger-Westphal Nucleus (EWN) of the posterior midbrain. The EWN neurons send impulses to the postganglionic neurons of the Ciliary ganglia whose axons innervate the pupilo-constrictor muscles (Fig. 40).
- CN VII preganglionic neurons are at the *Superior* Salivatory Nucleus, and they send synaptic connections to the neurons of three postganglionic ganglia: the pterygopalatine, sublingual and submandibular ganglia. The first supply the lacrimal and palatal mucosal glands. The second innervate the sublingual glands, while the third the submandibular glands
- CN IX shares the preganglionic neurons with CN VII, but it is at the *Inferior* Salivatory Nucleus, and the postganglionic neurons are at the Otic Ganglia whose axons supply the parotid gland.
- CN X preganglionic neurons at the Nucleus Ambiguus (NA) and Dorsal Motor Nucleus (DM) send lengthy parasympathetic efferent connections to the postganglionic neurons embedded in the smooth muscles of the heart, the bronchial tree, and the gastrointestinal walls. Postganglionic neurons supply inhibitory impulses---to the smooth muscles of the heart to cause bradycardia; to the bronchial wall to cause constriction; to the gastrointestinal system to cause hypermotility, and to the

sphincters of the bile and pancreatic duct to induce relaxation and release of bile and pancreatic enzymes.

The preganglionic neurons of the PSNS of the spinal cord come from the intermediate gray matter of S2-S4, and their postganglionic neurons lie very near or within the walls of the large intestines and genitourinary structures. The postganglionic neurons innervate the smooth muscles or the sphincters to produce the following physiologic effects: bladder contraction, urethral internal sphincter relaxation, smooth vessel wall relaxation, increased vascular perfusion of the penis and clitoris, increased intestinal peristalsis, and relaxation of the anal sphincter.

Sympathetic Nervous System (SNS)

The preganglionic neurons of the SNS lie within the Intermediate gray matter or Layer VII of the spinal cord that extends from T1 to L2, and their postganglionic neurons lie in the prevertebral and paravertebral chain of sympathetic ganglia. On both sides, the sympathetic ganglia divide into *superior, medial, inferior cervical ganglia; and sympathetic trunk ganglia*.

The sympathetic nerve from the *superior cervical postganglionic neurons* passes through the posterior apical portion of the lungs as they ascend to wind around the common carotid artery and internal carotid artery. At about the take-off of the ophthalmic branch of the internal carotid artery, the sympathetic nerve gives off branches to the *ciliary ganglia sympathetic* neurons to supply the *pupilo-dilator muscles, ciliary muscles* and *Muller's muscles* that participate in the elevation of the upper lids and the *sweat glands* of the face. The path of the sympathetic nerve of the superior cervical ganglia is at the posterior apical part of the lungs an area where malignant tumors like Pancoast's tumors can grow. The cancerous tumor can very well press and disturb the function of the sympathetic nerve and the brachial plexus. The sympathetic nerve affectation can cause **ptosis, miosis** (pupillary constriction) and **hemianhydrosis** (absence of sweat) collectively called **Bernard-Horner's syndrome** [53]. The brachial nerve compression and infiltration can be accompanied by pain in the axilla, scapula, shoulder and the ulnar distribution of the hand and this time referred to as **Pancoast-Tobias Syndrome**. Henry Pancoast, a radiologist, described the apical lesion in 1924 & 1932; J. Tobias from Buenos Aires described the tumor to be an invasive carcinoma and made the clinical correlation in 1932 [54,55].

The *middle cervical postganglionic neurons* supply the muscles of the heart, SA nodes, and the skin. The *inferior cervical ganglia* innervate the heart, bronchioles of the lungs and the esophageal sphincter. The *sympathetic trunk ganglia* from T4-L2 do not make synaptic connections with the paravertebral ganglia, but the axons pass through them and join the other fibers to form the greater, lesser and lumbar splanchnic nerves, then synapse with the postganglionic neurons of the *celiac ganglia, the superior mesenteric ganglia and the inferior mesenteric ganglia*.

The *celiac post-ganglionic neurons* innervate the stomach to decrease muscle activity; constrict pyloric sphincter; stimulate the adrenal medulla to secrete epinephrine and norepinephrine that would in turn stimulate the liver to release glucose; cause the smooth muscle of the renal vessel to constrict and decrease urine output; and innervate the smooth muscles of the intestine to decrease motility.

The *superior mesenteric ganglia post-synaptic neurons* send excitatory impulses to the smooth muscles of the small intestines and the ascending and large transverse intestines causing a decrease of motility.

The *inferior mesenteric post-synaptic ganglion neurons* send excitatory impulses to the smooth muscles of descending colon, sigmoid and rectum to cause a decrease of motility. The hypogastric plexus, which is a branch of the inferior mesenteric nerve, supplies the internal anal sphincter. This nerve stimulates the sphincter that triggers constriction and prevents anal spillage; innervates the urinary bladder smooth muscles to cause relaxation; transmits excitatory impulses to the internal urethral sphincter causing constriction that inhibits voiding; synapses with structures of the genitalia, like the vas deferens, epididymis and prostate gland, to cause ejaculation in males and vaginal contractions in females.

The ANS transmitters.

The nerve transmitters of preganglionic efferent SNS and PSNS postganglionic afferent are Acetyl Choline (ACh), while the postganglionic SNS transmitter is noradrenaline (NE) except the SNS that innervates the sweat gland which has ACh as a transmitter. These past two decades, Nitrous Oxide, a gasotransmitter and postganglionic PSNS transmitter to blood vessels and the heart is gaining prominence in cardiovascular protective functions [56,57].

The ANS nerve fibers.

The preganglionic afferent fibers are A-delta fibers while the efferent fibers are Beta 1 fibers. The postganglionic nerves, on the other hand, consist of unmyelinated C fibers for both efferent and afferent branches.

The ANS receptors.

Different afferent receptors transmit impulses to the dorsal ganglia, then to the spinal cord or to the brainstem that allows avenues for ANS connections and ANS appropriate responses. These afferent receptors are sensitive to mechanical, stretch, chemical or temperature changes. The efferent receptors of the postganglionic SNS neurons, on the other hand, are the following:

- o Alpha receptors of peripheral blood vessels that cause constriction and raise the blood pressure.
- o Beta 1 receptors that increase heart rate and contractility
- o Beta 2 receptors of the peripheral vessel's smooth muscles that cause relaxation in the bronchi, gastrointestinal tract, and other gut organs.
- o Beta 1 stretch receptors for atrial, ventricular, and coronary vessels that increase heart rate, myocardial contractility, and coronary dilation respectively.

The preganglionic parasympathetic (PSNS) vagal efferent receptors to the heart, on the other hand, are the:
Atrial, ventricular, and coronary receptors that cause decreased heart rate (bradycardia) decreased contractility, and coronary vasoconstriction.
Here are more examples of everyday situations that demonstrates ANS critical participation.

Fear responses of the ANS.

Imagine a wild dog with huge, sharp fangs and raging eyes running fast towards you! Your eyes see the image of the dog and send impulses that estimate the speed of the oncoming dog. The occipital lobes receive the picture from the eyes and interpret the data as a determined, angry dog rapidly running and growling ready to bite!! The occipital neurons then send impulses to the limbic system that provides meaning to the images as a threat! Fear immediately follows!! Some limbic system neurons send synaptic fibers to the hypothalamic sympathetic neurons, which in turn transmit descending impulses to the T1-L2 intermediate gray of the spinal cord where sympathetic preganglionic neurons reside. These neurons then send their axons to join the peripheral nerve, but separate immediately to synapse with the paraspinal sympathetic ganglia that house post-synaptic sympathetic neurons. These post-synaptic sympathetic neurons send efferent fibers to different parts of the body: to the pupillary-dilator muscles of the eyes to cause pupillary dilatation; to the heart to increase the rate of contraction (tachycardia); to the piloerector muscles that raise the hair; and to the smooth muscle of blood vessels causing them to constrict and increase blood pressure. All of these explain many of the body responses related to fear! After reaching safety, you notice that your heart starts to decelerate, and this is because the PSNS takes over to cause an opposite response.

Visual clarity maintained with static or moving images mediated by the ANS

Transformation of light stimuli into electrical impulses occur at the rods and cones of the retina. The electrical waves are transmitted to the ganglion neurons (Fig. 40). The ganglion cell's afferent axons synapse with the nuclei at the Lateral Geniculate Ganglia (LGG) where some neurons send efferent axons to the pretectal neurons at the superior colliculi of the midbrain. The pretectal neurons that transmit crossed and uncrossed axons to the Edinger-Westphal Nucleus (EWN) are parasympathetic neurons. These EWN presynaptic parasympathetic neurons send an efferent transmission to the post ciliary ganglia neurons whose axons supply the pupillary constrictor muscles and ciliary muscles that relax the lens. The constriction of the pupils that control entry of

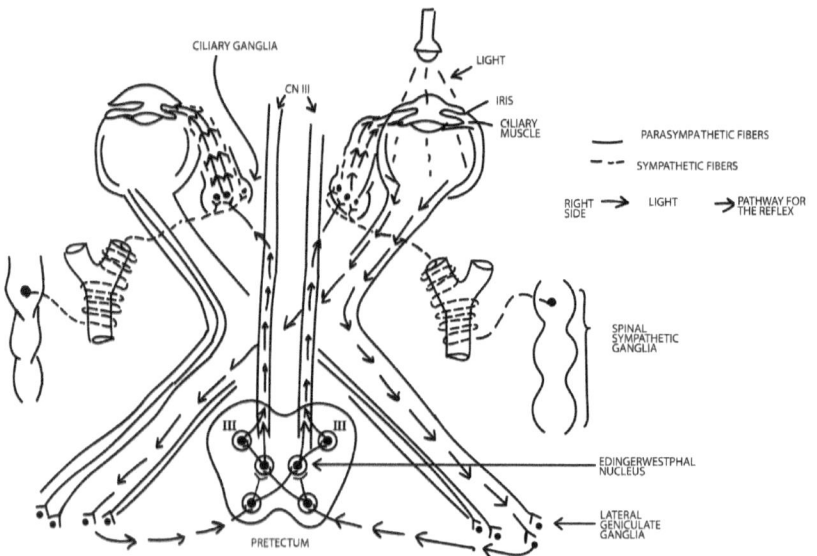

Figure 40. Anatomic pathway of pupillary reflex. Parasympathetic impulses pathways (arrows) from the ganglion cells of the retina, to pretectum, through CNIII, to Ciliary ganglia, then to pupil constrictor muscles. Sympathetic nerve impulses from the spinal sympathetic ganglia (broken lines), looping around the internal carotid artery, to ciliary ganglia, then to pupil dilator muscles.

light and the shape of the lens that projects the size and deflect the form of light to the retina contribute to visual clarity of images.

Some of the visual pathway neurons at the LGG send afferent fibers to the hypothalamus sympathetic neurons which also receive afferent impulses from the limbic structures. The sympathetic hypothalamic neurons then transmit depolarizing wave down to the sympathetic neurons located at the intermediate gray horn that extends from T1 to L2 of the spinal cord. The preganglionic sympathetic neurons carry impulses to the paraspinal superior, medial, and inferior chain ganglia that contain post-ganglionic sympathetic neurons. The post-ganglionic sympathetic neurons then send axons that wind around the internal carotid artery to reach the ciliary sympathetic ganglia where sympathetic branches supply the pupil dilator muscles to cause pupillary dilatation and the ciliary muscles to effect contraction of the lens that contribute to the degree of deflection of images to the retina.

The pupils and the lens are in constant adjustments even while asleep, and this is possible through the automatic and involuntary balancing of the PSNS and SNS to contribute to the clarity of moving images that will eventually reach the brain for processing.

Taste and salivation necessary for an appreciation of food that is mediated by the ANS

There are three cranial nerves that transmit specialized sensation from taste bud receptors that are present in the different parts of the oral cavity. These are CN VII, providing the anterior 2/3 of the tongue and the soft palate; CN IX, innervating the posterior 1/3 of the tongue; and CN X, supplying the base, the area around the tongue and the epiglottis. Like any sensory nerves to the brain, the transmitting neurons reside in the ganglia. The ganglia are the Geniculate Ganglion for CN VII, Inferior Glossopharyngeal Ganglion for CN IX, and Inferior Vagal Ganglion for CN X. The receiving neurons in the ganglia send impulses to the lower pons and upper medulla portions of Nucleus Solitarius where neurons, in turn, send axons that cross and join the medial lemniscus on its way up to synapse with the nucleus of the ventroposteromedial thalamus (VPL). The thalamic neurons forward impulses to the medial part of the postcentral gyrus (tongue and lips of homunculus) where taste is perceived and to the hypothalamus, amygdala, and insula where emotional and behavioral responses impact on the appreciation of taste.

The "taste" impulses from the hypothalamus send descending fibers to the preganglionic parasympathetic salivatory nucleus and, in turn, the neurons here send impulses to the postganglionic PSNS neurons at the pterygopalatine ganglia, submandibular and sublingual ganglia (CNVII), otic ganglia (CN IX), and inferior ganglia (CN X). The neurons in these ganglia supply the *lacrymal, submandibular, sublingual glands* (CNVII), *parotid glands* (CNIX), and *secretory mucosal pharyngeal glands* (CNX) respectively. These complete the cycle of appreciation of food and salivation to aid in chewing and digestion. Saliva is necessary for food mastication and for facilitation of swallowing. Now you know why and how taste and salivation became partners. To be a food gourmet your discriminating brain, together with cranial nerves I, VII, IX, and X, are essential.

Physiologic changes mediated by the ANS to meet the body demands during exercise.

Blood Pressure, Heart Rate, Respiration Regulations are essential to meet the body demands during exercise and at rest. During training, the muscle contractions' demand for oxygen increases. The lungs supply the oxygen needs and carried by the red blood cells to the muscles. The Hering Breuer Inflation Reflex is a neural control of respiration. Respiration is initiated by inspiratory alveolar inflation that causes stretching of the inhibitory afferent smooth muscle receptors (ISM) of the bronchial tree. The stretching transmits through the afferent Vagus nerve, inhibitory impulses to the Inspiratory Center (IC) of the medulla, blocking it along with the apneutic center of the pons (AC) causing the arrest of inspiration which is again followed by prolonged expiration -- this is the respiratory cycle. Every time the ISM receptors of the bronchial tree are stimulated by inflation of the alveoli, some of the inhibitory afferent stimuli synapse with neurons at the Nucleus Ambiguus (NA) and Dorsal Motor Nucleus (DM) and block them. The NA and DM neurons are inhibitory by nature and, if blocked, the impulses transmitted through the efferent vagus nerve stops the inhibitory effect to the heart rhythm causing increased heart rate. This reflex explains the associated heart rate increase during high oxygen demand, more frequent inspiratory-expiratory cycle (panting) and increased heart rate (tachycardia during exercise).

As the exercise progresses, body demand for oxygen increases, triggering the heart to pump faster and stronger and the blood pressure to go up. These body mechanisms cannot however continue unabated. Tolerance to physiologic responses to exercise is dependent on the preconditioning of the body to regular exercises. When the body demand for oxygen decreases and as the activity decelerates, the Carotid Body and Carotid Sinus Reflex are operant in the process of lowering heart rate and reducing blood pressure. The baroreceptors for CN IX are within the Internal Carotid and Common Carotid Artery bifurcation while the Chemoreceptors for CN X are at the Carotid Sinus and Aortic Arch. The baroreceptors are stimulated by stretch due to increased arterial blood pressure while low pH, pO_2 and pCO_2 stimulates chemoreceptors. The baroreceptors, when excited, send impulses through CN IX to Nucleus Tractus Solitareus (NTS) of the medulla. The neurons of the NTS, in turn, transmit pulses to the reticular formation of the medulla, hypothalamus. Preganglionic parasympathetic NA and DM. The NA and DM neurons send parasympathetic descending stimulus through the vagus nerve which is inhibitory and cause decreased heart rate and blood pressure.

The ANS, sympathetic and parasympathetic nerves are continually responding to the physiologic changes during exercise, when slowing down and when resting.

Case Story:

Mr. Ross is a 67-year-old retired financial adviser who is enjoying his retirement. While walking along the beautiful shore of Honolulu, he suddenly felt dizzy and collapsed. When he regained his senses, he related to the ER doctor that this was the fourth time that this happened since two years ago. His blood pressure while lying down was 110/70 and heart rate was 60/minute. After standing for two minutes, his blood pressure was noted to have dropped to 90/50 while the heart rate remained at 60/min. After five minutes, the blood pressure started to settle at 100/60. When asked about other autonomic body functions, he related that his bowel habit changed since two years ago from daily to once every three days and with the help of laxatives. He hesitantly admitted the absence of erection. He also said, "The most distressing really is my effort to void which requires me to strain and press on my bladder, and what is also disturbing is that I have to wake up four times at night to empty my bladder." He sweated only on his neck while the rest of the body did not sweat. A neurologist, about a month ago, advised him to submit for further workup because of a suspicion that he might have autonomic nerve dysfunction or dysautonomia due to diabetes for 15 years.

Clinical-anatomic Correlation:

Prolonged diabetes especially when poorly controlled causes microangiopathy of the peripheral nerves. Mr. Ross' peripheral autonomic nervous system took most of the brunt of the disease causing hypotension, constipation, erectile dysfunction, and bladder disturbance, perhaps aggravated by possible co-existence of prostatic hypertrophy. All of these problems are due to the affectation of the sympathetic and parasympathetic nerves from the complications of poorly controlled diabetes.

Neurological Examination:

When there is a suspected spinal cord or peripheral nerve injury or disease, the autonomic function can be involved, a reason that evaluation of the ANS function is essential. Historical data on symptoms related to postural changes, dryness of the mouth, the absence of sweat or unusual distribution of sweat, change of bowel movements, constipation, urinary, and sexual disturbances queried. Postural changes in blood pressure and evaluation of the heart rate from lying to the standing position are necessary. A drop of more than 20 mm Hg and 10mm Hg of systolic and diastolic pressure respectively and consistently suggest a possible ANS problem. The bladder should be palpated over the suprapubic (just below the umbilicus) to check for retention of urine. A rectal examination can evaluate the function of the anal sphincter. Feel the tone of the sphincter and the corresponding change during Valsalva's maneuver. Feel also for the laxity of the sphincter. Dryness of the affected areas of the skin and nail beds and disappearance of hair denote sympathetic dystrophy as a chronic complication of immobilization.

The absence of sweating in certain areas when they should be sweating denotes sympathetic dysfunction exemplified by Bernard-Horner's syndrome consisting of anhydrosis, miosis, and ptosis involving one side of the face. These are due to tumor destruction of the sympathetic nerve at the apex of the left lung (Pancoast tumor) disturbing the innervation to the sweat glands, pupillary dilators, and Muller's muscles of the upper lid. If appropriate, alizarin powder dust discoloration or iodine-starch discoloration mapping can be done to see the sweat distribution pattern of the entire body.

Clinical-anatomic Correlation and Localization of motor and sensory deficits.

First, determine which side is involved and determine their distribution. Is the distribution more proximal or distal? Or are they symmetric or asymmetric?

One-sided sensory deficit (hemisensory deficit) denotes a spinothalamic lesion where the upper and lower extremity tracts or connections are near each other, and this could be at the opposite thalamus or brainstem median lemniscus. If it is a *one-sided motor deficit* (hemiparesis or hemiplegia), the arm and legs are near each other is at the merging of the corticospinal tract at the internal capsule and throughout its descent, at the brainstem, before they decussate. If one extremity or a part of the extremity has a sensory deficit (monoparesthesia) or motor deficit (monoplegia or monoparesis), most likely the lesion involves the nerve or group of nerves innervating that dermatome or myotome. *Symmetric and proximal distribution of weakness* is indicative of primary muscle disease or myopathy. Examples of diffuse muscle affectation are hypokalemic myopathy or thyrotoxic myopathy. Diffuse pathologic lesions of peripheral nerve diseases are frequently symmetrical and distal in distribution. One example of diffuse pathology is in diabetic neuropathy where patients describe distal and symmetric "globe-and-stocking" type of sensory manifestations. Another example is Guillain-Barre Syndrome (GBS), which was what Mrs. Fox had, that involves all nerve roots and manifest symmetric and distal paresthesia initially followed by weakness. Polio, on the other hand, affects many areas of the CNS, particularly the motor neurons of the brainstem or the anterior horn cells with irregular distribution. *Pure motor weakness is manifested* and are *asymmetric* and *could be distal or proximal.*

Second, look for other accompanying involvements and their distribution, like sensory or autonomic nerve affectations, including the reflexes. Are this pure sensory? Are they mixed with motor and if they are, which is more dominant? Are they pure motor? Are the reflexes normal or abnormal? What are their distributions? Are there autonomic nervous system involvements like bladder retention, tympanitic abdomen, lax or increased sphincter?

A *pure sensory* deficit denotes a very focal pathology involving the spinothalamic pathway or an early involvement of small nerve fibers, as seen in painful neuropathies in diabetes. *Pure motor* weakness indicates anterior horn cell involvement, as in polio or motor neuron disease or amyotrophic lateral sclerosis. GBS or acute polyradiculitis *predominantly manifests motor weakness with few objectives or subjective sensory or symptoms*. The main characteristic of GBS is a loss of deep tendon reflexes. Spinal cord pathology as in *transverse myelitis (a disease affecting the entire cross section of the cord)* also involves the autonomic nervous system causing bladder and bowel disturbance, sensory deficits below the lesions and upper motor signs below the lesion but lower motor signs at the level of the pathology. During our student days we made simple clues to help us remember the characteristics of different diseases, like- Polio- **M** (motor); GBS- **M,s,-r** (a little sensory deficit and hyporeflexia); Myopathy-**M,c** (crampy sensation) and Transverse Myelitis- **M, S, A, R** (notice equally dominant sensory, A as autonomic function involvement and R as hyperactive reflexes below the lesion).

If there is a weakness, one should determine which muscle groups are involved and see if there is a myotomal distribution. Bilateral symmetrical pure motor weakness denotes myopathy especially if the reflexes are normal. The crampy sensation is a result of muscle disease, and therefore not a neural manifestation, but a nerve transmitted muscle discomfort usually brought about by anoxia. Motor neuron disease shows diffuse and irregularly distributed myotomal weakness in the early part of the disease.

Is the sensory and motor involvement consistent with the cord level and neural distribution?

Intersecting neuroanatomical functions points to the locale of the lesion. Presence of bilateral leg weakness (paresis), bladder and bowel dysfunction with a sensory level at T10 (umbilicus) and hyperreflexia below T10 all point consistently to a spinal cord lesion, transverse myelitis at T8-T10 levels.

Chapter VIII

The Cerebellum
(Functions: Balance, Voluntary Muscle Coordination, Visio-vestibular-spatial-proprioceptive Coordination, Cognition and Affect)

In the dying seconds of game 6, the NBA Finals in 1998 with Chicago behind by one point, Michael Jordan was being guarded closely. He and his opponents knew that the center of the game plan was on him. MJ ran behind a screen, then suddenly made a break, getting the guard off-balanced, allowing him much space for a pass. He received a quick pass, made two dribbles and before the guard could react, he made a jump shot at exactly a second before the buzzer. The guard was desperately making a jump for the ball as Jordan's right forearm flexed in fluid motion with the hand extending while holding the ball, then in a smooth but quick action, the forearm extended in a throw with the hand making a snappy flexion, hurling the ball to the air allowing destiny to take its course. Jordan's torso was perpendicular to the floor with fully extended legs and feet as the ball continued to float. Then as quick as the jump, both feet landed with the leg slightly flexed in perfect balance and at the same time, whoosh...the ball got in, thus the championship! The instant replay would show a kaleidoscope of bodies, eyes, heads, and even emotional coordination from the other players, the referees, and the fans. We were looking at the game oblivious to the fact that the cerebellum, basal ganglia, and the cortex had a lot of roles to play in this exciting drama.

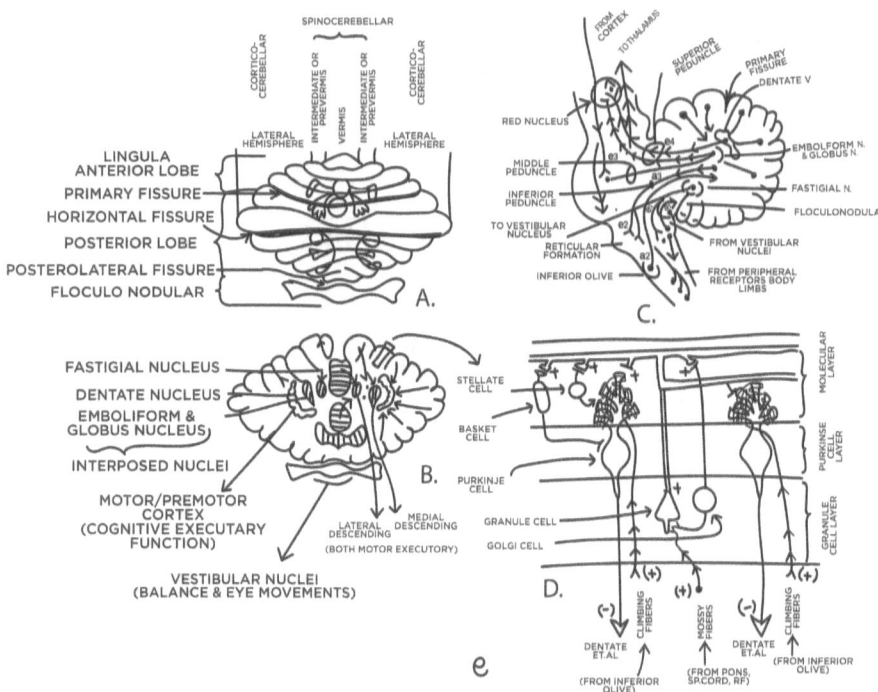

Figure 41. The Cerebellum. A. Parts of the cerebellum when unrolled and seen from above with homunculus. B. Horizontal cut of the cerebellum showing nuclei groups. C. Saggital cut showing peduncles and connections. Inferior peduncle, from vestibular nuclei to fastigeal nucleus (a1) and back (e1); from spinal cord and inferior olive to fastigeal nucleus (a2) and from fastigeal nucleus to reticular nuclei (e2). Middle peduncle, from pontine nuclear groups to Interposed nuclei (a3). Superior peduncle, from Interposed nuclei to red nucleus of the midbrain (e3); from dentate nucleus to thalamo-cortical neurons and red nucleus (e4). D. Histological components of the cerebellum and 3 cellular layers. Afferent excitatory fibers (arrow lines), mossy fibers to granule cells and climbing fibers to Purkinje cells. The only efferen axons within the cerebellum comes from the inhibitory Purkinje cells that connects with the cerebellar nucleus, cortex, subcortical structures and vestibular-spinal system.

The cerebellum consists of convoluted cerebellar hemispheres, deep nuclei, and white matter (Fig. 41-A). When seen from above, the division of the hemispheres appear into three zones: the medial vermis; just adjacent is the *intermediate zone;* then the left and right *cerebellar hemispheres.* On sagittal section (Fig. 41-C) the lobes are divided by the primary fissures into anterior and posterior lobes and, inferiorly, by the postero-lateral fissure [58].

On horizontal section (Fig. 41-B), in the middle of the white matter are islands of neurons on both sides and are grouped into three central nuclei arranged medial to lateral. Medially is the Fastigial nucleus, medio-lateral is the Interposed nuclei sub-grouped into emboliform and globose nucleus and most lateral is a grouping of the Dentate nuclei. This middle to lateral arrangement help understand the flow of efferent fibers from the lobes. Efferent fibers from the medial lobe, the vermis, send axons to the *Fastigial nucleus* (Fig. 41-B arrows), the Intermediate zone neurons send efferent axons to the *Interposed nucleus* while the large lateral cerebellar hemispheres send efferent fibers to the *large Dentate Nuclei.* All efferent outflows from the cerebellar lobes go through these three nuclei *except for the flocculonodular lobes that have direct connections with the vestibular nucleus at the pons.* It is for this connectivity that the Vestibular Nuclei in the pons and the cerebellar nuclei are considered part of the cerebellar system.

The white matter that consists of efferent and afferent axons within the cerebellum is connected to the brainstem by three peduncles (Fig. 41-C). The *inferior cerebellar peduncle (restiform body)* contains the afferent fiber (Fig. 41-C, a1,a2) and efferent fiber tracts (Fig. 41-C, e1,e2) from the medullary vestibular nuclei and the flocculonodular lobes primarily. The other afferent fibers that pass through the inferior peduncle are the *spinocerebellar fibers and reticular afferents from the medulla* (Fig. 41-C, a2). The *middle cerebellar peduncle (brachium pontis)* contains mainly *cerebro-cerebellar afferents* through the pons (Fig. 41-C, a3). The *superior cerebellar peduncle (brachium conjunctivum)* is the primary *efferent tract of cerebellar nuclei* and some afferent fibers from the *spinocerebellar fibers.* The axons from dentate nucleus synapse with the red nucleus and thalamocortical centers (Fig. 41 – C, e3, and e4 respectively).

Histologically (Fig. 41-D), the cerebellar cortex contains the innermost layer with tightly packed *granule cells*; the middle layer which has only the *Purkinje cells;* and the outer layer or molecular layer consisting of *axons of the granule cells,* many *dendrites of the Purkinje cells, interneurons, Golgi cells, basket cells and stellate cells.*

The connections show that the *Mossy fibers* come from the pons, spinal cord, reticular formation, and vestibular nuclei, and they give excitatory synapse with the cerebellar nuclei and hundreds of granule cells (Fig. 41-D, arrow line). The granule cells send excitatory axons to the outer layer that run parallel with the dendrites of Purkinje cells. The *Climbing fibers,* come exclusively *from the neurons of the inferior olive* and make axonal excitatory projections to the dendrites by wrapping around the dendrites of few Purkinje cells. *Outputs from all of these connections are solely through the Purkinje cells* that project *inhibitory connections with cerebellar nuclei* (Fig. 41-D, open arrow), to the cortical areas and the vestibular-spinal system.

There are three major functional interconnections derived from those described above that we can perhaps utilize to theoretically explain the actions demonstrated in the exciting and memorable buzzer-beating shot made by Michael Jordan for the NBA championship.

The vestibule-cerebellar circuitry, involving the flocculonodular lobe, and lateral vestibular nucleus which in turn sends efferent fibers to the vestibulospinal tract, could be responsible for the vestibule-ocular reflexes and posture maintenance. Jordan's extreme mobility while maintaining visual focus on the goal and making a well- balanced jump is a fascinating demonstration of the efficiency of this circuitry.

The spinocerebellar and cerebello-spinal circuitry is a complex integration of interconnections that influence finely coordinated and balanced movements. The ascending spinal fibers impulses to the cerebellar vermis and the intermediate zones ultimately reach the corresponding cerebellar nuclei -- fastigial nucleus and interposed nucleus. These cerebellar nuclei output project to; red nucleus which in turn project to the spinal cord as rubro-spinal descending fibers; vestibular nucleus which in turn project to the spinal cord as vestibule-spinal descending fibers; and reticular nucleus group which in turn project to the spinal cord as reticulo-spinal descending fibers. This complex circuitry is responsible for the integration of sensory inputs with motor commands to produce adaptive motor coordination. Michael Jordan, aided by a screen from his teammate, after seeing the imbalance of the guard that resulted, made a sudden well-balanced stop allowing him to receive the ball and make an immediate turn to face the goal in split seconds, dribbling twice to prepare the last jump for the championship. The sequence and series of movements in slow motion show, the flexion and extension of the right forearm and then the tonic snappy flexion of the hand that was holding the ball, at the same time the leg muscles doing a jump and, for a split second, stopping in mid-air as jump shots are, allowing him more control to hit the target. The rest is history. Well-oiled and efficiently coordinated multiple muscular systems integrated with his senses, the eyes to the opponent and the goal and the floor to stop and force a jump shot, the position of the body about space, and the body posture all made that fluid motion to get the championship trophy.

The cerebro-cerebellar system--the largest functional cerebellar system-- shows that the lateral cerebellar hemisphere, particularly the posterior lobe, receives cerebral afferent impulses from the pontine nucleus via the middle cerebellar peduncle. The neurons from the lateral lobes send impulses to the dentate nucleus, which in turn transmit electrical waves to the red nucleus and a large part to the thalamo-cerebrum complex via the superior cerebellar peduncle. This system is perhaps involved in the timing and planning of movements which can easily be shown by slow motion on television... the clock is about to expire, 3..2...then in a split second the jump-shot to history. This system is also responsible for the *cognitive function of the cerebellum* - a feature which probably integrates the more complex system of the effect of practice, physical make-up, and talent.

The cerebellum works through three functional systems: the cortico-cerebellar sensory/motor system, the vestibulo-cerebellar oculo-spinal system, and the cortico-cerebellar cognitive/affective system. The basal ganglia complex participates in almost all cerebellar functions. There is a recent suggestion that these three systems should be evaluated clinically [59,60].

Case Story:

Dr. R. Roth, 63 years old a cardiologist, had stopped monitoring his blood pressure for more than a year. While jogging at Central Park one morning, he suddenly experienced severe dizziness causing him to stop and fall. Dr. Roth struggled to stand repeatedly but failed because in every attempt his body would veer to the right causing him to fall. He vomited twice and was very anxious. Some joggers who witnessed the problem came to his aid and advised him to lie down and be still while calling for 911. When the paramedics arrived, his blood pressure was noted to be 210/110 while the heart rate was 92/min. He was immediately rushed to the nearest hospital while being given medicine to reduce the blood pressure by 20%. After 10 minutes, CT Scan was done and showed right cerebellar hemorrhage with an estimated volume of 10 ccs. He complained of a mild headache at the forehead and nape. He was cooperative, anxious and conversant. He preferred closing his eyes, and his verbal answers were loud and uncontrolled. His mental status examination was normal. Horizontal nystagmus with some rotatory component and fast component to the right was noted. He also showed clumsiness of the right hand especially when reaching out to objects; and on finger- to - nose test, he was missing the target and the tip of his nose. He could not tolerate standing because of his tendency to fall to the right. The was a mild weakness of his muscle tone on the right side but there was not weakness.

Clinical - anatomic Correlation:

If the homunculus represents muscle and sensory parts of the body at the cortical pre-central and post-central gyrus, the cerebellum also has body representations. The hands and feet are controlled by the lateral hemispheres, while the face and body parts, by the vermis and intermediate zones. In Mr. Roth's case, the cerebellar bleed mainly involved the right lobe, and this will explain the right-sided signs and symptoms of his stroke. Note that unlike the cortical homunculus where the body representation is from the opposite side, in cerebellar lesions the affected part of the body is ipsilateral or on the same side. Sensory-motor ataxia on the left side and vestibulo-ocular nystagmus are present. The behavior and cognitive function are normal. The cognitive/affective manifestations emphasized in the series of Schmahmann syndrome is not evident in this case.

Neurological Evaluation of the Cerebellar Function:

The basic principle is to remember that the cerebellum is responsible for fine coordination of muscle movements, visual balance, and position in space. When examining the person, there should be no preexisting problem that could alter the interpretation of the signs. Example of these is a weakness, spasticity or visual impairment.

Search for the presence of *ocular nystagmus* on primary gaze, lateral gazes, and upward/downward gazes. Rotatory and vertical nystagmus with the fast component to the same side of the vestibulo-cerebellar system pathology.

In *rapid pronation-supination,* the patient immitates the quick movements of both hands over the lap of the examiner. The speed and agility of the patient's hands are compared with that of the examiner. The slower and clumsy side is the abnormal side.

The *finger-to-nose test* is done by instructing the patient to use one finger to touch the tip of the index finger of the examiner then the tip of the nose of the subject, back-and-forth. While the patient is repeating the motion, the examiner is moving the "target finger" to different distances and angles to increase the chances of uncovering the abnormality. Compare each side. Watch out for *tremors or dysmetria,* especially at the end of the actions. Look for decomposition of movements, i.e. instead of a smooth motion of the shoulder, arm, forearm, hand, and finger, the patient exhibits movement of one joint after another to execute the command.

Romberg's test assesses the cerebellar, proprioceptive, and vestibular mechanism of the patient by letting the patient stand with feet together. Observe for imbalance. Then let the patient close his/her eyes to eliminate the vistibulo-ocular compensation; then look for the tendency to fall. The side where the direction of fall is consistent is usually the side of the pathology.

Walking in straight line can unmask the wide-based compensatory gait of cerebellar ataxia. The patient will find it difficult walking in a straight line and instead will compensate by widening the base of the stride. The patient with posterior column problems where proprioceptive sensation is lost and, vestibular dysfunctions where the sense of balance is affected, show wide-based pace too.

Explosive speech is an uncontrolled, irregular volume of phonation and rough syllabication of words -- a cerebellar dysfunction different from slurring or nasal twang. The type of speech is a disruption of the fluidity of word formation and volume of speech.

Lack of tone or hypotonia appears when there is paralysis or cerebellar lesion. In cerebellar dysfunction, however, there is the preservation of normal motor strength. Flexing the arm against resistance and sudden release can unmask this as a failure to control the return phase to the point that the arm might even hit the face of the patient.

Describe affect, behavior and mental status of the patient and inquire from family members if there are differences compared to the pre-disease state.

Chapter IX

Basal Ganglia
(Functions: Learning and Modulating Programmed Motor Acts)

A male teenager was trying to learn how to tap dance. During the first week, he struggled with the progressing sequence of tap steps. Persevering for another three months of frequent practice, he was already executing the different sequenced steps and this time was able to time the tap with the music. After a year, he could already perform different tap dances to four pieces of songs. His walking also changed, as they were now lighter and controlled together with more brisk movements of the upper extremities. The visio-spatial, vestibulo-spinal-cerebellar circuitry and the cerebro-cerebellar and basal ganglia circuitry are operant in the development of his skills.

The basal ganglia is an inscrutable subcortical structure closely linked to modulation of motor actions and recently to cognitive, emotional, learning, and memory functions as well. The complex functional interconnection that still has to be better understood has attracted many speculations as to its functions. We, however, will cover this briefly because there are indeed diseases attributed to basal ganglia dysfunctions, and their manifestations are worthy of recognition because they alter motor functions in the early phase of the disease and could very well mislead the examiner. Their manifestations, too, are unique and can very well be relieved by some treatment strategies.

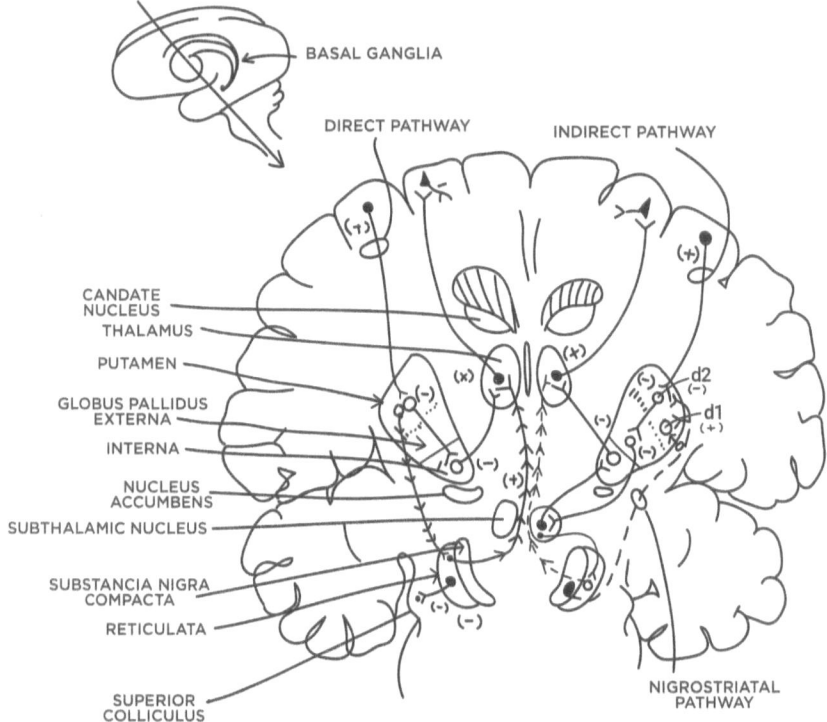

Figure 42. Basal Ganglia. A. Direct pathway. B. Indirect pathway. C. Nigrotriatal pathway from substancia nigra compacta to striatum, representing one side. Shaded neurons (circles) are stimulants while unshaded neurons are inhibitors.

The basal ganglia is a functional grouping of neurons consisting of nucleus accumbens, caudate nucleus, putamen, and globus pallidus (GP). These are collectively called **corpus striatum** (Fig. 42). Recently, the caudate nucleus and the putamen, because of the similarity of function, are jointly referred to as the *striatum* or *neostriatum*. The subthalamic nucleus (STN) located below the thalamus and the substancia nigra (SN) seen as a gray area in the midbrain is also an essential participant in the basal ganglia function. The globus pallidus subdivides into interna (GPi) and externa (GPe), and the substancia nigra into reticulate (SNr) and compacta (SNc). The nucleus accumbence (NA) lies ventral or below the striatum. The NA receives dopaminergic projections from Ventral Tegmentum and the limbic system [61].

The striatum and the STN are the chief input nuclei while the GPi and SNr are the output nuclei. The striatum receives projections from the cortex, SNc and the centromedial nucleus of the thalamus. The STN projects to both GPi and GPe and SNr. The Ventral Anterior Thalamus and Ventral Lateral Thalamus are the central recipients of basal ganglia output from GPi and SNr, and the thalamic neurons in turn project to the cortex.

The cortical projections to the striatum are excitatory glutaminergic. All of the basal ganglia participants in the interconnections have GABA transmitters that are inhibitory except the STN which has excitatory glutaminergic transmitters. The SNc, on the other hand, has dopamine as its transmitter, and it is excitatory to Dopamine type 1 striatal neurons and hyperpolarizing to Dopamine type 2 striatal neurons [62].

The functional model that regulates the motor system consists of the opposing direct and indirect pathways and the modulating influence of the nigrostriatal pathway that begins at the striatum, as shown in the schematic paths below. Cortical afferent fibers connected to the striatum have glutamine as a transmitter and is excitatory to the striatal neurons. The principal striatal neurons participating in the paths are the Dopaminergic type 1 (D1) and Dopaminergic type 2 (D2) neurons. The D1 neurons send impulses to the direct pathway while the D2 neurons carry impulses to the indirect pathway.

When cortical impulses excite the D1 neurons, these striatal cells are stimulated to send inhibitory impulses to the GPi and SNr neurons. The effect of these striatal inhibitory impulses is that they stop the GPi and SNr neurons from sending inhibitory impulses to the thalamus, thereby freeing the thalamic neurons to send excitatory impulses to various parts of the cortex.

Direct Pathway (Fig. 42 – left side):

Cortex (E)→ Striatum (I) → GPi and SNr (I)→ Thalamus (E) → Cortex

Excitatory cortical impulses to the D2 neurons cause these striatal cells to send inhibitory impulses to the GPe. The effect is stopping the GPe inhibitory neurons from sending inhibitory impulses to the STN thereby freeing the STN neurons to send excitatory impulses to the GPi and SNr. STN excitatory impulses result in stimulating the GPi and SNr inhibitory neurons to block the thalamic excitatory activities. The thalamic inhibition removes excitatory impulses to the cortex.

Indirect Pathway (Fig. 42 – right side):

Cortex (E) → Striatum (I) → GPe (I) → STN (E) → GPi and SNr (I) → Thalamus (E) → Cortex

The nigrostriatal pathway has a modulating function on the striatum, and this refers to the connection from SNc to the striatal dopaminergic neurons. The neurons of SNc transmit dopamine that stimulates D1 striatal neurons and inhibits striatal D2 neurons. The effect is a D1 or direct pathway dominance causing excitation of the thalamic and cortical neurons. Inhibition of D2 neurons removes the inhibitory influence to GPe, allowing the neurons to exert an inhibitory effect to STN, thereby releasing its excitatory influence to GPi/SNr. The subsequent result is disinhibition of the thalamus, allowing its neurons to transmit excitatory impulses to the cortex.

Nigrostriatal Pathway (Fig. 42- B):

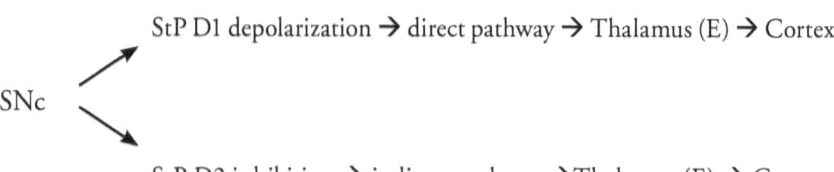

Clinical – anatomic Correlation:

In **Parkinson's disease (PD),** there is a deficiency of SNc dopamine transmitter. The effects are a decreased stimulation of D1 or direct pathway, causing decreased thalamic stimulation of the cortical system and a diminished inhibition of D2 or indirect pathway, resulting in similar lack of cortical stimulation. Both effects are manifested clinically as akinesia or poverty of movement and rigidity. In the early stage of **Huntington's disease (HD),** there is the selective destruction of D2 striatal neurons linked to the indirect pathway. The D2 destruction results in tilting the balance in favor of D1 direct pathway that allows thalamic stimulation of the cortex and clinically causes involuntary and unpredictable choreiform movements. Towards the end stage of the disease, the D1 or direct pathway neurons eventually get involved and the result this time is hypokinesia, a clinical observation in the late stage of HD. Neuronal degeneration in HD is not limited to striatal neurons. Cortical, neuronal degeneration is also prominent, manifesting clinically as dementia [63].

Recently, there are more interconnections defined that have challenged the popular model described previously. Aside from the influence on the motor act, the basal ganglia function seems to have expanded to selecting and enabling cognitive, executive, memory, and emotional programs stored in many parts of the brain to bring about appropriate acts. The striatum receives from the brain topographically arranged impulses divided into three sectors: The *sensorimotor sectors* from the premotor and sensory cortex; the *associative sectors* from the prefrontal, temporal and parietal association contributions; and the *limbic sectors,* that include the nucleus accumbens, from the hypothalamic and amygdala projections to the prefrontal area. The theory is that focused impulses associated with acquiring new sensorimotor actions result in presetting of a group of striatal neurons that is triggered only by the said action [64]. The hypothesis could perhaps explain the acquisition of skills by repeated practice (focused impulses) of the complicated steps and the exquisite coordination of the foot muscles of tap dance. The gradual development of coordination of various foot muscles to provide the desired taps that slowly progress to motion that harmonize with the rhythm of the music, and culminating in interpreting the music through foot taps, completes the transformation of the tap dance into an art form with the active participation of the basal ganglia. The theory is perhaps a classical way of showing how the sensorimotor, limbic, and cognitive sectors of the striatum coordinate the various inputs from the frontal cortex to learn different skills. The theory does not, however, isolate the critical participation of the cerebellum in the action described previously.

Clinical story:

Mr. Estrada, a 70 years-old retired policeman, complained, "I noticed that my walking is getting slower and with much effort, and my right hand has fine tremors. I could not determine exactly when this happened, but I would estimate that it called my attention about six months ago." The neurologist made him walk and noted that Mr. Estrada initiated the gait with initial shuffling and hesitancy of the feet, followed by small steps, and with the body, posture curved forward. The fluidity of flexion and extension of joints during walking was not present and instead replaced by a rigid barely perceivable flexion at the knees and ankles. The arm swing was absent, and tremors on both hands were obvious and of pin rolling type. When told to stop and come back, he exhibited a tendency to fall and was barely able to correct it, and it took four small steps to make a turn. His face was expressionless and devoid of a smile. When told to sit down, what was supposed to be a simple task was an arduous and slow maneuver coupled with a lot of hesitancy that culminated with passive fall of his buttocks to the chair, eliciting much relief to the doctor and the patient. He was instructed to stand up without support but was unable to do so without assistance. When the examiner alternately flexed and repeatedly extended the hand of the patient, the examiner felt a "cogwheel" sensation in the wrist joint during the act.

Clinical - anatomic Correlation:

Movement disorders are involuntary dysfunction of motor acts that disappear during sleep. They are broadly classified as **negative movement disorders** when the net effect of the basal ganglia disease is poverty of movements exemplified by the case of Mr. Estrada who was diagnosed to have Parkinsonism. **Positive movement disorders** are those where there is involuntary tonic or irregular movements or hyperkinesia typified by choreoathetosis, dystonia, and hemifacial tonic spasm. Movement disorders are best described when seen (look for them in YOUTUBE), though some subtle abnormalities may not be recognized. Clinicians should be able to detect basal ganglia related diseases because relief of symptoms is now achievable. The classical triad of PD which Mr. Estrada has consisted of tremors at rest, rigidity, and akinesia. These symptoms can very well be relieved by dopamine replacement treatment or use of dopaminergic drugs that mimic the action of dopamine and can result in the improvement of the quality of life. Recently, premotor changes are being identified as a harbinger of PD, thus opening a possible treatment strategy that would stop or delay the progression of the disease just like the current treatment of Alzheimer's Disease.

Neurological Examination:

Closely observe the patient while walking and when at rest. Look for spontaneous, uncontrollable movements and note body distribution (distal or proximal), muscle group involvement, absence or presence during sleep, aggravating or relieving maneuvers. Observe for facial and tongue movements too. A large population of the world own cell phones with video capability so taking cell phone video pictures (of course, with prior permission) of the spontaneous movements and their distribution is the best way of documenting the abnormal activities.

Common positive movement disorders are choreoathetosis, ballism, spontaneous spasms, and dystonia. **Chorea** consists of involuntary unpredictable, irregular, jerky movements of distal extremities which the afflicted often hide by merging them with voluntary and socially acceptable movements like scratching the head, gestures of afflicted hand when talking or playing around with pen or pencil. **Athetosis,** on the other hand, affects distal extremities or fingers and is characterized by irregular writhing, twisting, undulating movements. These are seen more often in combination as in **choreo-athetosis** which may progress to involve larger extremities termed ballism, and if one side of the body is affected the term is **hemiballismus,** and if only one extremity the term is **monoballismus. Blepharospasm** is a sustained tonic closure of the orbicularis muscles and the rest of the facial muscles, and in hereditary **blepharospasm** with persistent biting, this is described as **Meig's syndrome. Dystonia** is a tonic contraction of a group of muscles resulting in tonic posturing. An example of which is **cervical dystonia**, a tonic contraction of one of the sternocleidomastoid muscles causing tonic turning of the head contralateral to the muscles involved. **Tardive dyskinesia or oculogyric crisis** is an interesting side effect of central acting chlorpromazine or haloperidol drugs. The presentation is uncontrollable tonic and repeated head-turning to the side together with conjugate and tonic movement of the eyes to one side and tongue. Tardive dyskinesia has to be recognized by clinicians and health care providers because this can be entirely reversed by intravenous diphenhydramine which can immediately alleviate the panic and anxiety of both patient and relatives.

Chapter X

The Cerebral Cortex
(Functions: Memory, Learning, Language, Cognition, and Emotion)

A Reflection

I wonder how I started with "A,"
That reflection begins with a letter "r."
Why the "r" sounded rrrr, and why not sssss?
And how come an "e" followed "r"?

It is fascinating how I arrived at the series of letters--
They must have come from the alphabet that I sang.
Just suppose they are instead a series of squares, triangles, and other figures--
Could the sound and the series not differ at all?

My mom taught me the unique sounds for each letter
By the movements and shapes of my lips,
Fluidly fused with the opening of my mouth to produce those sounds.
It's funny to discover that my teeth are important
For the sound of the "F," and without the tongue,
the "L" will not sound an "L."

How come the word "reflection" made me imagine a mirror?
Yet...it is not only about seeing myself
For it can mean seeing my thoughts...seeing it?
Deeper thoughts? Oh, how language evolved!

This is a reflection of a reflection of
how my brain works...grammar, meaning, sound
Abstraction, the color of words, poetry, art, etc...etc...

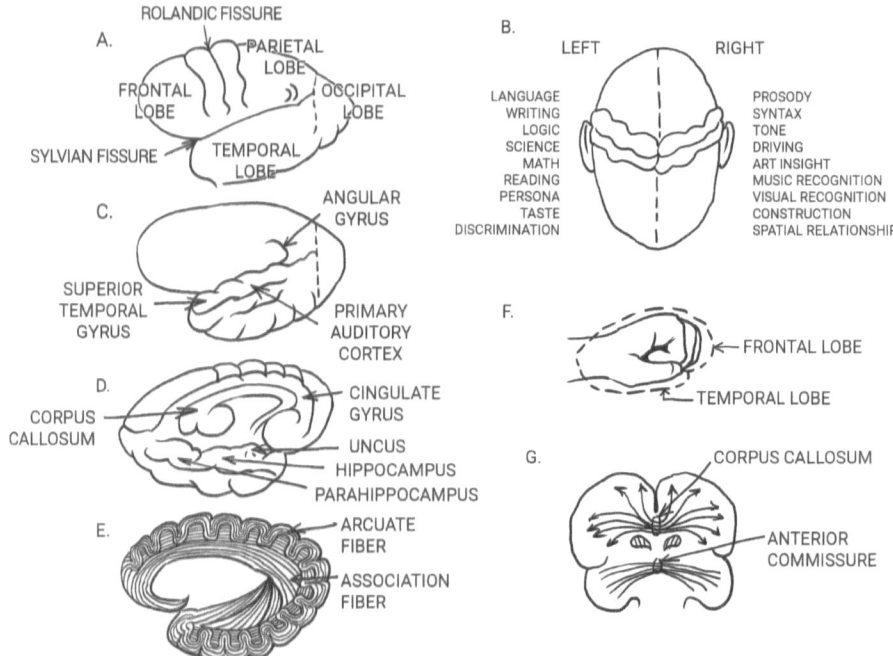

Figure 43. Gross anatomy of the brain. A. Rolandic fissure, Sylvian fissure and line perpindicular to end of Sylvian fissure, divide the brain into frontal, parietal, temporal and occipital lobes. B. Functions of the left dominant hemisphere and right non-dominant hemisphere. C. Parts of the lateral temporal lobe. D. Medial half of brain showing parts of the temporal lobe. E. Connecting fibers of the different regions. F. Fist to represent the brain for orientation, the thumb as temporal lobe. G. Crossing fibers to connect with opposite hemispheres.

The ***Cerebral Cortex*** is composed of *left, and right hemispheres* and each side are subdivided traditionally into four functional regions: the *frontal, parietal, temporal, and occipital lobes* (Fig. 43-A). There is a more detailed map based on cellular morphologic groupings marked as Brodmann area numbers to honor the remarkable man who made the study [65]. Brodmann identified 54 distinct areas. These numbered areas, however, were limited by individual variations of human brains and the difficulty of differentiating the cytoarchitectural differences. Many imaging studies and neurosurgeons still use these pioneering anatomic landmarks to guide in explaining manifestations of patients. The normal function of the brain is an integrated functional interconnection of these lobes and the Brodmann areas through arcuate and crossing fibers from the opposite side of the brain (Fig. 43-E & G). Assigning specific functions to these regions and laterality, therefore, is too simplistic, but for practical usefulness in the clinic, we can attribute some commonly accepted tasks to the different areas and parts of the cortex.

The concept of Dominant Brain. In general, the left side of the brain is often referred to as the *dominant hemisphere* (Fig. 43-B). This hemisphere is denoted to as "dominant" because it holds the *main mechanisms of language and other forms of communications in 95% of right-handed* individuals. Left-handed individuals still have their dominant hemisphere on the left side, but more of them have it on the right when compared to right-handed individuals. The concept of "dominance" does not, however, mean that all the necessary elements of language and communication are exclusive to the dominant hemisphere. The *non-dominant hemisphere holds the prosody of language or affects component of language.* These refer to the tone of speech, emphasis, stress, and exclamatory forms of language. This right hemisphere provides "color" to the function of the dominant hemisphere. The right side of the brain is also involved in multiple meanings in word formation. Integrating the left and right side of the brain will make the language of communication clearer and better expressed.

The left hemisphere is dominant for language and writing while the right brain is dominant for music, face recognition, drawing, and spatial relationships. Right-handed patients after corpus callosum sectioning (split brain that removes the inter-hemispheric connections) are better able to draw with their left hands than with their right hands because it is the right hemisphere that controls the left extremity. The right cortex has some functions that are superior to those of the left side, and the right brain is not just like the left hemisphere without language. An example of the superiority of the right cortex would be that split-brain patients can fit wooden blocks of different colors together to make a pattern better with their left hands than with their right hands, again showing that the right hemisphere is superior in spatial-perceptual tasks.

In conclusion, functions of the brain assigned to specific brain regions have considerable clinical importance. Localization of function can explain why some syndromes are characteristic of disease in particular brain regions. Nevertheless, *no part of the brain works in isolation*. Every part of the brain works in concert with every other part. When removing a part of the brain, the resulting behavior may reflect more the *adjusted capacities* of the remaining "parts" than the removed portions.

The temporal lobe is the thumb-like portion of the brain, if seen from the side or the lateral side, and consists of the superior, middle, and inferior lobes (Fig. 43 F). The primary auditory cortex located at the superior temporal lobe hosts the higher cortical integration of sound (Fig. 43C). The superior temporal cortex is where appreciation and discrimination of sound eventually happen. A lesion here may cause the *loss of the ability to give meaning to what is heard*, like the inability to identify the sound of rattling off a bunch of keys or the drop of a coin or a musician to correlate the written notes with the tune.

The posterior limit of this lobe is at the tip of the Sylvian Fissure which is an invagination created by the forward and inward folding of the temporal lobe during neuronal migration of the embryonic brain. If one looks at the medial or inner side of the lobe by gently splaying the brainstem away from it, one will see the *long parahippocampal gyrus*, and its anterior pole has a prominent round-shaped *hippocampus* with a slight indentation that separates the *uncus* (Fig. 43-D). These are all significant functional anatomic landmarks for memory.

Can you remember the breakfast you had this morning? One will not even take 5 seconds to be able to answer the question. But for somebody with early Alzheimer's disease, this could be an arduous task and irritatingly daunting, especially if the victim still remembers that he had breakfast but has no recall of what he had. How then does the brain recall what he ate that morning? The general physiology of memory formation consists of the appreciation of different stimuli through the senses and recognizing the information. The data are then processed (at this point memory is labile) then followed by consolidation of data. Storage of breakfast in different areas of the brain develops, and when asked about what he had that morning, stored consolidated breakfast data are retrieved and subsequently recalled.

The entire median portion of the temporal lobe, particularly the hippocampus, is now considered as an active participant in the *declarative type of memory*, specifically in *retaining new information of facts and events*. In this model, the hippocampus and the other structures of the medial temporal lobes participate in the early phase of memory formation or short-term memory. Consolidation of information sets intermediate or recent recall or long-term memory, depending on the volume of data and duration of storage before retrieval and recall. Storage of varied forms of memories occurs in other parts of the CNS. The temporal lobe, however, is assigned the general function of recall which can be evaluated at the bedside or the clinic [66, 67].

Learning begins with the ability to recognize new information from the motor and sensory stimuli which are then associated with retrieval of stored memories to provide meaning. These would require memory consolidation of short-term information, storage, and recall. The medial part of the temporal lobe, mainly the hippocampus is critical in this process. Hippocampal damage results in loss of short-term memory and failure to acquire new information. Learning the ABCs, sounds, intonation, and shapes and how they are spoken and written require a normal hippocampal function. However, the process of forming skills and habits seems to have a different pathway that involves the participation of the striatum. The different path for learning skills means that a patient with the inability to retain short memory can still learn ping-pong, painting skills, and even dance steps.

The medial temporal lobe components are active participants in the function of the limbic system that greatly influence behavior and emotional reaction to the surrounding environment. The *amygdala* output, in particular, results in hormonal, sympathetic and parasympathetic activation, behavior, motivation, and emotional changes about its reaction to the environment. The instinctive behavior for food, sex, flight, anger, fear, pleasant and unpleasant reactions to the internal and external environment are also some of the functions of the limbic system. The understanding of this system is fundamental to understanding human behavior, particularly in Psychiatry.

Clinical Story and Clinical - anatomic Correlation:

After a party of a cousin, John, a teenager who was driving but not wearing a seatbelt, hit his head against the windshield when his car was bumped from behind, causing loss of consciousness. When he awakened, there was a total absence of recollection of the party of the cousin nor the recall of his driving but was able to recognize his parents and where he was studying. CT scan revealed hemorrhages in both temporal lobes. The temporal lobes are encased by a rough sphenoid bone floor, predisposing it to injury in head acceleration accidents. The involvement of both temporal lobes explains the loss of memory of the events that transpired a few hours before the crash *(retrograde amnesia)*. When his parents left his bedside, the nurse was surprised to note that he did not remember that the parents visited him and that the doctor came and explained to him what happened. He was able to retain a long-term memory but not new information *(anterograde amnesia)*.

The doctor devised and kept ten series of tests or questions which he could repeatedly use to test long-term and short-term memories to check the status of his ability to recall. John was able to answer all questions and tests related to long-term memory like he was able to identify the family car from a picture, and he recognized the faces of relatives from a photo, his favorite teacher in school, and others. For short-term memory, he was unable to recall the food taken a few hours ago, the visitors who visited him, the color of medicines given to him and various objects shown to him. After a month, he was able to answer correctly eight out of ten questions and four out of five objects displayed to him after a minute and five minutes later. He even recalled the name of the secretary introduced to him during the last consultation a week before.

After about a year, he recovered all his ability to recall short-term memory. One afternoon while John was watching television, the sister was suddenly alarmed. She nervously described John, "His eyes and facial expression suddenly looked very angry." She continued, "... and chewing movements of the lips followed while his head moved to the left." In a trembling voice, "... and before I could do anything, he suddenly fell to the floor and went shaking and stiffening for about a few seconds. After the jerking, he seemed dazed and sleepy."

She just left him on the floor while calling 911 for help. After about a minute, she noted that he was awake but confused. When help arrived, he was already very much awake but tired. John shared the last thing he remembered before he lost consciousness, "I smelled something very foul and unpleasant then it became dark." The foul-smelling experience is typical of *uncinate fit,* the initial phase of temporal lobe seizure or partial complex seizures just before losing awareness. The event progressed quickly to generalized seizures. The source of the seizure discharges came from the temporal lobe injury sustained during the accident. The central termination of the olfactory bulb is in the medial temporal lobe and explains the experience of smelling a foul odor before the attack (please refer back to Chapter VI, Cranial N I). The other behavior witnessed, like the "angry look" and chewing movements, are typical of seizures emanating from the hippocampus and the limbic system. Some seizures involving the limbic system would relate to a "flashback "of experiences (Deja Vu), body distortions or other visual experiences, perhaps stored memories, released by the electrical discharges emanating from the medial temporal lobe that reached the occipital lobe's storage of visual imagery. Experiences just described localize the seizure foci to the temporal lobe, and it is for this reason that the patient is queried to detail the last that he can remember before losing consciousness. If the amygdala, which is part of the medial temporal lobe is the source of the seizure activity, experience of fear or dread, which is an emotional experience associated with autonomic manifestations like palpitation or sweating or gustatory experiences, are felt. The classification of seizure where the electrical discharges emanate from the temporal lobe is *temporal lobe seizure or partial complex seizures with secondary generalization.*

Neurological Examination:

Bedside testing of the temporal lobe function is possible. An example is letting the patient listen to common sounds and identifying them or making a distinction between the sounds of coins and keys. The term for inability to distinctly identify sounds is **auditory agnosia**. Memory functions, for old memory, most recently acquired and recent recall or ability to process memory are areas that need to be measured. Old memories are closely related to past experiences mostly meaningful in the life of the person. Names of grandchildren especially the first, the first job or the street where one lived are varied information that can test past or old memory. Showing five familiar objects and then after 1 minute or 5, 10, and 30 minutes test for recall of the five objects will roughly measure the ability of the patient to process and consolidate information for retrieval.

The **parietal lobe's** anterior boundary is the Rolandic fissure (Fig. 43-A). The postcentral gyrus is the main terminal of the ascending somatosensory fibers, and they are along its gyrus just like the motor homunculus. It is in the postcentral gyrus where interconnections with other areas of the brain happen to put meaning to the somatosensory impulses. After stepping on a lighted cigarette butt, the extreme noxious temperature is transmitted rapidly to the parietal area where the interpretation of the data is severe pain. The parietal lobe data are rapidly transmitted and integrated with other centers culminating in the immediate experience of fast and instantaneous localization of the stimulus and immediate decision to pull the affected foot to avoid further injury happens. The distance of the foot from the offending cigarette butt, the amount of flexion and extension of various muscles, the balancing of the body during the process, the eyes orienting the body in the surroundings, the severity of the pain and the appropriate verbal-emotional expression of s____t!!, and many more are integrated and initiated by the parietal lobe. Shapes and textures of objects, depth of distances visually and by tactile sensation find interpretation at the parietal lobe. The parietal lobe integrates the sensations from the outside world and responses to the various stimuli [68].

The parietal lobe is also commonly related to the genesis of language and communication. Much of these functions happen on the left side of the brain - the so-called dominant hemisphere. The precentral gyrus (Rolandic sulcus) is the anterior boundary that separates it from the frontal lobe. Language involves processing of different sensory stimuli (auditory, visual, somatosensory sensations) at the Wernicke's area which is located at the boundary of the parietal-occipital and temporal lobes of the dominant hemisphere (Fig. 44-A). The processed information is then sent to the angular gyrus (just above it), transforming them into common neural representation, then together with memory, it provides meaning at the Wernicke's area and then forwarded to Broca's area for verbal expression.

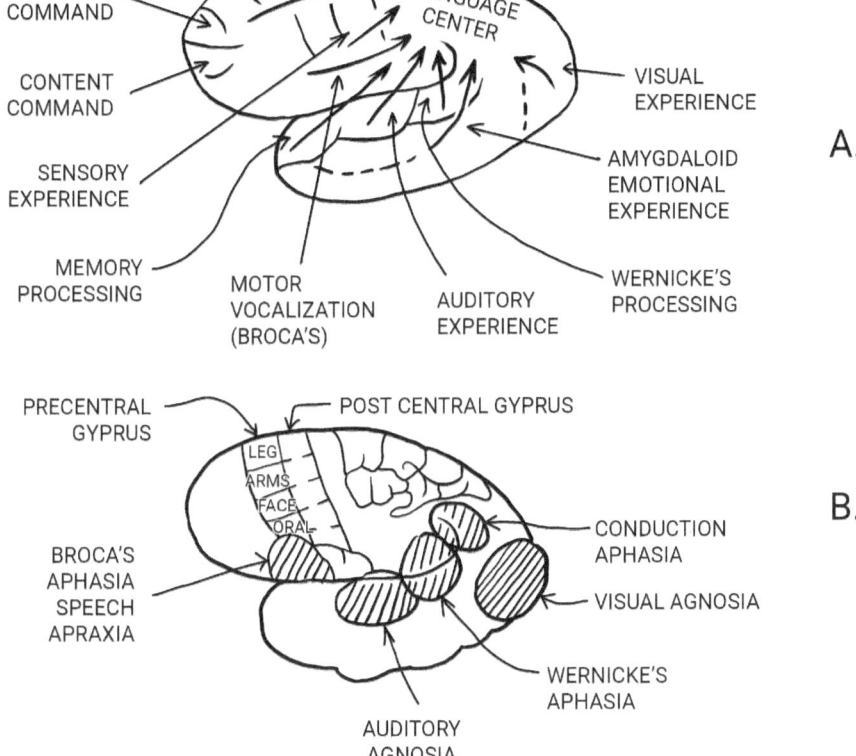

Figure 44. A. Dominant (left) parietal lobe showing contributions from different parts of the brain in language formation (arrows). B. Areas in the dominant brain with corresponding communication deficits when affected by strokes.

A language is a form of communication through words or symbols for words (e.g. heiroglyphics of ancient Egypt, 4000-1000 B.C.) or through actions or signs (e.g., hand language used by deaf and mute). Words link with sounds and meanings. **Grammar** is an acquired unique ability to make communication meaningful and better understood. Grammar is further subdivided into morphology, includes adding prefixes and suffixes following rules of combining words. **Phonology** is about standards of combining sound elements and **phonemes** into words. **Prosody** provides for instance patterns of intonation and stress. **Syntax** is processes of how to combine words and phrases to give a clearer meaning. The general term for disturbance of language communication is called **dysphasia**. Specific anatomic affectations can cause different language problems, and these are called **aphasias.**

Case Story:

Gina, a bubbly 46-year-old literature teacher, was noted by her son to be quiet and when prodded and asked, "Mom, what is the problem? Are you feeling bad? Mom, what is the problem..." she just stared at him. Alarmed, he immediately called his father who noted the same observation, prompting him to dress her for the hospital. By the time dressing her up was finished, she started talking, "Where is the dryer?" She said in her thought. She noted the bewildered and worried face of her husband and son and heard them say, "We are going to bring you to the hospital." She replied, "Why are you bringing me there?" Again, she understood but only in her thought...the facial expressions of her husband and son remained puzzled. At the ER, the husband anxiously related to the doctor, "She is saying weird things that we could not understand and were irrelevant or inappropriate, but she seemed not to know it." The doctor instructed Gina to repeat, "The renaissance man is Shakespeare." Gina responded, "I told them the dinner in the hospital is ready," but what was really in her thought was, "No, Shakespeare is not." She could understand but what she was expressing is entirely different from her intended responses, and she was unable to repeat what the doctor is saying.

Clinical – anatomic Correlation:

An embolic clot (a blood clot from a distant heart or blood vessel) can block a blood vessel to the brain and cause neurological symptoms.

The clot can temporarily block the big cerebral artery and, in the case of Gina, an initial block to the left main middle cerebral artery could explain her temporary inability to understand, express self, and recognize body senses and surroundings. The manifestation means a wide area of the left side of the brain suffered a limited or absence of blood flow. When the offending clot disintegrates as this often happens, distant and smaller blood vessels take the brunt of the disintegrated smaller emboli and produce different language abnormalities. When Gina finished dressing up, she started talking. As far as Gina was concerned, her thoughts and intended answers were correct, and she understood that she was going to the hospital. However, what words she was formulating did not match her thoughts and intended reply; that is why her loved ones were perplexed and worried. At the ER, the doctor tested her to repeat the sentence. She understood the statement, but failed to repeat the phrase and even replied with fluent sentence but inappropriate to the bewildered listeners.

Table IV. Types and differences of aphasia's

Type of Aphasia	Brodmann's Area	Comprehension	Expression	Able to repeat
Broca's Aphasia	44, 45	+	-	-
Wernicke's Aphasia	Posterior 22	-	+	-
Conduction Aphasia	39, 40 &/ or Arcuate fasciculus	+	+	-
Transcortical Motor	46	+	-	+
Transcortical Sensory		-	+	+
Global Aphasia	Anterior Speech area	-	-	-

Lesions (Fig. 44-B) involving the *left posterior superior temporal lobe* and *medial temporal lobe white matter* will cause **Wernicke's aphasia (fluent or sensory aphasia)**, where the patient can express self but is unable to understand sensory inputs, like questions or commands (Table IV.). If the lesion is a little posterior towards the left occipito-parietal-temporal lobe junction, the type of aphasia is **conduction aphasia** where the patients may be able to comprehend and talk; but they omit words or substitute sounds and show *profound inability to repeat sentences.* This latter condition is what Gina had, most likely a stroke involving the left parieto-occipital region. The *Broca's area* is at the left prefrontal area and base of the precentral gyrus (about the area where the mouth, tongue, and epiglottis which are muscles of articulation represented in the homunculus). Patients with a lesion that affects the Broca's area manifest **expressive aphasia.** In this type of aphasia, patients can understand but are unable to express themselves verbally and even in written responses. **Transcortical *sensory* aphasia** is a disturbance of the connection and some damage to the language area resulting in a Wernicke-like ability to talk and *unable to comprehend but can repeat sentences.* **Transcortical *motor* aphasia** is *like Broca's* aphasia, *but the patient can repeat sentences.* When the entire language area is involved, like obstruction of the take-off of the middle cerebral artery in the dominant hemisphere, it may result in a severe form of aphasia. **Global aphasia** is involvement of Broca's and Wernicke's area, resulting in the patient's inability to express and understand language - a very distressing and challenging problem for patients, families, as well as care providers [69,70].

Neurological examination:

In patients with expressive aphasia, the patient is unable to name objects shown but knows and understands them. How then do we know that they can understand? Show the patient five objects to identify and if unable to name the objects; we let them select from multiple choices. Table IV shows the types of aphasias and their differences.

The right hemisphere is vital in ***prosody,*** that is, putting the proper stress, tone, exclamation that provides color or appropriate meaning to sentences. The opposite of the Broca's area controls the *verbal execution of prosody* while that of Wernicke's area controls the *interpretation of the emotional sense and connotation of the statement.* A person who is unable to provide the appropriate tone and stress in a question will likely be misunderstood and can very well impact on communication and social adaptation. If the recipient of the conversation is unable to understand the exclamation point, fails to appreciate the emphasis, and misses the urgent tone, may lead to misinterpretation and inappropriate responses. A disaster in communication.

There are other language and communication problems. *Dysarthria does not belong to the group* even if it affects language expression and communication because the problem involves the muscles of articulation and not the language centers in the brain. *Speech apraxia* is the inability to execute a planned utilization of oral muscles to produce appropriate pronunciation of words. Some believe that Broca's aphasia is a speech apraxia because there are stroke patients with *Broca's aphasia* without apraxia, and this is because the affected Broca's area spared the insula. **Dyslexia** is a developmental or congenital inability to read, and writing difficulty and other problems related to language formation may accompany it. Children with dyslexia may have normal intelligence, be conversant, able to understand and acquire knowledge. This children can, therefore, be mistaken to have learning difficulties in school and can very well have failing grades in exams. The term for adult or acquired form is **Alexia,** and the common causes are strokes or traumatic brain injuries. The pathogenesis is suspected to be migration or a synaptic arrest involving the visual centers of the occipital lobes and the integrating areas in the parietal and temporal areas. In adults, the same areas can be involved in strokes or other injuries to the brain. **Agraphia,** on the other hand, is the inability to write and may co-exist with dyslexia or other aphasias [71,72]. Number concepts and how to use them can be affected by a lesion involving the angular gyrus (Fig. 43-C) and cause clinically, **acalculia,** the inability to do appropriate mathematical concepts, formulas, and solutions [73].

The occipital lobe is the back portion of the brain that begins at the posterior end of the Sylvian fissure (Fig 43 A). Visual impulses originating from the rods and cones of the retina terminate at the occipital lobe. The brain processes visual inputs of colors, edges, lines, motions, depths, contrasts, and shapes into different specific data which are then distributed to various predefined areas. The integration and analysis of the complex combination of information from the various areas of the brain, provide meaning to what the eye sees [74].

Seeing is an overlooked gift. After processing the visual data, the occipital lobe neurons then share this information, through the association fibers (Fig. 43 E), to predefined areas of the brain like the auditory and somatosensory areas, the limbic association areas and the prefrontal areas. The sharing provides many facets of visual experience (arrows in Fig. 45-A). We see the colors of the rainbow, the butterflies, the autumn leaves (occipital lobes) regarding being enthralled by their colorful beauty (limbic) and even appreciate and relate it to different canvasses of paintings depicting the visual experience (frontal lobe).

"Beauty depends on the beholder," is indeed visually accurate. The occipital lobes that process all the above visual experiences integrate them with various regions of the cortex, like the parietal lobe, in expressing into language what the eyes see. The final product of the utilization of all data is the appreciation of beauty, a few seconds of freedom from the distresses of the world.

There are, however, diseases that can impact on these perceptions. Cortical blindness is a disturbance of vision due to maladies or lesions involving the visual pathways and visual systems within the brain. Optic cortical pathway pathology produces superior quadrantic hemianopsia when involving Meyer's loop of the anterior pole of the temporal lobe and right or left hemianopsia when it is the contralateral occipital lobe (Please refer to Fig. 13). When the processing of visual impulses and integration with other parts of the cortex is disturbed, like lesions involving the occipital cortex and the association fibers, the interpretation, and utilization of the visual data are impaired. Failures of perception of visual sensation are called **visual agnosia**. The general term used for failure to interpret cortical sensory data are generally called **sensory agnosia,** and the different types are *visual agnosia, auditory agnosia, and somatosensory agnosia,* as shown in Fig. 44-B.

Case Story and Clinical – anatomic Correlation:

Mr. Omar, 60 years of age, is a very busy businessman who knew he had hypertension but had the wrong belief that the first sign of hypertension is a headache. One day, while having breakfast, he suddenly complained of blurring of vision. When seen at the ER, the neurologist was perplexed with the behavior of the patient who seemed to looked surprised with every person around him. The neurologist asked the patient to name the persons around him.

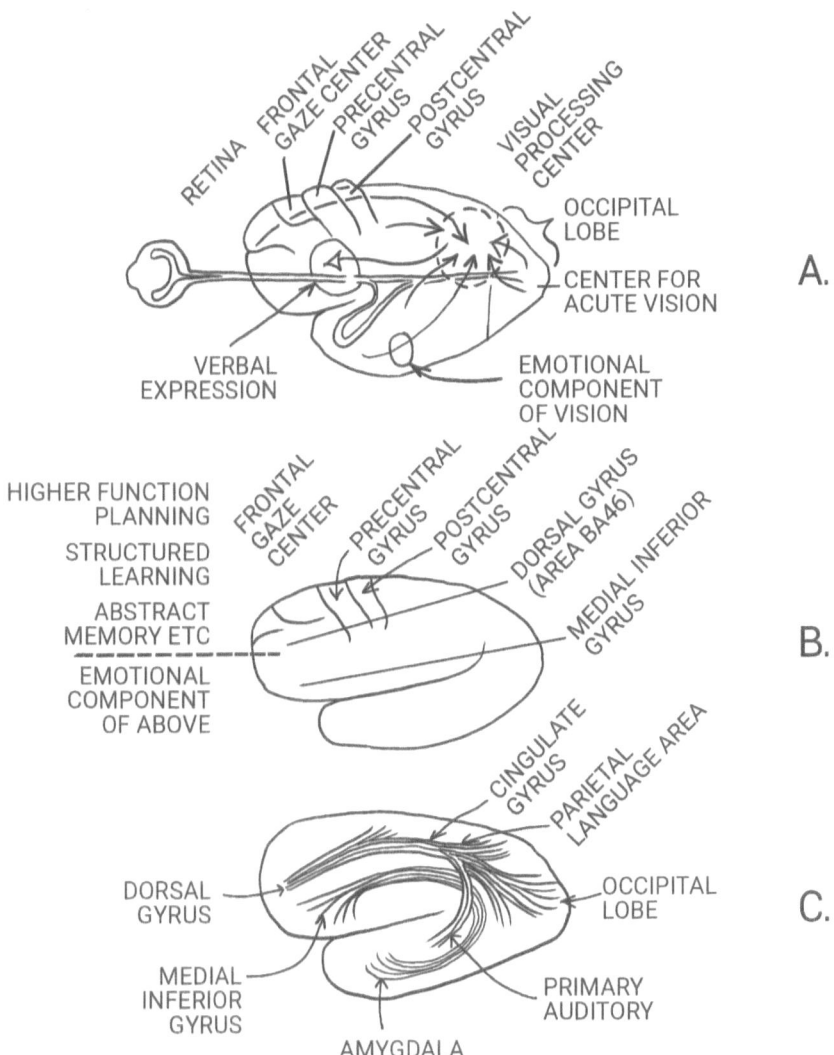

Figure 45. A. Occipital lobe termination of visual pathway from the retina and processing of parieto-occipital interpretation of visual experience (encircled with broken lines). Arrows showed participating regions of the brain to appreciate what is being seen. B. Frontal lobe functions. C. The fiber hemispheric interconnections.

He just smiled. Every time he hears the voice of the wife his facial expression is that of delight and conversant while holding her hand. The neurologist unraveled the failure to recognize the faces of the wife, the son, the mother and brother. He can describe their unique contours and acknowledge their voices. Inability to recognize faces is **prosopagnosia**, which is a form of visual agnosia. In Mr. Omar's case, the cause is bilateral inferior occipital lobe hemorrhage with some posterior temporal lobe involvement which was demonstrated by CT Scan [75].

Some other intriguing and fascinating forms of visual agnosias are:

1. ***Associative Agnosia*** is due to lesions involving the parietal cortex. The patient *can draw an object and identify the actual object by touch but is unable to name the object visually.*
2. ***Apperceptive Agnosia*** is a problem brought about by a lesion on the right occipitoparietal area and patients with this affliction will be *able to name figures but unable to draw it.*
3. An intriguing case is ***contralateral neglect***. A patient with this problem *fails to recognize left body images* and *cannot perceive the world on its left side*. The manifestation is brought about by a lesion at the *right parieto-occipital*. When told to draw a flower, the patient sketches the petals only on the right side and completely ignore illustrating petals on the left side and, amazingly not aware of it. Told to pick all the jigsaw puzzles scattered on the table, he would collect everything except those on the left side. The ability to imagine and recall visual images are vivid but when faced with the actual image, perception on the right is accurate, but tragically, the left is none existent. A patient with this affliction was able to describe his own house flawlessly while inside, but when brought outside, this time facing the entire structure, only the right side in his perception existed.

The **frontal lobe** consists of the precentral gyrus which is the initiator of motor movements (Fig. 45-B). Anterior to this motor strip is the superior and medial gyri where the location of frontal gaze center (FGC) or the frontal eye field is. Around the FGC is the supplementary eye field where the horizontal gaze coordination of the eyes is initiated and finely tuned to provide a single image even during movements. A lesion here produces a conjugate deviation of the eyes to the opposite side while electrical stimulation or seizures cause divergence of the eye contralateral to the stimulus. The mechanism of horizontal eye movement was discussed in more detail in Chapter VI-C. The position of the eyes during seizures or stroke should often be asked from the witness because these are evidence that may mean a focal problem.

Newborn babies would automatically open their mouths and start sucking when a mother's nipple touches the lips. Stroking any part in and around the mouth elicits the same response. We call this **sucking reflex**. Anything that strokes the palm evokes sustained *grasp* even when the stimulating hand is being pulled out. The similar reaction happens on stroking the plantar surface of the feet. As babies mature and their activities become purposeful and controlled, these infantile reflexes disappear. Adults do not have these. When diseases would involve the frontal lobes directly (eg., Hydrocephalus) or the brain is affected diffusely, causing significant cognitive decline and the mental function approaching that of an infant, these primitive reflexes may reappear, and we call these **frontal lobe release signs.** When the cognitive functions improve, these abnormal reflexes may disappear too.

The *prefrontal lobes receive widespread somatosensory, visual, and auditory association fibers.* The *limbic system that provides* emotion and instinctive action also deliver a rich connection to this part of the frontal lobe (Fig. 45-C). The prefrontal lobes, particularly the *dorsal gyrus (BA 46),* together with the *cingulate gyrus,* coordinates the requirements of higher intellectual functions like planning, structuring of learning, focused processing, abstract thinking, and memory. Visio-spatial memory, which usually answers the "where?" and visio-cognitive recall of colors and shapes are the functions of the *medial gyrus* which is just below the dorsal gyrus. The medial gyrus, the base of the frontal lobe, and the *orbitofrontal cortex* connect with the *amygdala and cingulate cortex* of the limbic system providing emotional components to the functions mentioned above [76].

The prefrontal cortex, which comprises approximately half of the frontal lobe in humans, is involved in *executive functions.* It integrates perceptual information, formulates plans and strategies for appropriate behavior in a given situation, and instructs the adjacent motor cortices to execute its computational product [77,78].

Case Story:

Mrs. Stewart, a 78-year-old well-dressed retired high school principal, was noted to lose her "mental faculties" gradually through the years. She used to write articles in different magazines and opinion pages of newspapers, but the first sign that there seemed to be a problem was an increasing number of misspelled words followed later by incorrect sentences. The change in her writing skills was dismissed by the family to be a beginning early Alzheimer's disease. Three months ago, she stopped writing because she could hardly complete a paragraph and even her choices of words during a conversation with the family were starting to be inaccurate. The daughter was alarmed when she started soiling her underwear and wetting the bed. The strange behavior prompted the neurological consultation. Her Mini-Mental Status Examination (MMSE), was abnormal and she was noted to have a wide-based gait with severe hesitancy to walk. There was a grasp reflex response upon stroking her palm, and all reflexes were hyperactive. A CT Scan showed a large right parasagittal (in-between frontal lobes) enhancing mass which was very characteristic of meningioma. Also, there was a significant shift of medial structures to the left. The mass was neurosurgically resected, and histopathology confirmed the mass to be a meningioma. She recovered her MMSE and her abnormal gait gradually. Three months after, the son attested that "my mom has completely recovered all that she lost."

Clinical – anatomic Correlation:

The gradual cognitive decline of this lady suggests that the inherently slow-growing meningioma was gradually pressing on both prefrontal lobes and the connecting fibers. The location of the homunculus for the leg and voluntary bladder and bowel controls are in the medial part of the precentral gyrus. These could have been affected, to explain the soiling, bed wetting, and the wide-based hesitant gait.

Neurological Examination:

There are many comprehensive or simplified validated examination strategies to test the function of the cortex in general and the different subdivisions. Some of the common simplified evaluation tools which utilizes a scoring method are the Mini-Mental Status Examination (MMSE) which evaluates the responses to orientation, registration, attention/calculation, recall and language items [79], and the Montreal Cognitive Assessment (MOCA) which measures visuospatial/executive functions, naming, memory, attention, language, abstraction, delayed recall, and orientation [80]. You will notice that the items in these examinations are testing the different functional subdivisions of the brain. The standard score for the former is 24-30 while the latter is 26-30. Socio-cultural and education variables need much consideration in interpreting the results of the tests. Some measures were developed to address these concerns.

An example is a study entitled "De-westernization of Dementia Screening Scale: a Philippine Experience," in which the tests considered the norms expected of a rural farmer who never went to school and whose life experiences were limited to the farm setting [81]. The study identified the inability of responders to solve simple mathematical equations, but when transposed to buying experiences, like the use of money currency in purchasing and computing for the change, they were able to answer correctly. The items covered by this test were behavioral activities of daily living, orientation/information, language, abstract thinking/judgment, memory, mental tracking, calculation, and praxis.

Before performing the chosen validated cognitive examinations, the general level of consciousness should be described first because, if it is indeed disturbed, the interpretation or reliability of the test will be difficult, if not impossible. If the patient is very much awake, attentive, and cooperative, then one may use any preferred mental status examination tool, and one can even use the same test to monitor the progress of the disease.

Much of the items in the different tests may not reveal all the dysfunctions mentioned above because they are but screening tools to tell us that something is going on in the brain. If the score is below the norm, there is a need to explore in greater detail the abnormalities noted. There might be a need to refer this task to a neurologist or a speech pathologist.

There are conditions where there is the absence of apparent structural damage or apparent genetic anomalies, yet aberrant behavior manifestation happens. These behaviors are **functional disorders or**

psychiatric disorders which fall in the realm of Medical Psychiatry. Functional imaging like Positron Emission Tomography (PET Scan) maps metabolic activities in the brain. PET Scan has demonstrated some metabolic changes described as hypo- or hypermetabolic in areas of the brain consistent with specific psychiatric disorders. These metabolic changes may be related to transmitter lack or excesses. The predominant neurotransmitter in the prefrontal region is dopamine, and among people with schizophrenia, where there is a lack of dopamine, their brain has been found to have hypofunctoning prefrontal cortical regions. In patients with severe depression, there is hypermetabolism in the subgenual cingulate area. These findings which still have to be fully understood emphasize the fact that there are indeed apparent functional changes that are happening in schizophrenia which is different from that of depression and these strongly suggest "organicity" of psychiatric disorders.

Chapter XI

The Functional Anatomy of Sleep and Consciousness

After a hard day's work, you went into a deep slumber and woke up refreshed and ready to face another day. How different was your sleep from a comatose patient? Are you sure that for every sleep you will wake up the following morning? Scary questions, aren't they? While listening to a boring neuroanatomy lecture at noon, your mind started drifting, then your senses clouded and eyelids closed to usher a relaxing sleep that got arrested when your posturing muscles suddenly gave way. The cycle continued despite the valiant struggles to keep awake, and while comfortably slouched in the auditorium seat you started to sleep into a stupor and started to snore. Why was it so difficult to stay awake?

Sleep is characterized by predictable cycles while coma either does not have these or only portions of the sleep stages may be simulated. The associated physiologic and EEG changes are not consistent in comatose patients. Most importantly, comatose patients are unarousable or need the application of strong stimuli to elicit elementary or straightforward responses.

At that noontime lecture, you just went through different levels of "unconsciousness," but in sleep physiology, they are **Non-rapid eye movement (NREM)** and **Rapid eye movement (REM) stages**. The NREM has *N1, N2, and N3 stages (some are staged to N4)* while REM has *parasympathetic mediated tonic component and sympathetic mediated phasic components* [82,83,84].

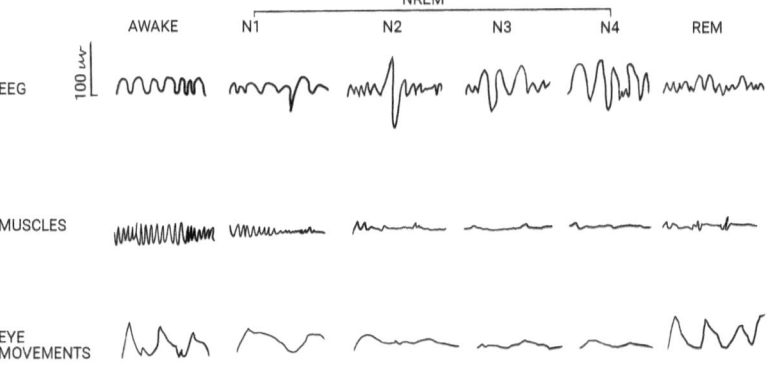

Figure 46. Electroencephalogram (EEG), muscle and eye movement recordings and changes at different stages of sleep.

Different depths of sleep and degrees of responsiveness to external stimuli are the characteristics of **NREM stage** (Fig. 46). The muscle tone is the same with wakefulness, but the heart rate, blood pressure, and respiration are low. Also, there is a reduction of cerebral blood flow and cerebral activity. The typical electroencephalographic (EEG) patterns show an initial decrease in amplitude and frequency, then gradually as the sleep deepens, the tracing is replaced by higher amplitude and lower frequency (theta to delta) and also marked by the appearance of K complexes.

REM characteristic is the presence of rapid eye movement and atony (absence of muscle tone). The blood pressure and heart rate are higher with varying degrees of fluctuations. There is increase respiration interrupted by occasional stoppage and cough suppression. Cerebral blood flow increases as well as cerebral metabolism in sensory-motor areas. Electroencephalogram shows desynchronized patterns, "sawtooth" wave forms, theta activities at 3-7 cycles per second, and some alpha activities. It is in this stage where dreams occur.

The depth of NREM sleep and the characteristics of REM sleep fluctuate during an eight hours sleep period. N1 stage occupies 2-5%, N2 stage 45-55% while N3 stage 5-15% of the period of sleep. N3 stage often occurs in the first 1/3 of sleep and REM stage in the last third of sleep. REM stages occur four to five times during the period of sleep, initially shorter and become longer towards the end of sleep (10 to 120 minutes). The switching of the sleep stages is influenced by a *pontine neuronal system* that sends outputs to the lower brainstem and spinal cord (to explain atonia and autonomic activities during REM). Also, the other outputs from the pontine neuronal system reach the forebrain and the cholinergic system of the thalamus, a projection that activates the characteristic patterns seen in the electroencephalogram. The loss of tone of the muscles during sleep may cause sudden fall of the hand that supports the head and the relaxation of the upper airway to cause snoring as what happened to you during the neuroanatomy lecture.

The fatigue of the day's work or the boredom of the lecture may have decreased sensory perception that could lead to sleep, that is why it is so difficult to keep awake. Sleep will not readily happen, however, because there are also many reasons to be awake. The described struggle to sleep and keep awake suggests that there are awake and sleep control mechanisms which perhaps are operant in *cyclic sleep pattern or circadian*

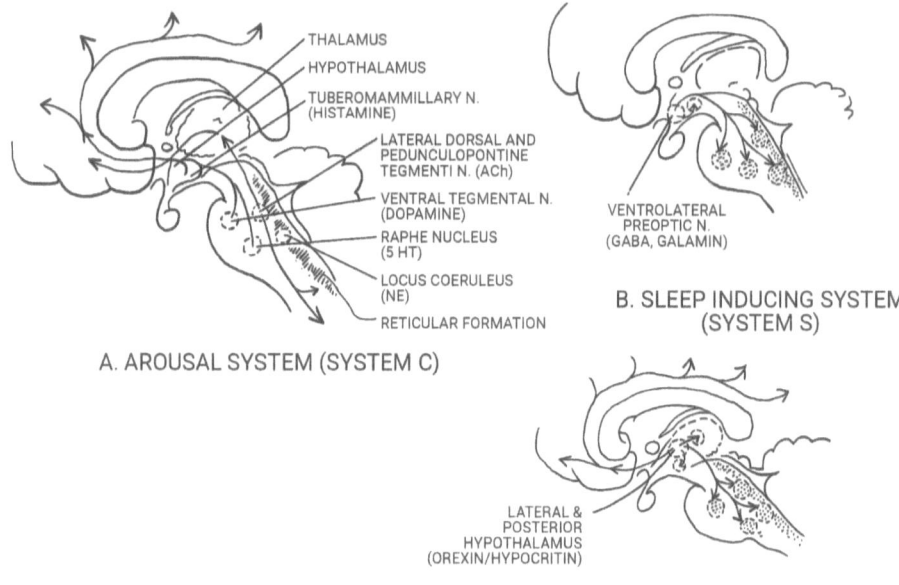

Figure 47. Participating structures in sleep cycle. A. Arousal System C. Ascending impulses (arrows) from different brainstem and tubero-mamillary structures and their respective transmitters for *maintainance of wakefulness*. Peduncular tegmentum also send descending impulses to the spinal cord. B. Sleep Inducing System S. Inhibitory transmitters GABA and galamin from ventrolateral preoptic nucleus to arousal system (arrows) *inducing sleep*. C. Lateral and posterior hypothalamus orexin stimulating the arousal system.

rhythm. An internal pacemaker or a "switch" exists, and this would decrease sensory inputs to the cortex to allow sleep. A popular candidate for this *"switch"* is the *anterior part of the hypothalamus (particularly the* **ventrolateral preoptic nucleus, VLPN***)*, which is found to be active during sleep. Neurons here secrete transmitter *GABA and galanin* that initiate sleep by *inhibiting the arousal regions* of the brain (Fig. 47-B). The regions responsible for arousal, on the other hand, are the **tuberomammillary nucleus (TMN)**, **lateral hypothalamus, locus coeruleus, dorsal raphe, laterodorsal tegmental nucleus**, and **pedunculopontine tegmental nucleus** (Fig. 47-A). **Circadian rhythm** is brought about by the *sleep cycle inducing system (***system S***)* and *arousal maintaining system (***system C***)*. The TMN nucleus is particularly important because it *projects cholinergic impulses to the intraluminal thalamus which in turn sends a transmission to the cortex.* Inhibition of TMN causes *brainstem, and cortical dissociation (system S) or loss of fluid coordination and the effect is sleep disturbance.* The brainstem arousal system transmitters consist of monoamine transmitters, *noradrenaline, histamine, serotonin, and dopamine* (system C). System C receives excitatory impulses from the *posterior and lateral hypothalamus*, particularly from *hypocretin or orexin secreting neurons* (Fig. 47-C).

Lack of excitatory hypocretin or orexin or their inhibition results in difficulty in maintaining wakefulness. This seemingly complex physio-anatomic mechanism of sleep assures us that if one is healthy, our "inner clock" will wake us up. It is however easy to imagine how circadian rhythm and control of sleep and wakefulness can be disturbed by mental distresses, poor sleep habits, drugs, and diseases.

Hypocretin or orexin neurons, which are excitatory, participate in the regulation of the sleep-wake cycle, and their absence or lack can cause **narcolepsy** which is an excessive brief period of daytime sleepiness. Sometimes, narcoleptics when at the brink of sleep, manifest episodes of brief hallucinations accompanying brief sleep incidents (hypnagogic hallucination). Their night sleeps often interrupted by brief wakefulness (sleep disruption), and occasionally, sudden inability to move or speak (**sleep paralysis**) happen while still awake. **Cataplexy** is a sudden loss of muscle tone causing limbs, neck muscles or jaw to drop usually triggered by sudden prolonged laughter or other outbursts of emotion. The hypocretin level is also low in cataplexy, but it may or may not accompany narcolepsy. Various medications can enhance or block the different transmitters of sleep and may cause hypersomnolence, insomnia or other forms of sleep disturbances. Lesions involving the anterior hypothalamus may cause insomnia. Different participating systems in the sleep-wake cycle, particularly the brainstem, hypothalamic, and cortical arousal system can very well be disturbed by diseases and produce various sleep pattern abnormalities.

Case story:

Mr. Brown was a 42-year-old stage and television director. He handled three to four projects at the same time and shuttled from one set to another. The director took a lot of coffee to make him awake but did not indulge in drug stimulants like amphetamines or cocaine. He knew that his sleep was very irregular and he slept most of the time briefly on every set he went. He took antihypertensive medicines but did not monitor his blood pressure. One morning, while reading a script, his vision doubled, he felt dizzy, his right side became limp, weak, and he was unable to swallow his saliva and coughed vigorously to bring out the phlegm. His wife brought him to the ER where a stroke team diagnosed him to have left pontine infarction. His blood pressure was noted at the ER to be 170/100. The stroke specialist told Mrs. Brown, "Your husband, is finding it very difficult to sleep, so we have to sedate him."

Clinical – anatomic Correlation:

Mr. Brown lived a stressful life and, most importantly, a sleep-deprived life. He has a poorly established circadian sleep rhythm. These factors took its toll on the cardiovascular state that predisposed him to stroke. His blood pressure was noted to be high despite the maintained antihypertensive medicine. His sleep pattern was disturbed, so the attending doctor found it necessary to sedate him to allow rest.

Sleep is a biological necessity. Disturbances in sleep, like sleep deprivation, cause endocrine and immunologic derangement. Cognitive and executive functions of the brain also suffer from inadequate sleep. Various cardiovascular diseases, like myocardial infarction or strokes, are risks associated with abnormal cardiovascular and pulmonary physiologic changes related to different stages of sleep.

Case story:

Mr. J. Course was a 78-year-old retired accountant and a known hypertensive and diabetic. He was taking a diuretic, beta blocker, and calcium blocker for hypertension and long-acting insulin injection for diabetes. He complained of a toothache that prevented him from chewing his food. That night, he was seen to mumble unintelligible words incessantly, wet his pants and at the same time, felt drowsy. When called by name, he opened the eyes widely but briefly, then went back to mumbling and drowsiness. Alarmed by the sudden change in behavior his family brought him to the ER where his blood sugar was found to be low at 50 mg/dl and low serum sodium of 129 meq./L. His peripheral smear showed a high count of 15,000 white blood cells with 80% predominance of neutrophils indicative of infection. Dextrose with 50% glucose (D50) was administered immediately, and intravenous line of D5NSS started to correct the low serum sodium gradually. Intravenous antibiotics were given simultaneously given. Shortly after giving D50 the patient was more awake and can follow simple commands. When hyponatremia was corrected, and infection controlled he recovered his usual self.

Clinical – anatomic Correlation:

Consciousness consists of elements of *arousal (wakefulness) and awareness (of self and environment)*. The anatomic substrate of arousal is composed of the brain stem rostral reticular formation, reticular activating system, and subcortical hypothalamic and thalamic structures, while awareness is the hierarchal integration of cortical structures and subcortical structures as well. Affectation of any of these structures will result in mixed degrees of cognitive and affective functions and changing levels of sensorium. They are almost the same structures participating in the sleep-wake cycle. The difference is that when diseases affect the systems that control consciousness, other CNS structures are involved, providing us with more complex manifestations aside from changes in sensorium.

Behavior changes (this is what Mr. Course manifested) like, restlessness, difficulty in sleeping, and confusion precede changes in sensorium like, clouding, drowsiness, stupor, and coma. Behavioral changes precede changes in sensorium because the brainstem is relatively resistant to metabolic insults. The exception is that, when the brainstem is involved directly by diseases, like a stroke, early manifestation is a change in sensorium. The popular terms used to describe levels of sensorium, like drowsy, clouded, stupor and coma, have clinical meanings that differ from one examiner to another. Drowsiness may accompany confusion; clouding may have some mixing of awareness and disorientation; stupor may include inappropriate verbalization and degree of coma can be varied as well. How then will we determine if a patient with disturb sensorium is getting worst or getting better? The considerable variability in the interpretation of these popular terms may cause a confusing assessment that may impact on medical decisions. Patients with different degrees of cognitive decline and sensorial changes respond correspondingly to **graded stimuli** provided. Describing the different grades of stimuli and the detail of the corresponding responses can afford a more useful tool for bedside assessment. This form of examination gives a more meaningful interpretation of the state of cognition and sensorium of patients with disturbed consciousness.

Brainstem structures recover faster to allow essential functions like respiration, stable blood pressure, and other autonomic functions, to continue. Patients in a coma who survive a severe traumatic injury or hypoxic encephalopathy usually start to awaken after about a month, an indication of recovering brainstem functions but not necessarily cortical activities. Patients who are in an awake state but without awareness are in a **vegetative state (VS)** because the cortical functions still have to recover or permanently damaged. If the cortical functions fail to improve in a month, it is said to be in a **state of persistent vegetative state,** and after three months, **permanent vegetative state**. When more signs of recovery occur after two weeks of injury and are reproducible or sustained, examples of which are blinking of the eyes or pressing of the hand upon instructions, the term used for the transition is a **minimally conscious state (MCS).** Recognition of MCS is critical as this signals a need for continuous and aggressive management because there is still a chance of improvement, survival and even a favorable functional outcome. The neuroanatomic clinical meaning is that the thalamus and its connections to the cortex and the limbic system are perhaps starting to work. As improvement continues, simple to complex functions emerge in a hierarchal fashion -- regaining of the activity is a sequential order of recovery of thalamic-limbic system expression first, then basal ganglia and sensory cortex manifestations, followed by the motor, executive, emotional, and cognitive behavioral changes [85,86,87,88]. Fortunately, Mr. Course's behavioral changes and drowsiness were recognized early to be due to the combined effect of low sugar, low sodium and infection permitting fast and complete recovery when the causes were normalized.

Focal lesions involving the cortex and subcortical structures will disturb consciousness depending on their size and location. When the volume is large enough to cause compression of neighboring structures, increased pressure, or diffuse abnormal reactivity of the vascular system, cognitive decline is manifested and often with different degrees of changes in sensorium. Lesions directly involving the reticular activating system in the brainstem often depress sensorium with cranial nerve involvement and long tract signs.

Neurological Examination.

Evaluating the neurological status of a patient with different levels of altered consciousness is always a challenging experience, a daunting task, and can even be dreadful to many. The difficulty is compounded by barriers to neurological evaluation, like intubation tubes, nasogastric tubes, intravenous lines, and monitor connections. The neurological examinations taught to medical students are often on normal persons or cooperative patients. Examining patients with altered consciousness requires a good knowledge of functional neuroanatomy of consciousness and sleep (which by now you must have possessed and can always read again) to allow reasonable interpretation of observed responses [89].

The **vital signs** that are routinely taken by the nurses should be evaluated carefully for their medical and neurological meanings.

Blood pressure (BP) should be valued in three ways: 1. As a physiologic friend that responds appropriately to the demands of the body parts, like if one is running; 2. As a pathologic foe that can cause harm and destroy body parts if ill-controlled, like producing a stroke; 3. As an alarmist that requires immediate and critical attention for it is sounding a warning of an impending catastrophe that requires decisions to lower it down or bring it up and to look for the causes.

The third way of looking at the blood pressure is very relevant in a critical care setting. Blood pressures can rise in increased intracranial pressure -- a **Cushing's reflex**. Harvey Cushing, in 1901 described systolic rise of blood pressure associated with increased intracranial pressure. Subsequently, Cushing observed that the increase in blood pressure accompanied increase respiratory rate and decreased heart rate, a triad that carried his name -- the Cushing's triad, an ominous sign of an impending herniation. When the offending problem continues to cause increased intracranial pressure, the triad can very well reverse to dangerous drop of blood pressure, deceleration of respiratory rate and slowing of heart rate. "Vital signs" are indeed vital in saving lives.

In cerebrovascular infarction, atherosclerosis or blood clot blocks entirely or partially the blood supply to the affected area. As a compensatory mechanism the **arterial collaterals,** which are small branches of blood vessels arising from neighboring blood vessels, open in response to hypoxia to help diminish the damage. Sudden drops or fluctuations of blood pressures can disturb further the blood perfusion dynamics around the stroke and may affect the outcome [90,91]. Cerebral vascular perfusion possesses an **autoregulatory mechanism** that ensures oxygen flow to the brain. In healthy individuals, when blood pressure goes down or up, an immediate adjustment in cerebral flow happens to provide constant blood perfusion to the brain. There is, however, a limit to this mechanism. When BP is below 60 or above 120 mean arterial pressure, the autoregulatory mechanism does not work or is inefficient. The regional area of cerebral infarction in strokes show the absence of autoregulation, making blood pressure control critical. Should hypertension in cerebral infarction be controlled or allowed to seek its level? When should hypertension be reduced? And by how much? Handling of elevated blood pressure in acute ischemic stroke patients require close monitoring of their effects not only to the brain but to other body organs like the heart and kidneys. If reperfusion treatment (e.g., rTPA infusion) is indicated, keeping the blood pressure below 185 systolic and 110 diastolic is essential in the treatment protocol. In patients with co-existing myocardial overload problems, the elevated blood pressure can be lowered gradually to normal. In general, blood pressure of 220 systolic and 120 diastolic will need gradual reduction.

Blood pressure may go down when the brain stem function is affected, but one should be quick also to look for other causes like sepsis, dehydration or hypoglycemia because abnormal BP interpretation and management are different. BP monitoring, therefore, requires an understanding of the etiology of its behavior, a vital requirement.

Temperature rise could mean there is a systemic infection or this could be a meningeal inflammation by infection or subarachnoid hemorrhage. Centrally acting drugs can trigger malignant hyperthermia or hypothalamic pathology that affects the thermoregulatory center.

The *heart rate* increases during fever, pain, circulatory collapse, sepsis, and many other causes. Heart rate can increase during a *nonconvulsive seizure* or with inotropic agents. One must watch out for arrhythmias that could appear in increased ICP.

Increases in *respiratory rate* may indicate extracranial causes like acidosis, pneumonia, and airway obstruction or may indicate cortical or brainstem dysfunction. Vital signs, therefore, are not "routinely" recorded and given less attention. They are called "vital," so they have to be correctly done, and if abnormal, should be considered as an alarming signal that requires prompt evaluation and intervention by the physician.

The technique of neurological examination of patients with disturbed consciousness or sensorium consists of the following:

1. Observation of spontaneous movements and behavior
2. "Trick maneuvers."
3. Describing the graded stimulus and the responses
4. Grading or Scaling of neurological status like Glasgow coma scale
5. Cranial nerve examinations to assess the function of the brainstem
a. Observe the pattern of respiration (Fig. 48).

Cheyne-Stokes Respiration is a decrescendo and crescendo breathing with apnea (absence of respiration) in between. The pattern associated often with diffuse cortical pathology but sometimes can be seen in normal elderly persons.

Central Neurogenic hyperventilation is deep and rapid breathing suggestive of brainstem problem.

1. Observation:

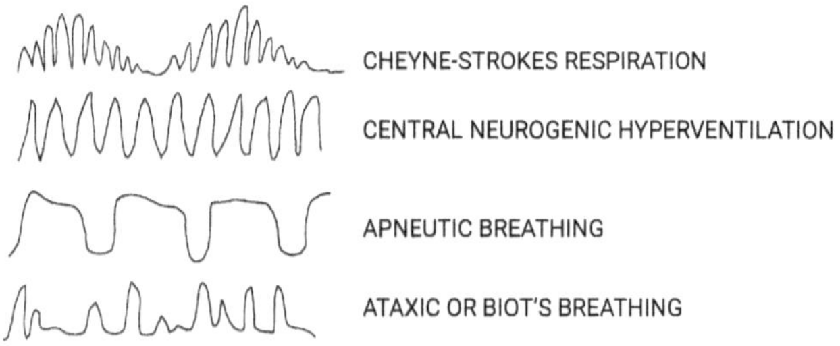

~~CHEYNE-STROKES RESPIRATION~~
CHEYNE-STROKES RESPIRATION
CENTRAL NEUROGENIC HYPERVENTILATION
APNEUTIC BREATHING
ATAXIC OR BIOT'S BREATHING

Figure 48. Recordings of different breathing pattern abnormalities.

Apneustic breathing is a gasp of inspiration that is held briefly then followed by expiration, often seen in patients with pontine and medullary lesions.

Ataxic or Biot's respiration is an irregularly irregular depth of inspiration and expiration With periods of brief apnea seen in lesions involving the medulla.

Note: The types of breathing pattern described above are ominous signs that will require immediate evaluation by the doctor. If Cheyne-Stokes was not present before and appears only recently, then it is a pathologic sign that needs a prompt and accurate diagnosis and treatment.

b. Observe for spontaneous motor movements or posturing. Spontaneous decerebrate or decorticate posturing, sometimes on one side, can be mistaken as a seizure. In **decorticate posturing,** the head is hyperextended while the *upper extremities are hyper flexed* with the hand internally rotated and in fist form and the lower extremities hyperextended (Fig. 49). **Decerebrate posturing** is just like decorticate posturing, but the only difference is that the *upper extremities are hyperextended,* and the hand externally rotated and in fist form. Sternal pain and other strong stimuli could elicit the posturing. Both posturing are grave signs that require vigilant observation and aggressive management, especially in head-injured patients, because of a chance of survival and even a favorable outcome. Decorticate posturing means the involvement of a large part of the cortical structures but not the diencephalic (hypothalamus and thalamus) and brainstem structures. When decorticate posturing changes to decerebrate positions, this can be interpreted as deterioration or progression of the clinical status because this means that the diencephalon and the brainstem are already affected. Decerebrate posturing however can be seen in bilateral cortical problems without brainstem involvement emphasizing the need to consider additional clinical parameters, like signs of brainstem involvement and the etiology of the neurological problem, before prognosticating.

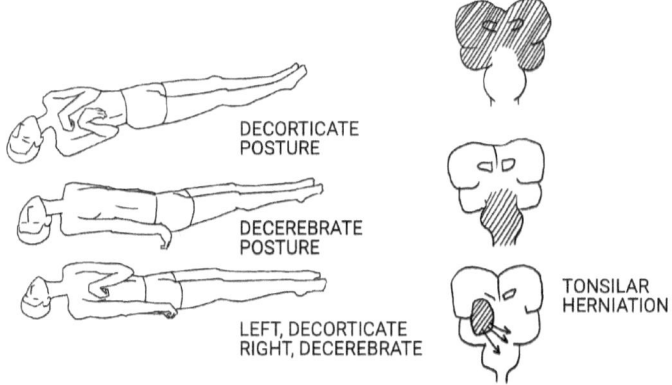

Figure 49. Posturing and corresponding areas of the brain affected.

Limited or absent movements of one side or one extremity speaks of paresis or paralysis. Splinting of the extremities due to pain can be mistaken as weakness so one should look for signs of inflammation or swelling and tenderness in the area or even elicit pain by moving the seemingly weak limb. An exaggerated lateral deviation of one foot when compared to the opposite side means that the tone of the former is weak.

When a patient scratches a particular area that itches or uses bed covers because of a cold room, both mean that the patient can appreciate the need to address the itch and the cold appropriately. These actions can be interpreted as a form of cortical function though it may not be a high and complex cognitive function.

There are many more observable differences that one can discover by just imagining and comparing your neurological self with patients who are lying down. Pay particular attention to the position and tone of extremities, limitations of movements, eye-opening, blinking and reactions to sounds.

c. Observe for spontaneous eye movements like eye-opening. Observe the primary position and robing of the eyes. The eyes can be deviated *conjugately* to one side "towards" the cortical location of the lesion but "away" in the brainstem-pontine lesion (Fig. 50-A). If there is a focal seizure, the eyes will deviate "away" from the source of the cortical electrical discharges. The primary eye position may be deviated downwards as in "sunset sign," indicative of increased intracranial pressure from hydrocephalus or pressure downwards on the superior colliculi by a hematoma above it. You may see a rhythmic down beating of both eyes or "*ocular bobbing*" which is indicative of pressure from above or below the superior colliculi by either an intracerebral hematoma or a large infarct (Fig. 50-B).

d. Observe for spontaneous swallowing, gag or coughing which are functions of Glossopharyngeal nerve (CN IX) and Vagus nerve (CN X). These can be observed especially during suctioning.

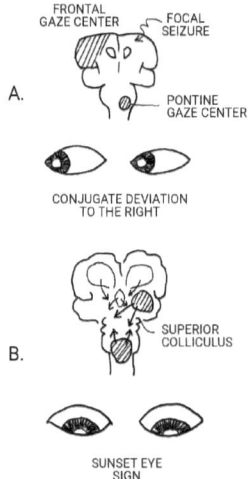

Figure 50. Characteristic positions of eyes. A. With *lesions* affecting the gaze centers or with irritative electrical activities like *focal seizures* (arrows). B. Pressures to the superior colliculus from pathologies above or below.

2. "Trick maneuvers" are commonly done in awake but uncooperative or restless patients.

If the patient can see and follow the examiner or the light while moving around and observing how the eyes follow the direction toward the stimuli, this will enable the examiner to make a rough assessment of the function of the extraocular muscles. If the eyes deviate conjugately to one side, the eyes may follow the direction used by the examiner but will not be able to cross the midline towards the opposite side.

One maneuver is ringing a bell or making a loud sound from different areas of the room and observing if the patient moves the head towards the direction of the noise. The sound stimulus is to check if the patient could hear and can localize the source of the noise.

Calling the name of the patient (the sweetest sound) and observing any form of consistent responses is an indication of self-awareness. Repeat the call and look for consistency of reaction. Watch out for an emotional response to the sound of a loved one.

There are many imaginative stimuli that one can create to trigger reproducible responses. The stimuli and responses, however, have to be described and recorded so that the maneuver can be repeated and observed for any deterioration or improvement. In children, playing a favorite song or letting a cat meow can be the stimuli that can elicit some form of auditory response.

3. Describing the graded stimulus and response.

> Graded stimuli can range from: Describing conversational calling of name and asking questions that require simple responses, to the deafening "call of name" besides the ear; describing the frequency of prodding to elicit even a minor response; describing light touch to shrug to eliciting pain. Then, describing in detail responses of the patient to the graded stimuli. Remember to repeat the same triggers and adjust according to the clinical status. The stimuli chosen by the examiner shall be fixed and repeated as frequently as possible and may change according to responses. Responses should be described or with the advent of smartphones; video recorded everything.

Examples of varying graded verbal stimulation and sensory stimulation.

When a patient readily responds by looking at the source of the call of his name, and then the following day, one has to *increase the vocal volume* significantly to get his attention, this is a sign of deterioration, if consistent. In the succeeding days, a pattern of declining sensorium can be described as -- a verbal *volume that is almost shouting,* then a *shout accompanied by a light shrug,* then in the absence of a verbal response, only *sternal pain elicits a reaction.* To continue this hypothetical scenario with the same patient, this time, a sternal pain (pressing on the sternum with knuckles) evokes restlessness and attempts to get hold of the source of pain. The following day, while doing the same maneuver, purposeless movement of the hands was obtained – all of these indicate a deteriorating sensorium. As the condition continues to deteriorate, response to sternal pain changed to a decorticate posturing, then decerebrate posturing. Patients can very well undergo any of the scenario described above. Recovery usually follows the same sequence but in reverse. The "graded stimuli and response" examples show that deterioration and improvement, to a certain degree, has a hierarchal pattern and this is brought about by the relative sensitivity of the different brain structures to metabolic insults.

Forced eye-opening and giving verbal commands. Sometimes patients may have **lid apraxia**, that is, their eyes stay close and unable to open voluntarily. With eyes shut, the observer can mistake the patient to be in a coma or is continually asleep and therefore in a poor neurological state. One should ask permission from the patient before *manually opening the upper lids.* If the patient is conscious, the movements of the eyes will be voluntary and can be meaningful. You can do eye stimulation while holding on to the lid. Informing the caregivers of these observations and encouraging them to do the same maneuver while talking to the patient will give much reassuring comfort to the conscious patient knowing that he/she is understood and that communication is possible. Another condition that may explain the difficulty in opening the eyes might be a bilateral midbrain infarction causing a **locked-in syndrome** where the cortex still functions but there is paralysis of eye movements. The above maneuver will significantly provide reassurance to the patient who will then know that people around him are aware that he is "alive." When there is resistance to "force-opening" of the lids, this may be a voluntary resistance in pseudo-unconscious patients and hysteria.

"One-step, two-step, and more complex commands." Holding the hand and commanding the patient to "press the hand," and he follows, is a one-step type of response. It is similar to telling the patient to open the mouth or putting out the tongue. One can further increase the command to two-step command like "press my hand and put out your tongue." You can further make a more complex command like, "press my hand, put out your tongue, and move it in and out." The more combination of commands and the execution more complex and the patient can follow them, the better the neurological status.

4. Glasgow Coma Scale and Other Measures.

Table V shows the **Glasgow Coma Scale (GCS).** GCS is the most popular scale used in evaluating levels of consciousness because of its simplicity and reproducibility. The scale was introduced in Glasgow, Scotland during a gathering of traumatic brain injury specialists. The purpose of the meeting was to adopt a standard and simplified measuring instrument so that intervention outcomes will have validity and universality, especially in multicenter studies. The GCS was subsequently found to be a valid, and valuable tool in non-trauma related diseases like strokes, and other neurological illnesses causing disturbance of sensorium. The GCS, however, has its limitations [92, 93]. These are:

Table V. Glasgow Coma Scale

Best Motor Response	
Obeys Commands	6
Localizes Pain	5
Normal flexion	4
Abnormal flexion	3
Extension	2
Nil	1
Verbal Response	
Oriented Speech	5
Disoriented Speech	4
Words Only	3
Sounds only	2
Nil	1
Eye Opening	
Spontaneous	4
To command	3
To pain	2
Nil	1

a. Inconsistency in inter-observer reliability;
b. Concerns over its predictive value in brain injury patients undergoing modern neurointensive care like deep sedation and hypothermia;
c. The impossibility of assessing the verbal score in intubated patients.
d. In addition the exclusion of brainstem reflexes and subtle deterioration or improvements may still belong to the same grade, like localizing and lateralizing shall be similarly scored as 5 and following one- to two-step commands shall be similarly scored as 6.

Other measures were designed to address some of the limitations like **Full Outline of Unresponsiveness Score (FOUR)**, a coma scale consisting of four components: eye response, motor response, brainstem reflexes [94,95], and respiration pattern. Investigators from the Mayo Clinic propose the use of FOUR. Other popular measures are the **NIH Stroke**

Scale (National Institute of Health Stroke Scale) and Modified Rankin Scale [96,97]. Uses of these standardized measures are important for research purposes as if the hospital is compiling a registry for future or current studies.

5. Cranial nerve examinations to assess the function of the brainstem.

The *size of the pupils and the degree of reactivity* to light are evaluated and compared with each other. The normal pupillary size and reactivity are continuously changing due to the use of the eyes for near and far vision and light perception. The parasympathetic (PSNS), and sympathetic Nerve (SNS) nerves control the pupillary reactivity. The PSNS constricts the pupils (**miosis**) while the SNS dilates the pupils (**mydriasis**). The PSNS exits the midbrain together with CN III then separates from the CN III bundle to supply the ciliary muscles of the pupils. The SNS descend from the hypothalamus and exits the spinal cord to synapse with the superior, middle and lower sympathetic ganglia.
The SNS arising from the superior sympathetic ganglia innervates the dilator pupilae muscles of the pupils.

When there is pupillary dilation due to uncal herniation as described in Chapter VII-C, the parasympathetic nerve to the ciliary muscle is weakened or paralyzed causing the sympathetic nerve to dominate thus, the dilatation of the pupil usually on the side of the herniation (Fig. 51-C).

Lesions involving the descending SNS tract at the brainstem allows dominance of the parasympathetic nerve, in effect causing the pupil to constrict on the side of the lesion. Pinpoint pupils are seen in morphine toxicity (Fig. 51-B), severe metabolic diseases, and brainstem lesions that affect both descending sympathetic nerves (Fig. 51-A).

Ice caloric test is a diagnostic procedure utilized to evaluate the function of the labyrinthine pathways to the brainstem and the evaluation of the extraocular muscle movements in semi - or comatose patients. With the head of the patient flexed at 30* from the horizontal plane and after making sure that the ear canal is patent and the eardrum is intact, instill

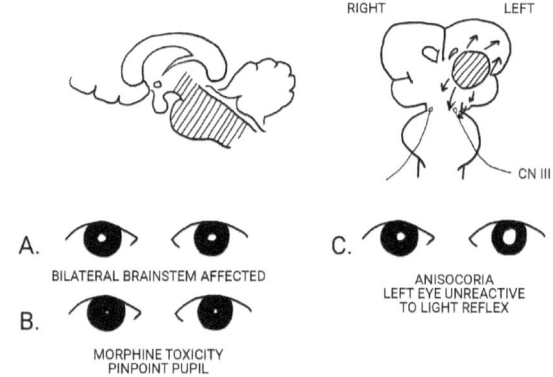

Figure 51. Pupillary sizes and correlation with clinical conditions.

ten cubic centimeters of cold water into one ear then observe the movements of the eyes. If the labyrinthine organ and its brainstem connections are intact, the response of the eyes to the cold stimulation is a movement of both eyes conjugately toward the stimuli (Fig. 52). Repeat the test on the other ear at least five minutes after emptying the first side. The ice caloric test is a very important maneuver to determine if the brainstem is still showing some functions in the evaluation of brain death and also to determine the extent of the lesion that has affected the horizontal gaze movements at the brainstem level. The test for vertical gaze movements requires instillation of cold water on both ears at the same time. With the head flexed forward during cold stimuli to both ears, the expected movement of the eyes is upward. With the head flexed backward during the procedure, movement of both eyes downward. One can also use a *doll's head maneuver* which is done by observing the movement of both eyes when turning the head to one side. The response is usually a conjugate movement away from the direction of head rotation. The test evaluates the vistibulo-ocular reflex (VOR) of patients in coma. The reflex involves the labyrinthine apparatus and the brainstem
and cerebellar interconnections; therefore, just like the caloric test, it evaluates brainstem function.

The corneal reflex examination in a cooperative patient is done by instructing the patient to look upward and lateral, while a wisp of cotton is applied to the cornea by the examiner (Fig. 53 – A). In a comatose patient, gently and lightly open both eyelids or taping both lids but just enough to make the eyes visible and using a wisp of cotton, touch the edge of the cornea and look for a blink response (Fig. 53). The afferent arm of the reflex is the sensory ophthalmic branch of the Trigeminal Nerve (CN V) while the efferent motor arms are from both Facial Nerves (CN VII) that supply the orbicularis muscles of both eyes to cause both lids to blink. The examination evaluates the status of the cranial nerves V and VII and also the brainstem nuclei.

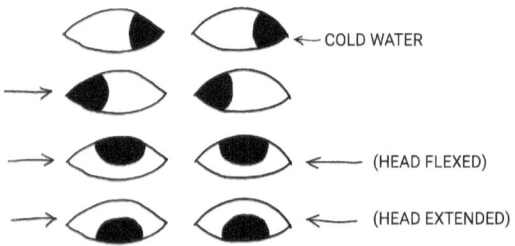

Figure 52. Reactions of the eyes in comatose patients during ice caloric test. Arrows show side of stimulation.

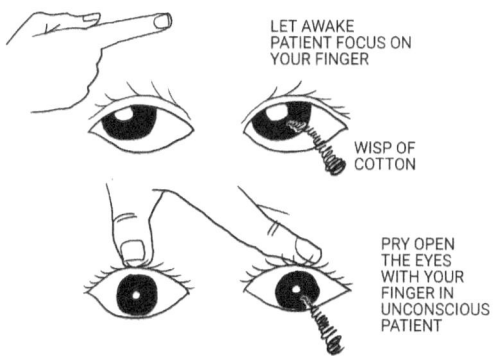

Figure 53. Maneuvers in testing for sensitivity of the cornea in awake and unconscious patients.

Important reminders:

1. The different maneuvers should be repeated frequently to establish reproducibility and reliability.
2. Record by writing or by cell phone video (this needs legal permission) the responses to the tests and various neurological examinations. The data established can be used as a way of monitoring the progress of the patient's clinical status.
3. Subtle changes can mean deterioration that will require immediate action on your part or improvement which gives a welcome hope for the patient's loved ones.
4. Interpretation of the test results will require a good knowledge of functional neuroanatomy and clinical correlation. Frequent evaluation of patients will lead to confidence in the understanding of the signs.
5. Patients with quadriplegia and ocular palsies can very well be mistaken as comatose when they might be very awake (e.g., Locked-in). So, all the people around, especially the doctors and the support teams should give the same respect as for regular patients. Every time you touch the patient or do something to the patient, you should always ask permission first, then explain what you will be doing. Even when the patient is genuinely unconscious, you do the same thing because what the patient does not feel, the loved ones will, especially when the test can trigger discomfort or pain.
6. Many of the examinations described above are also done in the NIH Stroke Scale but are mostly quantified and standardized for research purposes.
7. Always consider the contribution of sedative drugs, the possibility of seizures, and normal physiologic sleep when interpreting the reactions and signs.

Chapter XII

Cerebrospinal Fluid Circulation

Imagine the brain as immobile, rigid and wrapped by the dura. Every time we bump our head accidentally, or a football player does a header on the ball, or even when one does a simple jump for joy, the brain, and cellular structures will absorb all the body and head vibrations and other energies caused by the momentum. These simple activities could destroy the delicate interconnections of the brain, rip off the tiny vessels, destroy the cells and cause disturbances of the thinking processes or even cause seizures. Fortunately, there is a cerebrospinal fluid that bathes the brain and the spinal cord and fills up the ventricles and protects the CNS structures from the direct impact of mechanical forces by diffusing or dispersing this unwanted energy. There is, however, a limit to this. If the power is excessive, mechanical damage to CNS structures can still happen.

The Papyrus of Smith of 1600 B.C. showed ancient writing by an Egyptian physician, Imhotep, around 3,000 B.C., describing intracranial fluid inside an injured head. The papyrus is the first written document ever written about intracranial cerebrospinal fluid. Hippocrates from Kos (460-370 A.D.) and Claudius Galen from Pergamon (130-200 A.D.) thought that "animal spirit" with its mental functions was within the cerebral ventricles. This influential belief was carried for centuries until the 16th century, during the Renaissance period, when heretical belief toned down and allowed human postmortem studies. Nicolo Massa (1536) described cerebrospinal fluid (CSF) within cerebral ventricles.

Domenico Cotugno (1764) discovered the CSF through experimental postmortem research during the autopsies and described CSF in the subarachnoid space around the spinal cord. Francis Magendie, in the first half of the 19th century, coined the name "cerebrospinal fluid" and discovered the method of CSF pressure measurement, thus the start of the study of CSF dynamics [98].

The cerebrospinal fluid (CSF) volume is 70-120 cc and churned out at a rate of 0.3 to 0.5 cc/min or 500-700 cc per day. This 99.2 percent of water allows the brain to float. Otherwise, the 1400-1500 mg weight of the brain will have in its base dead neurons and compressed blood vessels. It also bathes the brain and spinal cord and contributes to the nutrition of the brain, maintains homeostasis by preserving intracranial pressure, provides antibody protection, and participates in waste cleansing. Tapping the CSF fluid is done by doing lumbar puncture at L1-2 lumbar space in infants and L2-3 to L4 spaces in adults. Intracranial pressure is measured by connecting a spinal manometer to a three-way stopcock that in turn, is connected with the spinal needle. CSF fluid is allowed to flow passively to the manometer, and when the flow stops, the level of the fluid is the pressure in millimeter water unit. Normal pressure is 180 to 200 mm water.

Case Story:

Dr. J. Monroe is a 48-year-old volunteer Canadian doctor in Africa. One day, he developed a cough, headache, and fever; then the following day he was noted to be restless, disoriented, and with neck rigidity. The primary consideration was meningitis. The lumbar tap done had a high cerebrospinal fluid opening pressure of 300 mm water. CSF analysis showed mildly elevated protein, low sugar, and 590 cells which were mostly polymorphonuclear cells. Gram staining showed gram-negative diplococcal organism, so Dr. Monroe was started immediately on appropriate intravenous antibiotic. CSF culture after 48 hours yielded Neisseria Meningococcal growth. After 14 days of treatment, he recovered except for left-sided deafness.

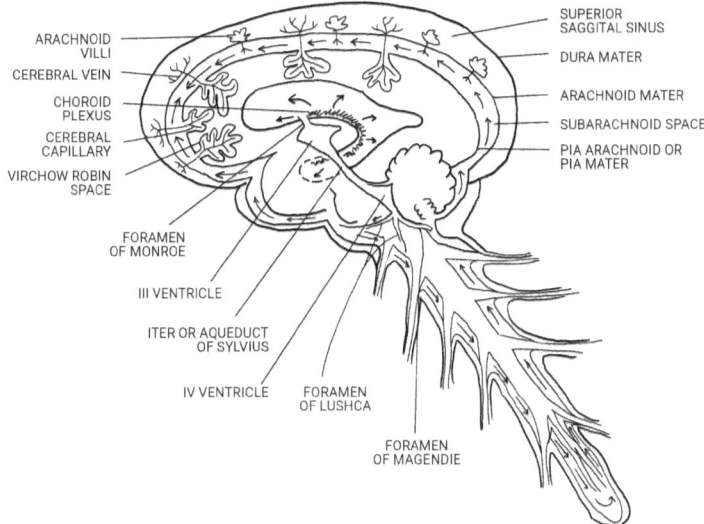

Figure 54. Cerebrospinal Fluid (CSF) Circulation. Production at the choroid plexus, arrows showing brain and spinal cord pathways until absorption by the arachnoid villi.

A year after the infection, Dr. Monroe complained of generalized headache which was tolerable at first, but through the month it became severe and disturbed his sleep. Because of the history of meningitis, the considerations were hydrocephalus and increased intracranial pressure. A CT Scan of the head showed an enlargement of the lateral ventricles, the third ventricle, and the fourth ventricle. A consideration was a communicating type of hydrocephalus which is a sequela of past meningitis. A neurosurgical insertion of a ventricular shunt to the lateral ventricle afforded relief of the headache.

Clinical - anatomic Correlation:

Infections of the brain and supporting structures are reflected in the cerebrospinal fluid. Increased white cell count with a predominance of lymphocytes or polymorphonuclear cells, decreased sugar and increased protein in the CSF usually indicate a bacterial infection. Red blood cells due to a subarachnoid hemorrhage from a ruptured aneurysm or bleeding arterio-venous malformation can show in the CSF. Infectious organisms like Cryptococcus, Mycobacterium tuberculosis, and bacteria (like what Dr. Monroe had) can be isolated in the CSF by special stains, immunofluorescence, PCR, microfiltration, cultures and animal inoculation. CSF fluid can also be studied to help understand diseases better by identifying and quantifying antibodies in multiple sclerosis, tumor cells in lymphoma and tau protein in dementia.

The ependymal cells of the *choroid plexus* which lie inside the *lateral ventricles and the fourth ventricle* produce the CSF (Fig. 54). An alternate hypothesis has challenged the traditional belief that the choroid plexus is the primary source of CSF. The alternative theory is that the CSF reaches the brain through a direct circulatory route via the subarachnoid space-pia mater and Virchow Robin Space junction [99]. The systolic pulsatile contraction of intracranial vessels and pulmonary respiration are the main drivers of CSF circulation from the frontal to the occipital sides of the ventricles. From both lateral ventricles, the CSF passes through the *foramen of Monroe* to the third ventricle, from here the CSF passes through the *central Aqueduct* to the *fourth ventricle*. CSF then flows to the *cisterna magna* through the *foramen of Megendie* and the anterior and lateral space of the brain stem and to the spinal cord through the *foramen of Lushka*. Absorption of the CSF to the circulation is through the *arachnoid granulations* that empty to the *Superior Sagittal Sinus;* however, there is growing evidence that the return of the CSF to the peripheral circulation may also happen through perivascular and extracellular spaces, cranial nerve lymphatic system, cervical lymphatic, dural venous plexus and parasaggital dural venous plexus [100].

Obstruction of the connecting ducts disturb the flow of CSF and can cause the **non-communicating or obstructive type of hydrocephalus**. An example of this is obstruction of the iter or central aqueduct (the iter connects the third ventricle to the fourth ventricle) by the pressure from the cerebellum in Arnold Chiari Malformation in children or by tumors in the brain stem. If it is the absorption mechanism that gets impaired, the type of hydrocephalus is called **communicating hydrocephalus** (the CSF circulation pathways are intact or "communicating"). Inflammatory diseases like bacterial meningitis that disturb the absorption capability of the arachnoid villi cause CSF to accumulate and produce increased intracranial pressure and hydrocephalus. Communicating type of hydrocephalus was what happened to Dr. Monroe a year after meningococcal meningitis.

Clinical Evaluation of Increased Intracranial Pressure from Hydrocephalus

When there is increased intracranial pressure (ICP) due to hydrocephalus, structures of the cortex around the enlarging ventricles, like the white matter, the cortical gray, and the vascular system, can be displaced causing headache as an early manifestation. As the pressure continues to build up, neurological deterioration follows. These could be *disturbance of cognition* or symptoms of dementia, change in sensorium and other neurological signs described below:

Frontal lobe signs like grasping and sucking are called *primitive reflexes* because they are typically seen only in babies. As the frontal lobes mature, the ***primitive reflexes*** get suppressed and are manifested only when the frontal lobe function is disturbed by large tumors, hydrocephalus, and infection.

The leg positions of the homunculus lie in the medial or saggital parts of the precentral gyri of the frontal lobes. These areas are between and a little above the heads of the enlarging lateral ventricle, predisposing these structures to pressure effect. The manifestation is a *gait disturbance or gait apraxia of Bruns, a tribute to the first person who described the gait in two cases with frontal lobe tumor in 1892* [101]. The gait is described as difficulty initiating the first step of walking in the absence of weakness and cerebellar signs. Typically, their base on walking is a little broad and shuffling of gait may merge with the initial step. Patients with this problem can walk when there is no conscious effort to do it and this, can be demonstrated by letting the patient walk and get an object around him. In Parkinsonism the gait hesitation or gait shuffling appears to be persistent even when there is no awareness of the initiation of walking.

Just below the homunculus of the legs are the center for voluntary control of the *bladder and bowel* sphincters. Hydrocephalus can press on these centers causing *bowel and bladder retention and incontinence.*

The subarachnoid space of the optic nerve being continuous with the subarachnoid space of the brain also receives the brunt of the increased pressure. The increased pressure compresses the venous and arterial vessels of the optic nerve reflecting the effect to the disc as a swelling, which can be seen by fundoscopy as *papilledema*. Also, there are retinal venous congestion and rupture of microvessels seen as retinal hemorrhages. These are classical objective evidence of increased intracranial pressure in the clinic.

The quadrigeminal plate gets pressured also by the hydrocephalus to cause *"sunset sign"* in children.

The above signs are late signs of hydrocephalus, and as such, CT Scan will show, dilatation of the ventricles, perhaps with some thinning of the cerebral mantle, and the surrounding periventricular white matter with edema.

Fortunately, the diagnosis of communicating hydrocephalus in Dr. Monroe's case was detected early. Immediate ventricular shunting intervention relieved him of the severe headache and prevented neurological deterioration.

Chapter XIII

Cerebral and Spinal Blood Circulation

Our understanding of the functions of the human brain were mostly made by correlating neuropathologic lesions caused by strokes with specific areas of the brain. The scientific process which seemed odd was made long before the advent of modern imaging machines, like the CT Scan and MRI. It was like unraveling the functions of the different parts of the brain, "stroke by stroke," studying what each stroke does to a person. As early as the 16th century, the so-called "circle of Willis" was already described in brain dissection and the label, "circle," was credited to Thomas Willis for expounding on the hemodynamics of the anterior and posterior interconnections of the major cerebral vessels. He also established **neurology** as a distinct discipline in medicine, making him the Father of Neurology. It was in this century that the 2400 years old Hippocratic diagnosis of apoplexy, which meant, "being struck down by violence," was discovered by Jacob Wepfer to be due to intracerebral hemorrhage and blockage of the blood vessel to the brain. Subsequently, the term "stroke" took over the term apoplexy. The consequence of these observations and understanding led to the identification of the cerebral blood vessels and the corresponding territories they supply; recognize neurological deficits or abnormalities manifested by the affected areas; speculate and understand the normal functions of the parts of the brain provided by the blood vessels. [102].

Stroke is the most common neurological disease and the third most common cause of mortality worldwide. Our patients in this modern time are fortunate because early imaging studies and early therapeutic interventions can now minimize the potentially debilitating damage caused by a stroke in selected cases. Also, these advances allow a better understanding of the disease that leads to better preventive measures. It is, therefore, imperative for all health care providers to recognize stroke syndromes by understanding the vascular supply to the brain in general and by identifying the vascular territories they supply and correlating this with functional anatomy. Ugh! This three-step process is easier said than done. It is like saying, "Identify the different cerebral vessels, and what they supply, then know the functions of those territories." History tells us that it took centuries for scientists to discover the vascular territories supplied by the different vessels and they are still learning more with modern imaging studies. So why should we remember the vascular supplies, functions of the territory they supply and recognize the resulting abnormalities on neurological examination? It is not as formidable as it seems. We are the fortunate generation to benefit from the centuries of discoveries that provided us with a better understanding of how the circulation and the brain work. The earlier chapters discussed the functions of the different brain areas and brainstem structures. So by now you more or less have good knowledge of the how the various structures of the brain, work and if vaguely remembered, you will know which section of this book will help you recall and understand. This chapter will help you comprehend (please do not memorize) the specific areas of the brain that are nurtured by particular blood vessels. Once you have become familiar with the blood supplies to the different territories, we will make some simple generalizations that will help you recognize most of the stroke syndromes that will ultimately lead to early recognition of stroke and decision making. Always remember, when a stroke occurs, time is gold!

In the previous chapters, we studied the clinical functions of the different structures of the central nervous system "tract by tract and station by station." We emphasized that involvement of a particular anatomic structure in diseases like strokes can alter their functions and are subsequently manifested in a patient. Blood supply to the CNS structures often covers more than two functional structures so that participation of these vessels results in syndromes many of which named after the persons who first described them or the areas of the brain affected or the names of the blood vessels involved in the stroke. Many of the original

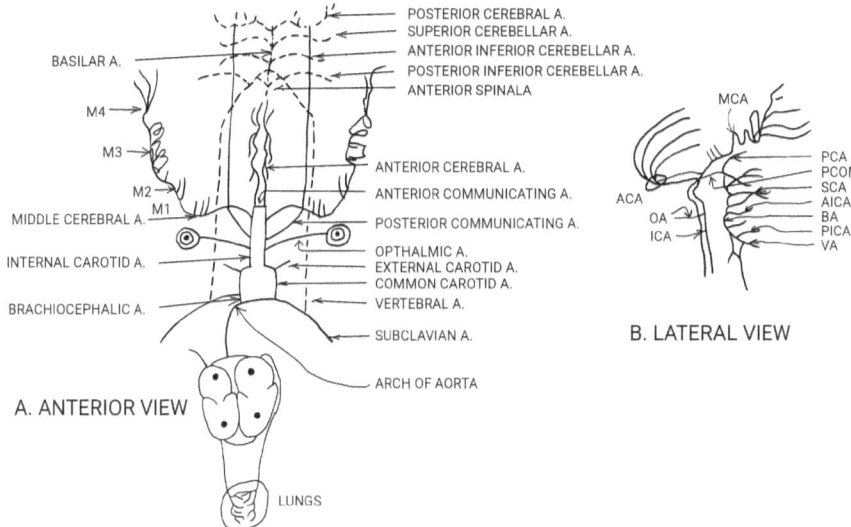

Figure 55. A. Line cartoon of cerebral circulation from the heart. Anterior circulation (solid lines) and posterior circulation (broken lines). B. View from the side.(MCA-middle cerebral artery; ACA-anterior cerebral artery; OA-opthalmic artery; ICA-internal carotid artery; Acom-anterior communicating artery; PCom-posterior communiating artery; PCA-posterior cerebral artery; SCA-superior cerebellar artery; AICA-anterior-inferior cerebellar artery; BA-basilar artery; PICA-posteriro inferior cerebellar artery; VA-vertebral artery.

syndromes characterized may vary or may not be completely present, perhaps because of the presence of collaterals that take over to supply the area rendered hypo-perfused by the main blood vessels or because of common vascular anomalies of the cerebral vessels. **Collateral vessels** serve as a compensatory mechanism that provides an alternate source of blood supply to areas of the brain when blood vessels are unable to provide adequate blood supply. The posterior communicating artery of the Circle of Willis is one large vessel that can act as collateral when either of the anterior or posterior cerebral circulations gets impaired. Other sources of collaterals are the branches of the External Carotid Artery (ECA).

The Heart.

Strokes that impair cerebral circulation may have its causation attributed to events or diseases of the heart. It is, therefore, an excellent dictum to always imagine the cerebral blood flow to begin from the heart. When there are defects in the walls or valves of the heart, blood elements like fibrin and platelets are triggered to coalesce and form *thrombi or clots*. When a part of the thrombi or the entire thrombi dislodges the many detached clumps are called *emboli* that shower the systemic circulation. The irregularity of the heart or atrial fibrillation can also trigger clot formation and embolization. One of the recipient organs of embolic clots is the brain. Lodgment of embolic clots depends on the size of the lump and the diameter of the cerebral blood vessels. The mechanism described is a **cardio-embolic stroke** because the source of the embolic clot is the heart.

Case Story:

Mr. Luber, a 65-year-old, Chief Executive Officer (CEO) of a construction company, suddenly experienced severe chest pain during the board meeting. A colleague quickly made a 911 call! The ambulance paramedic noticed him to be pale, cold, and clammy. He was immediately injected IV Morphine which dramatically gave him much pain relief. Just before they arrived at the hospital, Mr. Luber developed irregularity of the heart, then cardiac arrest. Immediately, the paramedic instituted cardio-pulmonary resuscitation (CPR).

The arrhythmia was noted to be paroxysmal ventricular tachycardia (irregular contraction of the ventricle), so appropriate medicine was provided. Resuscitation continued, then after about three minutes he recovered his consciousness but was not responsive to questions. The cardiac team of the hospital was able to correct the arrhythmia, improved cardiac circulation, and treated the myocardial infarction. A transthoracic 2D-echo cardiogram showed anterolateral wall myocardial infarction. The cardiologist noted a worrisome complication. Right-sided motor weakness and inability to answer questions. The cardiologist asked, "Do you have pain?... What is your name?" Mr. Luber just blankly looked at him and the surrounding. The observed deficits prompted the cardiologist to consider cardio-embolic cerebral infarction. Thus referral to a stroke specialist was made. After confirming the presence of ischemic infarction in the left middle cerebral territory, the cardiologist and the stroke specialist agreed to give intravenous thrombolysis, by using recombinant thromboplastin activator (rt-PA) after explaining the risks and benefits to the family. Three months after discharge from the hospital, the patient was up and about. A few naming difficulties in his language remained, but he was still able to continue his work as CEO.

Clinical - anatomic Correlation:

Adynamic (non-moving) walls in myocardial infarction, just what Mr. Luber had, can predispose to the formation of thrombus which can, in turn, dislodge and cause an embolism. Myxoma, a cardiac tumor, may have a part of the mass detach and produce *tumor embolism*. Signs and symptoms will depend on which vessel the embolus lodges. In Mr. Luber's case, he had an embolic stroke involving the main left middle cerebral artery, causing global aphasia at first. There are other cardiogenic causes of strokes. Cardiac *dysrhythmias, valvular defects, and cardiac failure that significantly lower cardiac output* can result in low brain perfusion which may cause loss of consciousness, transient dizziness or even focal deficits like weakness or sensory deficits. *Non-valvular atrial fibrillation* can trigger clot formation within the heart, and if the clot dislodges cardio-embolic infarct can result. Venous thromboses from the legs can detach and cause pulmonary embolism, and if there is a hole in the wall of the heart, like *patent foramen ovale or ventricular septal defect,* the emboli may bypass the pulmonary artery and go through the anomaly to reach the brain. This mechanism is called *paradoxical embolism*. Rheumatic carditis with the valvular disease can trigger thrombus formation that can dislodge and cause embolic infarcts. Subacute or acute bacterial endocarditis causes infected valvular vegetation and thrombus formation which can detach and cause septic thrombo-embolic infarcts.

Mr. Luber's case emphasizes an assertion, that when a stroke happens, the myocardium should always be considered as a factor in stroke pathogenesis and, therefore, examined thoroughly. Besides, cardiac diseases, mainly, myocardial ischemia is a common co-morbidity of strokes and a common cause of sudden death. A significant number of patients who have strokes die of cardiac causes and not due to stroke.

The Branches of the Aortic Arch (Fig. 55).

The *Left Common Carotid Artery (CCA)* and L*eft Subclavian artery (SCA)* arise directly from the aortic arch. On the *right side, the Brachiocephalic Artery (BCA)* is the one that takes off from the aorta (Illustration 55-A). The BCA will then branch into the *Right Common Carotid artery* and *right Subclavian artery*. The subclavian arteries provide the *Vertebral Arteries (VA)* branch on each side. The Common Carotid arteries branch into *Internal Carotid (IC) and External Carotid arteries (EC)*. If there is subclavian artery stenosis or obstruction just before the take-off of the vertebral arteries and you exercise the arms, which are supplied by your subclavian artery, blood flow intended towards the VA is instead diverted to the upper limb, causing symptoms related to the posterior circulation; this is the **subclavian steal syndrome** (literally stealing blood from the VA). Manifestations of loss of consciousness, dizziness, visual impairment, imbalance, double vision, facial numbness or motor weakness may occur singly or in combination that provides a picture of affectation of the different structures of the brainstem.

The Posterior Circulation (Table VI).

This circulation supplies the brainstem, cerebellum, the thalamus and medial portion of temporal lobes and the occipital lobes on both sides. When both *vertebral arteries* leave the subclavian artery, they pass through both transverse foramen of C6 to C2 spinal vertebra *to merge* at the level of the foramen magnum to form the *basilar artery* (broken line in Fig. 55-A). The vertebral artery on each side gives off anterior branches that merge to form the *anterior spinal artery* that supplies the anterior part of the cervical spinal cord [103,104].

Clinical – anatomic Correlation:

The anatomic pathway of the vertebral artery through the transverse foramen predisposes this vessel to neck injuries that may cause *vertebral artery dissection* or *compression* which in turn produces posterior circulation ischemic syndromes.

Just before the branching of the anterior spinal artery, the VA gives off the *Posterior inferior cerebellar artery (PICA),* which is the blood supply to the *lower half of the cerebellum and lateral and back portion of the medulla* (Fig. 55-B).

Case story:

Mrs. Johnston, 85-years-old, is a strong and very active retired pharmacist who, upon waking at 5:30 A.M., suddenly experienced dizziness, numbness on the *left* side of the face, and numbness on the *right* side of the body (crossed sensory deficit). She also started struggling with how to handle her saliva, and every time she attempts to swallow paroxysmal coughing often follows. She staggered and held on to the wall in going out of her room to call the son who was sleeping on the other side of the room. She struggled in forming the sound of the word, "Tonngmmy, Tonngmmy, pleee wek upphh." She spoke with nasal twang during word formation. Tommy noted the distress from the face of the mom, so he rushed her to the ER. An immediate MRI of the brain demonstrated, hypodensity (infarct) involving the lower half of the cerebellum and the left lateral posterior medulla.

Clinical – anatomic correlation:

Mrs. Johnston had an obstruction of the PICA, causing *Lateral Medullary Syndrome or Wallenberg Syndrome or Dorsolateral Medullary Syndrome.* The typical syndrome consists of the crossed-hemisensory deficit (i.e. left side facial numbness and right or contralateral hemisensory deficit of the extremities), dysphagia (difficulty handling the saliva)/dysphonia (nasal twang), Horner's Syndrome (pupillary constriction, ptosis and absence of sweating), ataxia (staggering and needing to hold on to something) and *sparing* of the corticospinal tract (lack of weakness, the patient is still able to walk). The lateral medullary syndrome is the most common syndrome of ischemic infarction involving the brain stem.

The first branch of the basilar artery is **the anterior inferior cerebellar artery (AICA)** that supplies the posterior pons and part of the cerebellum. The **internal auditory artery** that supplies the acoustic and labyrinthine apparatus most of the time originates from the basilar artery and occasionally from the anterior inferior cerebellar artery. A stroke involving internal auditory artery can manifest as acute and severe dizziness with deafness – a very important differential diagnosis for the more common Benign Postural Vertigo and cerebellar infarction. Typical AICA Syndrome consists of facial weakness, deafness, and numbness at the same side of the branch involved.

The other branches of the **basilar artery,** as it ascends, are small diameter **short circumferential branches and penetrating or paramedian** vessels that supply the corticospinal tract and cranial nerve nuclei in the brainstem. The pontine participants to the horizontal gaze mechanism as described in Chapter IV-C are the pontine gaze center (PGC) or paramedian pontine reticular formation (PPRF), CN. VI, Median Longitudinal Fasciculus (MLF) and CN III. If a block or rupture of any of the basilar artery penetrating branches to the pons happen, the descending motor and ascending fibers can be affected to cause paresis or numbness. The descending sympathetic tract can also be involved, allowing the parasympathetic nerve to dominate and results to pinpoint pupils. The other cranial nerve nuclei can be affected to produce corresponding sign and symptoms, but the most typical is the presence of various extraocular muscle weakness.

Case story:

Mrs. Cheng, a 72 year- old grocery owner in Chinatown, New York, was brought to the ER because of dizziness. Dr. Lu, the ER doctor, asked what her problem was, and she said, "When I woke up this morning, I was seeing double, was dizzy and felt like vomiting." Dr. Lu took her blood pressure, heart rate, and respiratory rate and was found to be normal. He then asked, "Do you have numbness or weakness in any part of the body or difficulty swallowing?", Mrs. Cheng replied, "None." Dr. Lu then examined her eye movements and noted that on horizontal movement, both eyes did not move inward and as a matter of fact, both eyes deviated outward, or they looked apart from each other. He then asked, "Mrs. Cheng, do you have diabetes?" and she worriedly replied, "I am on treatment for diabetes for more than seven years now." MRI of the brain showed minute hypodensities around the periventricular white matter which are commonly found in her age group. The brain stem did not show any hypodensity. She was confined at the acute stroke unit for close observation and treatment.

That afternoon, a repeat eye examination done by Dr. Lu revealed that the right eye was not moving at all while the left eye deviated to the left side. This time there was subjective complain and objective numbness on the right side of the face but none in the body. There was no weakness. A repeat MRI showed small lower pontine infarction midline and more on the right. Transfemoral angiography showed atheromatous vertebro-basilar and anterior circulation arteries.

There was no more progression of the neurological signs, and after four days Mrs. Cheng went home.

Clinical – anatomic Correlation:

To understand the intriguing eye signs, please review the horizontal gaze mechanism discussed in Chapter VI-C, and this is appreciated much more by drawing the structures that were involved and following the connections as shown in Figure 18. (Investing time to do this will result in a lasting understanding of the different eye signs). Involvement of the PGC or PPRF can produce conjugate gaze away from the lesion unlike superior prefrontal affectation where the direction of the eyes is towards the side of the affectation. The classic **internuclear**

ophthalmoplegia (INO) manifests as bilateral medial nerve palsy or inability of both eyes to move medially or toward the nose, because of lesions involving both median longitudinal fasciculus (MLF); this was the initial problem of Mrs. Cheng. INO is commonly due to obstruction of paramedian vessels in the elderly and diabetics, and an important differential diagnosis is multiple sclerosis in young female patients. **One and a half syndrome** can happen with the involvement of the take-off of both MLF and one of the CN VI nucleus; Mrs. Cheng developed this subsequently after admission. The MRI of Mrs. Cheng's brain correlated with a lower pontine infarction and angiogram showed that most likely the cause was athero-thrombosis of the penetrating vessel of the basilar artery which is difficult to demonstrate in an angiogram. Sometimes a unilateral midbrain lesion can catch the exit of CN III, producing same side medial rectus palsy and contralateral weakness (**Weber's Syndrome**). Analysis and understanding of the ocular muscle movements will provide clues that will determine if the problem is anterior or posterior circulation.

Top of the basilar artery branches are the superior cerebellar artery (SCA) and the posterior cerebral artery (PCA) that connects to the anterior cerebral circulation via the *posterior communicating artery (PCom)*. Embolic or atherosclerotic obstruction of the basilar artery at its top can very well affect the areas supplied by the SCA and the PCA. The *SCA* provides blood to the superior cerebellum; the superior cerebellar peduncle and part of the middle cerebellar peduncle; the dentate nucleus; the inferior colliculus; the pineal body; the medial, and lateral lemniscus; part of the Cranial V nucleus; and the *tela choroidea* of the III ventricle. The *PCA* supplies the medial temporal area and the occipital lobe, midbrain peduncle and the thalamus.

Clinical Vascular Syndromes:

Affectation of the *SCA* may produce a complex syndrome of ataxia, upper extremity tremors, facial numbness, vertical gaze palsy, and some ocular signs. Obstruction to the *PCA*, on the other hand, produces symptom and signs of inability to assimilate new information (**amnesic**) and contralateral hemianopsia respectively. If the left inferior occipital-parietal area gets involved, Gerstmann Syndrome, consisting of **finger agnosia** (inability to recognize fingers), **acalculia** (difficulty comprehending or utilizing mathematical information), **right-left disorientation** (inability to distinguish between right and left) and **agraphia** (inability to write information) may happen. If the right side gets involved, *visual neglect* may manifest. Involvement of perforating vessels at the tip of the basilar artery can cause various thalamic syndromes and midbrain peduncular behavioral changes, like a *visual or auditory hallucination* and contralateral hemiplegia.

Case Story:

Mrs. Posadas, a 50-year-old housewife, suddenly experienced for the first time a severe pain over the right occiput that radiated to the right nape, neck, and right shoulder. It was so painful that in distress, she shouted for help from a neighbor who then called for 911 help. At the ER, she was in anguish and pain but was able to cooperate. The ER doctor noted the right pupil to be dilated; there was a mild weakness in moving the right eye towards the nose, and there was mild ptosis. A short-acting opioid was administered straightaway to provided relief from pain and sedation. The emergency CT angiogram revealed a right posterior communicating artery aneurysm. A ruptured right posterior communicating artery aneurysm with broad base required an emergency craniotomy and clipping. She survived the dreadful threat to life and recovered the function of the right eye. She lived without a trace of pain.

Clinical – anatomic Correlation:

Aneurysms forms at arterial junctions and the most common sites are at the posterior communicating-posterior cerebral artery junctions and the anterior communicating-anterior cerebral artery junction (Fig. 55). The posterior communicating artery (PCom) and posterior cerebral artery (PCA) aneurysm often lie just above the Cranial Nerve III, predisposing it to compression or irritation resulting in dilatation of pupils and sometimes ptosis and medial rectus weakness at the side of an aneurysm. The CN III signs just described provided the clue of an aneurysm at the PCom-PCA junction.

The Anterior Circulation

The left common carotid artery emanates directly from the arch of the aorta while the right common carotid artery comes from the brachiocephalic artery. The **common carotid artery** bifurcates into **internal carotid** and **external carotid arteries**. This bifurcation is a common site for the formation of atherosclerosis. This information is necessary because atherosclerosis can enlarge and may obstruct the vessels. Atherosclerotic plaques, especially the rough plaques, elicit clot formation and possible dislodgement to cause embolism, an **artery to artery embolism**. The external carotid artery provides vascular supply to extracranial structures like the thyroid gland, ears and salivary glands. Another important branch is the **meningeal artery** that supplies the temporal side of the meninges. The meningeal artery is clinically relevant because when there is a linear fracture of the temporal bone, the trauma may result in injury to this meningeal artery and cause epidural hematoma -- a deadly consequence of head trauma if treatment gets delayed. The external carotid branches are essential sources of collateral vessels that lend support to the anterior circulation in cases where atherosclerosis block the internal carotid artery and intracranial vessels.

The *internal carotid artery* enters the skull just at the back of the tonsils and posterior pharynx, predisposing it to injuries from pointed objects placed in the mouth of children. It then makes an anterior bending in front of the pituitary gland (carotid siphon) and gives out the *ophthalmic artery*. Embolic clots sometimes can block this vessel temporarily and produce transient blindness called "amaurosis fugax," an urgent warning that a possible major stroke can happen. Immediately after this branch, the internal carotid artery siphon gives off medially, the *inferior and superior hypophyseal arteries* supplying the pituitary gland. The internal carotid artery then penetrates the cavernous sinus and gives off three major branches: (a) the *anterior cerebral artery (ACA)* that courses forward and medially to meet with the opposite anterior cerebral artery and get connected at the base by the *anterior communicating artery (ACom)* which is one of the most common sites of aneurysm; (b) the *posterior communicating artery (PCom)* that connects with the *posterior cerebral artery* to complete the anterior and posterior circulation, thus completing the *circle of Willis* (Fig. 55). (The posterior communicating and posterior cerebral arteries give off small penetrating branches that supply the thalamus.) (c) The *middle cerebral artery*, which is not part of the "circle," branches off from the lateral part of the internal carotid artery to supply most of the internal capsule and basal ganglia and lateral surface of the cortex.

The first portion of the *anterior cerebral artery (A1)* gives off medial lenticular penetrating vessels and the *recurrent artery of Heubner* that supplies the inferior part of the caudate head, the anterior limb of the internal capsule, and the most medial and anterior portions of the Globus pallidus. The next branches extending anteriorly *(A2)* are the *medial orbitofrontal artery*, and a little distal is the *frontopolar branch*. These vessels supply the olfactory cortex, gyrus rectus, and medial orbital gyrus. The anterior cerebral artery continues upward and gives off the *calloso-marginal artery* that moves forward and sways backward along the cingulate sulcus. The ACA continues to form the *pericallosal artery (A3)*. These vessels give off branches that supply the anteromedial parts up to the superior medial parietal lobe of the cortex (Fig.55-A).

Clinical-anatomic Correlation:

In the homunculus, the leg and the bladder and bowel voluntary motor control are at the medial portion of the prefrontal gyrus. The higher form of functions resides in the frontal lobe, and primitive reflexes are stored and suppressed in the area. **Frontal lobe signs** are constellations of dysfunctions associated with lesions affecting the frontal lobe and can manifest on the opposite side. Frontal lobe signs are: 1. grasp and sucking reflex; 2. lower extremity weakness with *sparing or less affectation of the arm and face*; 3. *bladder and bowel incontinence*, if both sides are affected; 4. *gait apraxia* (loss of walking skill acquired during childhood); 5. *motor aphasia* (loss of ability to form words gathered through time); 6. *personality changes*; 7. *planning and strategy formation dysfunction*; 8. *apathy*; 9. *abulia* (loss of speech); 10. *poor working memory*; 11. *disinhibition;* 12. *emotional lability;* 13. *sociopathy;* 14. *sexual disinhibition*; and 15. *lack of concern for others*. These are the varied manifestations in anterior cerebral artery obstruction. They could manifest in varied combinations. Profound *akinetic mutism* (awake but not aware of environment) may reveal when both anterior cerebral arteries are infarcted.

The *posterior communicating artery (PCom)* takes off from the IC just before the ACA and MCA branches and extends posteriorly to link with the posterior cerebral artery (PCA). The other way to describe the PCom is that it arises from the PCA as its first branch from the basilar artery, considered the P1, where perforating vessels supply the anterior thalamus through the anterior thalamo-perforators or polar *or tuberothalamic artery*. The other structures it provides are the hypothalamus, the optic chiasm, and mammillary body.

The PCom is a primary collateral for posterior and anterior circulation needs. *Pcom infarct syndromes* are rare and consist of any combination of alteration of sensorium, loss of speech, personality change, disorientation, visual field defect, and thalamic aphasia for left-sided lesion while hemi-neglect or alien hand present in right thalamic infarct. Some would attribute the syndrome to PCA.

The *middle cerebral artery* (MCA) is the largest branch of ICA. The MCA branches laterally and horizontally. The first portion *(M1)* is the horizontal segment that gives off *lenticulo-striae vessels* that supply the basal ganglia and the posterior limb of the internal capsule. It proceeds laterally as the insular or Sylvian segment *(M2)* that provides the insula and divides into temporal and parietal branches, then into cortical branches *(M3)* that supply the lateral side of the cortex. The MCA *does not* supply the superior frontal and superior parietal gyrus, median temporal gyrus and the occipital lobe [105].

Several cortical branches *(M4)* supply largely the lateral gyri of the frontal, temporal, and parietal lobe and these are the following structures with their corresponding supplies: (Please do not memorize. Just know that the MCA cortical branches have these extensive branches supplying almost 2/3 of the cortex).

1. Frontal lobe:
   a. Orbitofrontal branch - Inferior frontal gyrus
   b. Prefrontal arteries - inferior and middle frontal gyrus
   c. Pre-Rolandic artery (precentral) - posterior part of the middle and inferior frontal gyri and lower part of the precentral gyrus
   d. Rolandic arteries (central) - posterior pre-central gyrus and inferior portion of the post-central gyrus

2. Parietal lobe:
   a. Anterior parietal arteries - anterior parietal area
   b. Posterior parietal arteries - posterior parietal and supramarginal gyrus
   c. Angular artery - angular gyrus, supramarginal gyrus, posterior superior temporal gyrus, and parietooccipital arcus
   d. Temporo - occipital arteries - superior and inferior occipital gyri

3. Temporal lobe:
   a. Temporopolar arteries - polar and anterior lateral portions of the temporal lobe
   b. Anterior temporal arteries - same area as above
   c. Middle temporal arteries - a superior and middle part of the middle temporal lobe
   d. Posterior temporal - posterior portion of the temporal lobe and perforating arteries to insula

Clinical -anatomic Correlation:

Remembering all of these branches and the corresponding areas that they supply is a daunting task to master. You do not have to memorize these vessels and the areas that they correspondingly supply. Just understand that there are diseases that can very well affect a single branch or two or more branches, especially in embolism. In the earlier part of this book, we described the different anatomic brain structures and their corresponding functions. These various structures can be affected singly or in combination in stroke, causing changing dynamic *syndromes or manifestations*. The involvement of several parts of the CNS is exemplified by cerebral embolism, when often, the embolus can lodge in the main branch, and when the natural lysis of clot happens, it can very well disintegrate into smaller emboli, some of which can significantly block distant arterial branches. The lysis of the clot occurred in Gina, the teacher (Clinical Story, p. 105). There are occasions when only one cortical branch to the posterior parietal can be affected, and in this case, if the involvement is on the left side, conduction aphasia without hemiplegia or hemisensory deficits can manifest.

The most common MCA syndromes due to strokes are:

1. Involvement only of the perforating branch which can cause lacunar infarct that manifests as *pure motor paresis*
2. *Contralateral hemiplegia or hemiparesis*
3. *Contralateral hemisensory deficit that* may include discriminatory abnormalities
4. *Hemianopsia* opposite to the lesion, usually with other cortical manifestations
5. *Broca's aphasia* for frontal branches involvement; *Wernicke's Aphasia* for temporo-occipital artery branch involvement; *Conduction aphasia* for parietal branches involvement, particularly the angular arteries. All of these on the left side; *contralateral hemineglect* if the right parietal is involved
6. *Conjugate deviation of the eyes* towards the lesion if the frontal branch is mainly affected
7. When the main trunk of the MC, all of the above syndromes may manifest, and for the aphasias, a Global Aphasia. Global Aphasia is a terrible type of aphasia because understanding and communication are severely affected. Elemental responses to the conversation are the only thing that remains. For example: If asked, "How are you?" It will be answered by "yes" or "oh," or gaze or a smile that is devoid of meaning.

Special Clinical Correlates for Stroke Recognition:

The most important task for health care providers is to be able to recognize transient ischemic attacks (TIA) and strokes. What follows then is to determine which vascular territory is involved. Is it the *anterior circulation* or *posterior circulation?* Then, decide which imaging study is appropriate. Should it be an MRI or a CT scan with angiography or a combination of both? Is 4-vessel cerebral angiography necessary? What treatment intervention is suitable for a three hour or 4.5 hours or 6 hours "golden periods?" The **"golden period"** is an estimated time borne out of stroke ischemic infarct research where the chances of a good outcome can be achieved with the least risk of hemorrhagic complications when using thrombolytic agents to reestablish blood flow. The thrombolytic agent is rTPA (Actylase). Should the patient be referred immediately to Neurosurgery or acute stroke facility? In exceptional cases, thrombolysis can still be given within 24 hours after posterior circulation stroke [106]. There are treatment strategies currently being studied, like intraarterial thrombolysis done within the six-hour period for anterior circulation; or if reconstitution of blood flow fails, then clot retraction can be done.

We have detailed the functions of the different structures of the central nervous system and the blood supplies to these structures for you to understand their relationships and be able to appreciate the symptomatology and signs. We will now try to simplify our approach by describing signs and symptoms that will make us determine if it is the anterior circulation or posterior circulation that is involved. The most characteristic of strokes or TIA is the *acuteness of onset*, literally like a "stroke of lightning."

The *long descending corticospinal* and *ascending spinothalamic tracts* can be affected in anterior and posterior cerebral circulation strokes to cause hemiparesis or hemisensory deficit. Because these are readily involved in a stroke, for localization purposes they serve as the "vertical lines" and the intersecting "horizontal lines" are the involvement of the functions of the cortex, cranial nerves in the brainstem and spinal cord. Where they intersect is the location of the lesion.

One should remember that single or isolated manifestations can commonly present as a TIA or a stroke. One could however surmise if the anterior or posterior circulation is the one involved.

1. *Pure motor hemiplegia or hemisensory deficits* are usually due to lacunar infarcts which are tiny lesions hitting the corticospinal or spinothalamic tracts respectively, and this is generally due to small vessels or perforating branch involvement. The MCA perforating branch obstruction can cause pure hemiparesis, and usually, there is a *leg and upper extremity dissociation,* where the upper extremity is weaker than the lower extremity because the ACA is the blood supply to the leg area in the brain. The most common cortico-spinal tract involved is usually the *internal capsule;* so most often this involves the *anterior circulation*. The most common site however for the spinothalamic tract

involvement is the *thalamus*, which involves most likely the *posterior circulation*.

2. *Transient monocular blindness* or "amaurosis fugax" involves the ophthalmic artery branch of the internal carotid artery, and therefore it concerns the *anterior circulation*.

3. *Sudden homonymous hemianopsia or" hemi blurring*" may point to one side of the occipital lobe involving the posterior cerebral artery and, therefore, the *posterior circulation*.

4. *Sudden vertigo or dizziness that may be accompanied by nausea and vomiting* and is not aggravated by head movement may be due to unilateral inferior cerebellar infarct; thus *posterior circulation* disturbance should be suspected.

The above-isolated manifestations may present in combinations and the form of a transient ischemic attack (TIA), evolving stroke or part of the completed stroke. An example of TIA is short-lived right side hemiplegia that disappears and replaced by dysphasia; this is highly indicative of an embolic activity.

The following syndromes are suggestive of anterior circulation strokes:

a. Language disorders like the *aphasias* (Broca's and Wernicke's) with or without contralateral hemiplegia and hemisensory deficit or contralateral homonymous hemianopsia, Global aphasia (inability to understand and express) with right-sided hemiplegia with or without disturbance of sensorium

b. *Agnosias*, abnormalities in interpreting sensory inputs like visual agnosia, auditory agnosia, difficulty identifying faces (prosopagnosia) with or without contralateral hemianopsia. Another example is finger agnosia, an inability to recognize fingers

c. *Apraxia*, abnormalities in performing acquired motor acts like ideational apraxia, which is an inability to perform an imaginary act of brushing teeth; constructional apraxia, failure to make a simple drawing like intersecting lines; Gait apraxia, difficulty to execute gait sequence in walking; agraphia, inability to write information; and acalculia, difficulty in comprehending or utilizing mathematical information

d. *Behavioral or personality changes* that may be accompanied by hemiplegia or hemisensory deficits or a combination of primitive reflexes like grasp and sucking reflexes; apathy; personality; abulia or loss of speech; lack of ability to plan; poor working memory; emotional lability; sociopathy; sexual disinhibition; and lack of concern for others

e. Right- left disorientation or left side neglect together with or without hemianopsia.

f. Conjugate deviation of the eyes towards the side of the lesion or opposite of the paralyzed limb.

The following are suggestive of posterior circulation strokes:

a. *Crossed signs.* Ipsilateral facial numbness or motor paralysis and contralateral hemisensory deficits or paralysis. Ipsilateral and cranial nerve affectations and contralateral hemisensory deficit or hemiparesis.
b. *Vertigo, dizziness, unsteadiness or tendency to fall to one side, nystagmus, and ataxia.* Lateral medullary or dorsolateral Wallenberg syndrome consisting of *dysphagia/dysphonia, crossed hemisensory deficit, ipsilateral facial palsy and contralateral hemisensory deficit, Horner's syndrome, sparing the corticobulbar tract*
c. *Cranial nerve manifestations* in combination with or without hemiplegia, hemisensory deficit, or even visual field abnormalities. Internuclear ophthalmoplegia (bilateral medial rectus weakness), 1 ½ syndrome (complete ophthalmoplegia and contralateral medial rectus weakness), CN III involvement and contralateral hemiparesis (Weber's). Diplopia or double vision is a common manifestation together with resultant dizziness

Table VI. Posterior Circulation Syndromes and Involved Structures

SYNDROMES	SIGNS/SYMPTOMS	STRUCTURES INVOLVED
Lateral Medullary Syndrome; Dorsolateral Medullary or Wallenberg Syndrome	Anhidrosis, miosis, ptosis (Horner's Syndrome) (Cross sensory deficit) ipsilateral facial numbness and contralateral numbness	Descending Sympathetic tract, Ipsilateral Spinothalamic and Trigeminothalamic tract
	Ataxia, Vertigo, Nystagmus	Inferior cerebellar peduncle, Dieter's and other nuclei, nodular lobe, inferior cerebellum, Ipsilateral
	Dysphagia, Dysphonia Sparing of corticospinal, no paralysis	CN IX & X of Nucleus Ambiguus Lesion is dorsolateral does not involve the ventral portion
Anterior Inferior Cerebellar Artery Syndrome	Ipsilateral hearing loss, facial paralysis and loss of facial sensations to all modalities.	Lateral and inferior portion of the pons,
	Ataxia Vomiting Nystagmus	middle cerebellar peduncle, flocculus and other lobules of cerebellum
Superior Cerebellar Artery Syndrome	Vomiting, Nystagmus, Ipsilateral ataxia, tremors, explosive speech, dysmetria	Superior cerebellar peduncle and lobules and dentate nucleus.
	diplopia	Midbrain dorsal tegmentum CN IV
	Anhidrosis, miosis, ptosis (Horner's Syn)	Descending sympathetic tract Lateral Lemniscus
	Contralateral deafness	Spinothalamic tract
	Contralateral numbness	
Top of the basilar artery syndrome Rostral brainstem infarction syndrome (Posterior cerebral artery +/- Superior Cerebellar artery Syndromes)	Unresponsiveness, hypersomnolence, hallucination, behavioral abnormality	Midbrain tegmentum, peduncle
	Vertical Oculomotor dysfunctions, pupillary changes, small, slow or fix, ocular convergence	Midbrain pretectal
	Hemianopsia, Amnestic dysfunction, Acalculia, Agraphia, finger agnosia, right left disorientation, for right side-prosopagnosia, visual neglect	Median temporal lobe and occipital lobe: Thalamus Lateral thalamus, contralateral
	Hemisensory deficits	Contra-Lateral thalamus
	Motor dysfunction often absent	

d. *"Locked-in"* state of preserved consciousness with quadriplegia and cranial nerve signs suggestive of complete pontine and lower midbrain infarction
e. *Acute disturbance of consciousness,* especially if accompanied by any of the following: double vision, vertigo, ataxia, hemiparesis or hemisensory deficits
f. *Contralateral homonymous hemianopia with macular sparing* together with disturbance of memory, sometimes with peduncular hallucination (visual bright colored hallucination). Vertical gaze palsy may be present.
g. *The sudden hemisensory deficit with left thalamic aphasia or right thalamic alien hand or disorientation or personality change*
h. *Dysphagia, dysarthria, hoarseness, and dysphonia* with or without hemiplegia or hemisensory deficits.

Always remember that aside from the syndromes described, the brainstem is recognized as a vital center because here resides control to essential functions for survival. These are wakefulness, swallowing, respiration, cardiac reflexes, blood pressure control, micturition, and of course, upward and downward tracts to the motor and sensory functions. Any of these essential functions can very well be affected together with the posterior circulation syndromes described above.

Review frontal lobe signs (p. 265) and MCA syndromes (p. 268) and suggestive posterior circulation syndromes (p. 271). Now you can recognize anterior and posterior circulation strokes.

Spinal Cord Blood Supply

The main arterial supply to the cord (Fig. 56-A) comes from the *anterior spinal artery (ASA)* which is medially located and gives off *the central artery* and *the two posterior spinal arteries (PSA)*. The ASA supplies two thirds of the spinal cord, including the base of the posterior column, while the PSA provides the posterior third of the gray matter, the rest of the posterior column, and the edges of the anterior and lateral white matter (Fig. 56-B). The ASA at the upper cervical spinal cord comes mainly from the vertebral artery while the

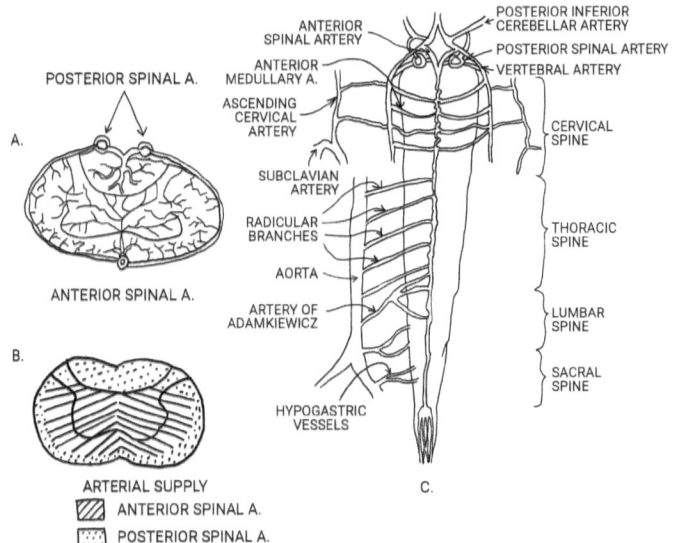

Figure 56. Arterial blood supply to the spinal cord. A. Cross section showing the paired posterior spinal arteries (PSA) and single anterior spinal artery (ASA). B PSA supplies posterior column, posterior part of gray matter and edges of the cord while ASA supplies the inner white matter and anterior 2/3 of the gray matter. C. Arterial branches contributing to ASA at different levels of the spinal cord.

PSA comes from the posterior inferior cerebellar arteries, VA and C2 blood vessels [107]. The ASA and the PSA at the lower portions of the cervical are richly innervated by *radiculo-medullary arteries* coming from neck vasculatures that originate from the subclavian arteries. The segmental vessels from the aorta which includes the *Artery of Adamkiewics* are the sources of radiculo-medullary vessels that supply the thoracic segment and the upper lumbar areas (Fig. 56-C). The lumbosacral parts, on the other hand, are provided mainly by *pelvic or hypogastric arteries* [108].

Clinical-anatomic correlation:

Rich collaterals contribute significantly also to the spinal circulation like the *extensive epidural arterial network, pial plexus, and the paraspinal muscle arteries*. This rich anastomoses and collaterals make spinal infarction rare, even if there are obstructions at the contributing vessels. *The thoracic spinal cord, however, does not have a rich collateral system* and also have long inter radicular vessel sources thus making it vulnerable to stroke like the *Anterior Spinal Artery syndrome*. Other diseases involving the vessels are vascular myelopathies, leukemic infiltrations, intermittent spinal claudication, arterio-venous malformations, and inflammatory arteritis.

The Venous Drainage of the CNS

Blood from the CNS structures will have to flow back to systemic circulation for oxygenation. Outside the brain, the veins have valves that favor flow towards the direction of the heart. For centuries, the vascular system was seen as a continuous tube with the heart at the center. About the 16th century, the venous system of the CNS was found to differ from the other parts of the body because its walls are made of *dura mater and are valveless*. The *spinal venous plexus is likewise without valves,* and this characteristic extends outside the spine to the *prostatic plexus*. The valveless venous plexus could perhaps explain the propensity of prostatic carcinoma to metastasize to the spine [109].

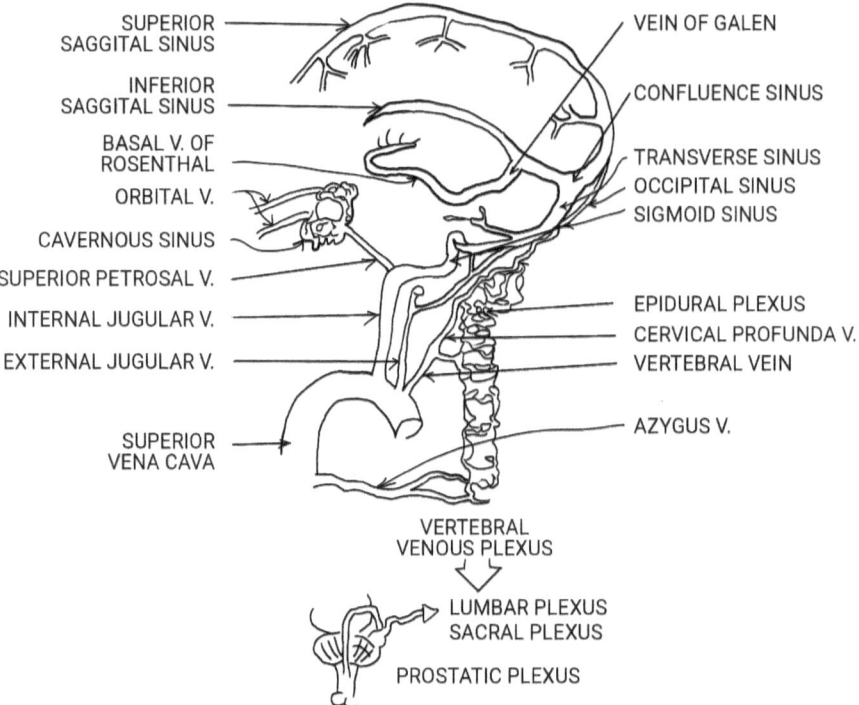

Figure 57. Venous drainage of the brain and upper spinal cord and various draining extracranial veins—Jugular veins and Epidural plexus and vertebral vein.

The venous drainage subdivides into the superficial and deep system (Fig 57). The superficial system drains the surface of the brain through the *Superior Sagittal Sinus (SSS),* located in between the two hemispheres. The arachnoid villi that absorb the CSF penetrate the pia and the dura to drain at the SSS. Blood flows posteriorly and inferiorly to the *torcula* where the two *transverse sinuses* meet; laterally and inferiorly these sinuses curve in an S-shaped curve as the *Sigmoid Sinuses* which continue to form the *Jugular veins*. The jugular veins drain into the superior vena cava which finally brings back venous blood to the heart.

The deep structures are drained via the *thalamo-striae vein* that flows to the *internal cerebral vein*, then to the *vein of Galen*, and the *straight sinus*. Just beneath the SSS is the *inferior sagittal sinus* that drains to the *straight sinus* which is a confluence of sinuses. The straight sinus then drains to the *transverse sinuses.*

The *cavernous sinus* is a confluence of the venous pool at the lateral sides of the *selae turcica* (where the pituitary gland sits). It receives drainage from *superior and inferior ophthalmic veins, sphenoparietal sinus, inferior petrosal sinus, and basilar venous plexus*. It drains to the *sigmoid sinus* thru the *superior and inferior petrosal sinus*. Each side of the internal carotid artery traverses the cavernous sinuses, and the cranial nerves that pass through are CN III, IV, VI and CN V1, V2.

The "final" common pathways for cerebral venous drainage are mainly through the bilateral jugular vein. Studies, however, have demonstrated what has long believed that the spinal venous plexus during sitting and standing positions receive much of the cerebral venous drainage [110, 111].

Clinical-anatomic correlation

With the veins being valveless and bidirectional, it is easy to imagine that prostatic carcinomas characteristically metastasize to the bone of the spines. The absence of valves in the venous plexus could also explain Schistosoma parasites or perhaps the eggs reaching the brain, or tumor metastasis without pulmonary lesions [112].

Clinical Story:

Mrs. Reyes, a kindergarten teacher, 33 years old was on her 32nd week of pregnancy when she complained of a generalized headache the morning of Sunday. She could not tolerate the pain, so she took paracetamol 500 mg which afforded mild relief and allowed her to attend church service. When the service was about to end, Mrs. Reyes suddenly fell and lost consciousness and was noted by the husband to turn her head to the left and with the eyes deviated to the left too. Before she could be raised to be seated, she went into generalized shaking for about a minute, followed by generalized limping of the body.

The husband immediately rushed her to the hospital, and along the way, she was found to be restless. The ER doctor, Dr. Luther, noted that she was already awake but confused. The left upper and lower extremities were weak at 2/5 to 3/5, there were no appropriate responses to questions; there was no neck rigidity. The funduscopic examination did not show papilledema nor retinal hemorrhages; the extraocular movements were intact; there was no facial asymmetry; blinking was spontaneous; upper extremities showed normal reflexes while the lower extremities were with hyperreflexia, and bilateral Babinski signs were present. She was immediately given intravenous antiepileptic drugs. CT Scan of the head with contrast showed edema and small hyperdensities suggestive of small hemorrhages surrounding the sagittal sinuses; empty delta sign, a venous clot, was present near the junction of the superior sagittal sinus and transverse sinus. Magnetic Resonance Venogram (MRV) done confirmed sagittal sinus thrombosis. The patient was anticoagulated. She gradually recovered and discharged on the third week with normal cerebral function and improved left-sided weakness at 4/5. Her pregnancy reached maturity at 40 weeks, and after briefly discontinuing the anticoagulant, labor was induced, and she delivered a healthy 7-pound baby boy. She recovered completely.

Clinical – anatomic Correlation:

Cerebral Venous Thrombosis (CVT) or obstruction of the veins by blood clots could occur because of possible infection, hypercoagulation, traumatic head injury, hyperhomocysteinemia, oral contraceptives, and pregnancy. The typical manifestations are a headache, seizures, hemiplegia, and fever. Complications like venous infarct, hemorrhage, subarachnoid hemorrhage, increased intracranial pressure, aseptic meningitis, Dural AV fistula, progressive psychiatric diseases, and recurrent seizures are possibilities. The most common of the CVT is the sagittal sinus thrombosis which Mrs. Reyes had, with pregnancy as the predisposing factor.

The other cerebral sinuses and the deep venous system can have thrombosis too. Cavernous sinus thrombosis are commonly associated with infection of the face, particularly around the nose where the angular veins drain to the cavernous sinus. Another cause can be sinus infections. In addition to headache and hemorrhage, proptosis of the involved eyes, papilledema, and involvement of CN III, IV, VI, and V1V2 may happen because these cranial nerves pass through the cavernous sinus. It is for this reason that when there is an infection in the face and nose, antibiotics should be given to prevent this complication which has a high mortality rate.

SUMMARY

We dissected the CNS by stations and substations, by tracts, and by many other connections (neuroanatomy). Along the journey, we described how the CNS controlled our day to day physical and mental activities (*neurophysiology*). We were reminded regularly to emphasize on understanding the mechanisms and not memorizing. To enhance understanding, tracing the tracts and connections in the illustrations, while reading, was encouraged. We then defined the dysfunctions, deficits or hyperactivities that resulted from injuries and diseases that affect the function of the different parts of the CNS (*pathophysiology*). We discussed simple bedside examinations to uncover aberrant CNS functions (*neurological exam*). The corticospinal and spinothalamic tracts served as the imaginary functional "vertical lines" while the "horizontal lines" were the functions of the cortex, brainstem cranial nerves and spinal cord. Where manifestations intersected that is where the lesion is (*localization*). Neuroanatomic structures need to have clinical relevance, so several case examples were matched with particular CNS parts. The mechanisms of the manifestations in the case examples were illuminated and expanded to include other possible diseases that can mimic the syndromes (*clinicopathologic correlation and differential diagnosis*). The cerebrospinal fluid (CSF) that bathed the brain provided protection and nourishment to the CNS. Diseases of the brain are reflected in the CSF and can be collected and analyzed to identify pathogens, inflammatory and immunologic reactions. The CSF circulates in the subarachnoid spaces of the brain and the spinal cord and gets absorbed in the brain lymphatics, arachnoid villi, and cerebral venous system and returned to the peripheral circulation. The route of the CSF circulation or its absorption can be blocked to cause hydrocephalus and increased intracranial pressure (ICP). Tumors, cerebral edema, and other space-occupying lesions could also show typical signs and symptoms of increased ICP. Stroke, which is the most common neurological disease was used as a takeoff point to discuss the blood supply to the CNS. We highlighted the heart, not only because it is the central pumping station of the circulation, but because the stroke mechanism can very well emanate from cardiac diseases. The anatomy of the main intracerebral blood vessels and their corresponding CNS territories supplied were identified. Various syndromes brought about by blockage or rupture of particular blood vessels were described. Anterior circulation and posterior circulation syndromes were outlined to enhance stroke recognition. The venous drainage from the brain and spinal cord were detailed, and diseases affecting the veins and their manifestations were described.

Conclusion. If the illustrations were laid on top of one another, it would show complex subways of interconnecting stations and tracts—the different structures of the brain and the nervous systems interconnected, interdependent, interactive and integrated into a circuit that makes us humans. The basketball skills of Michael Jordan, the tenacity and strength of tennis legend Rafa Nadal, the speed and power of Novak Djokovic and the rhythmic grace of the tap dancer—all different in their genes and chosen crafts but the same integrated circuitry of the central nervous system addressing and adapting to their needs. When one moves an index finger it is not only the pyramidal neurons at the precentral gyrus that caused the movements of the muscles of the index but a contribution of the cerebellum, the entire brain, the basal ganglia, the spinal cord, the peripheral nerves and the muscles. As we gaze at the distant sunset and look at its reflection in the sea; and as we see and recognize the smiling faces of our friends; and as we feel the warmth of the sun and the tender touch of a loved one; and as we lick and taste the unique flavor of an avocado ice cream; and as we are reading this book and the many examples of daily activities that we do -- the CNS is bursting with zillions of electrical discharges, complex and finite mathematical system integral -- complete to make us uniquely human. A human with delicate neural control system, vulnerable to injuries and diseases. We as health providers are now ready to care for them.

BIBLIOGRAPHY

I wish to cite all the known and mostly unknown noble members of the neuroscience community who have generously encoded, and are still encoding, information to my nervous system for more than thirty five years. This book is an integrated synthesis of all that I have read, heard, skilled, researched, taught and cases seen --- about neurology.

1. Jozefowicz RF. Neurophobia: the fear of neurology among medical students. Arch Neurol 1994;51:328 –329.
2. Hadley G, Evans R, Yang L, Santini V, De Luca G. Expert Patient Tutors: The Eradication of Neurophobia. Neurology Apr 2018, 90 (15 Supplement) P2.011
3. San Luis AM, Magpantay CD, Quebral J and Villamor M. Experiences and Perceptions of Medical Students on Neurology Curriculum: A Reminiscing Focus Group Discussion of Graduates. Submited for publication January, 2019 UERMMMCI Health Sciences Journal.
4. The Royal Swedish Academy of Sciences. Studies of G-Protein-Coupled Receptors. The Nobel Prize in Chemistry 2012 is awarded to Brian K. Kobilka and Robert J. Lefkowitz.
5. Lefkowitz, RJ. Nobel Lecture: Brief History of G-Protein. https://www.nobelprize.org/nobel_prizes/ chemistry/laureates/lefkowitz-lecture pdf.
6. Penfield, W. and Boldrey, E. (1937) Somatic Motor and Sensory Representation in the Cerebral Cortex of Man as Studied by Electrical Stimulation. Brain: A Journal of Neurology, 60, 389-443. https://doi.org/10.1093/brain/60.4.389
7. Van Gijn J. The Babinski sign –a centenary-. Universities' Utrecht (publication dept.). Heidelberglaan 8, 3584 CS Utrecht. 1996.
8. Mehndiratta MM, Bhattacharyya KB, Bohra V, Gupta S, Wadhwa A Babinski the great: Failure did not deter him. Ann Indian Acad Neurol. 2014 Jan;17(1):7-9. doi: 10.4103/0972-2327.128522.

9. Thomas, L. The nocifensor system of nerves and its reactions. British Med J. 1937.431-435.
10. Light, AR. "Nocifensor" System Re-Revisited. Focus on Two Types of C Nociceptor in Human Skin and Their Behavior in Areas of Capsaicin-Induced Secondary Hyperalgesia. J Neurophysiology. Jun 1, 2004.
11. Brand, P W and Yancey, P. The gift of pain. 1st Ed., 1993.
12. Melzach R, Wall PD. Pain Mechanisms: a new theory. Science. 1965 Nov.19; 150 (3699): 971-979.
13. Katz J, Rosenbloom BN. The golden anniversary of Melzack and Wall's gate control theory of pain: Celebrating 50 years of pain research and management. Pain Research & Management : The Journal of the Canadian Pain Society. 2015;20(6):285-286.
14. IASP Taxonomy, Part III: Pain Terms, A Current List with Definitions and Notes on Usage pp 209-214, Classification of Chronic Pain, Second Edition, IASP Task Force on Taxonomy, edited by H. Merskey and N. Bogduk, IASP Press, Seattle, ©1994.
15. Williams ACC, Craig KD. Updating the definition of pain. Pain, 2016. Vol. 157-11, p 2420-2423.
16. Saunders C. Introduction: history and challenge. In: Saunders C, Sykes N, eds. The Management of Terminal Malignant Disease. London, Great Britain: Hodder and Stoughton; 1993:1-14.
17. Davis MC, Griessenauer CJ, Bosmia AN, Tubbs SR, and Shoja MM. The Naming of the Cranial Nerves: A Historical Review. Clin. Anat. 27:14–19, 2014. Published online 9 December 2013 in Wiley Online Library (wileyonlinelibrary.com). DOI: 10.1002/ca.22345.
18. Lopez-Elizalde R, Campero A, Sanchez-Delgadillo T, Lemus-Rodriguez Y, Lopez-Gonzalez MI and Godinez-Rub M. Anatomy of the Olfactory Nerve: A Comprehensive Review with Cadaveric Dissection. Clinical Anatomy 31:109–117 (2018)
19. Thong YH. Primary amoebic meningoencephalitis: fifteen years later. Med J Aust. 1980 Apr 19;1(8):352-4.
20. Seo HS, Jeon K, Hammel T, Min BC. Infuences of olfactory impairment on depression, cognitive performance, and quality of life in Korean elderly. Eur Arch Otorhinolaryngol (2009) 266:1739–1745
21. Li X, Lui F. Anosmia. [Updated 2018 Feb 9]. In: StatPearls [Internet]. Treasure Island (FL): StatPearls Publishing; 2018 Jan-. Available from: https://www.ncbi.nlm.nih.gov/books/NBK482152/

22. Dragoi V, Tsuchitani C, Chapter 14: Visual Processing: Eye and Retina, Neuroscience Online neuroscience.uth.tmc.edu. Department of Neurobiology and Anatomy, The UT Medical School at Houston. Ed., John H. Byrne.1997
23. Briggs F. Mammalian Visual System Organization. Oxford Research Encyclopedia of Neuroscience Subject: Sensory Systems Online Publication Date: Feb 2017 DOI: 1093/acrefore/9780190264086.013.66
24. Dragoi VV. Chapter 8: Ocular Motor Control. Neuroscience Online neuroscience.uth.tmc.edu. Department of Neurobiology and Anatomy, The UT Medical School at Houston. Ed., John H. Byrne.1997
25. Sharpe, J and Wong, AM. Anatomy and Physiology of Ocular Motor Systems. Walsh & Hoyt's Clinical Neuro-opthalmology, 2005. Chapter 17:809-885. cdmbuntu.lib.utah.edu/utils/getfile/collection/EHSL-NOVEL/id/1809/.../1550.pdf
26. Tewfik, TL Chief Editor: Arlen D Meyers, MD, MBA Trigeminal Nerve Anatomy. emedicine.medscape.com/article/1873373-overview. Medscape. Jun 19, 2013.
27. Huff T, Daly DT. Neuroanatomy, Cranial Nerve 5, Trigeminal (CN V) [Updated 2018 Jan 18]. In: StatPearls [Internet]. Treasure Island (FL): StatPearls Publishing; 2018 Jan-. Available from: https://www.ncbi.nlm.nih.gov/books/NBK482283/
28. Myckatyn TM and Mackinnon SE. A Review of Facial Nerve Anatomy. Seminars in Plastic Surgery. Vol. 18, No. 1, 2004.
29. Vin Gijn, J. Charles Bell (1794-1842). J Neurol. 2011 Jun; 258(6): 1189-1190.
30. Gray L. Chapter 12: Auditory System: Structure and Function. Department of Communication Sciences and Disorders, James Madison University. Neuroscience Online neuroscience.uth.tmc.edu. Department of Neurobiology and Anatomy, The UT Medical School at Houston. Ed., John H. Byrne.1997
31. Alberti, P. The anatomy and physiology of the ear and hearing. In B. Goelzer, C. Hansen, & G. Sehrdt (Eds.), Occupational exposure to noise: Evaluation, prevention, and control. 2001. pp. 53-62. Geneva, Switzerland: World Health Organization. Retrieved from http://www.who.int/occupational_health/publications/noise.pdf
32. Gray L. Chapter 13: Auditory System: Pathways and Reflexes. Department of Communication Sciences and Disorders, James Madison University. Neuroscience Online neuroscience.uth.tmc.edu. The UT Medical School at Houston. Ed., John H. Byrne.1997

33. Gray L. Chapter 10: Vestibular System: Structure and Function. Department of Communication Sciences and Disorders, James Madison University. Neuroscience Online neuroscience.uth.tmc.edu. Department of Neurobiology and Anatomy, The UT Medical School at Houston. Ed., John H. Byrne.1997.
34. Jones SM, Jones TA, Mills KN, Gaines GC. "Anatomical and Physiological Considerations in Vestibular Dysfunction and Compensation." Seminars in hearing 30.4 (2009): 231–241. PMC. Web. 4 Sept. 2018.
35. Gray L. Chapter 11: Vestibular System: Pathways and Reflexes. Neuroscience Online neuroscience.uth.tmc.edu. Department of Neurobiology and Anatomy, The UT Medical School at Houston. Ed., John H. Byrne.1997.
36. Walker HK, Chapter 63: Cranial Nerves IX and X: The Glossopharyngeal and Vagus Nerves. Clinical Methods: The History, Physical, and Laboratory Examinations. 3rd edition. Walker HK, Hall WD, Hurst JW, editors.Boston: Butterworths; 1990.
37. Matsuo K and Palmer JB. Anatomy and Physiology of Feeding and Swallowing – Normal and Abnormal. Phys Med Rehabil Clin N Am. Nov 2008; 19(4): 691–707.
38. Pearce JMS. Wallenberg's syndrome. J Neurol Neurosurg Psychiatry 2000, 68, 570 doi: 10. 1136//nng.68.5.570
39. Hayashi F, Coles SK, McCrimmon DR. Respiratory Neurons Mediating the Breuer–Hering Reflex. Prolongation of Expiration in Rat. Clinical Investigations. Respiration 2001,68:140-144
40. Tryfon S, Kontakiotes T, Mavrofides E, Patakes D. Hering-Breuer Reflex in Normal Adults and Patients with COPD and Interstitial Fibrosis. Clinical Investigations Respiration 2001; 68: 140-144.
41. McAllen RM, Shafton AD, Bratton BO, Trevaks D and Furness JB. Calibration of thresholds for functional engagement of Vagal A, B and C fiber groups in vivo. Bioelectron. Med. (2018)1(1), 21-27.
42. Castoro MA, Yoo PB, Hincapie JG, et al. Excitation properties of the right cervical vagus nerve in adult dogs. Exp Neurol (2011) 227, 62-68.
43. Campos D, Rieger A, Mohr H, Ellwanger JH and Borba Jr AM. Anatomy and evolution of accessory nerve: cranial or spinal. Morphol. Sci., 2011, vol. 28, no. 4, p. 222-227
44. Kubin L, Jordan AS, Nicholas CL, Cori JM, Semmler JG, Trinder J. Crossed motor innervation of the base of human tongue. Journal of Neurophysiology (2015), 113 (10) 3499-3510; DOI:10.1152/jn.00051.2015
45. Fritz MA, Kang BJ, Fox TP, Bhatia NB, MD, Mandel SM. Iatrogenic Hypoglossal Nerve Palsy. 2014 Practical Neurology. Jan/Feb. pp. 13-16.

46. Ramchandren S, Gruis KL, Chervin RD, et al. Hypoglossal nerve conduction findings in obstructive sleep apnea. Muscle & nerve. 2010;42(2):257-261. doi:10.1002/mus.21690.
47. Certal VF, Zaghi S, Riaz M, Vieira AS, Pinheiro CT, Kushida C, Capasso R, Camacho M. Hypoglossal nerve stimulation in the treatment of obstructive sleep apnea: A systematic review and meta-analysis. Laryngoscope. 2015 May; 125(5):1254-64. Epub 2014 Nov 12
48. Gillespie MB, Soose RJ, Woodson BT, Strohl KP, Maurer JT, de Vries N, Steward DL, Baskin JZ, Badr MS, Lin HS, et al. Upper Airway Stimulation for Obstructive Sleep Apnea: Patient-Reported Outcomes after 48 Months of Follow-up. Otolaryngol Head Neck Surg. 2017 Apr; 156(4):765-771. Epub 2017 Feb 14.
49. Dafny N, Chapter 3: Anatomy of the Spinal Cord. Department of Neurobiology and Anatomy, UT Medical School at Houston. Neuroscience Online neuroscience.uth.tmc.edu. Ed., John H. Byrne.1997
50. Bhattacharyya KB. The stretch reflex and the contributions of C David Marsden. Annals of Indian Academy of Neurology. 2017;20(1):1-4. doi:10.4103/0972-2327.199906.
51. Purves D, Augustine GJ, Fitzpatrick D, et al., editors. Neuroscience. 2nd edition. Sunderland (MA): Sinauer Associates; 2001. The Spinal Cord Circuitry Underlying Muscle Stretch Reflexes. Available from: http://www.ncbi.nlm.nih.gov/books/NBK10809/
52. Chawla J. Autonomic Nervous System Anatomy. emedicine.medscape.com/article/1922943-overview Medscape. Chief Editor: Ramachandran TS. Updated Aug 12, 2013
53. Pearce JM. A Note on Claude Bernard-Horner's Syndrome. J Neurol Neurosurgery Psychiatry. 1995 Aug; 59(2): (88,19)
54. Foroulis CN, Zarogoulidis P, Darwiche K, et.al. Superior sulcus (Pancoast) tumors: current evidence on diagnosis and radical treatmentJ Thorac Dis. 2013 Sep; 5(Suppl 4): S342–S358.
55. Panagopoulos N, Leivaditis V, et.al. Pancoast tumors: characteristics and preoperative assessment. J Thorac Dis. 2014 Mar; 6(Suppl 1): S108–S115.
56. Schultz HD. Nitric Oxide Regulation of Autonomic Function in Heart Failure. Current heart failure reports. 2009;6(2):71-80.
57. Ahmad A, Dempsey SK, Daneva Z, Azam M, Li N, Li PL and Ritter JK. Role of Nitric Oxide in the Cardiovascular and Renal Systems. Int. J. Mol. Sci. 2018, 19, 2605; doi:10.3390/ijms19092605 p.1-23.

58. Knierim J, Chapter 5: Cerebellum. Neuroscience Online neuroscience.uth.tmc.edu. Department of Neurobiology and Anatomy, The UT Medical School at Houston. Ed., John H. Byrne.1997
59. Manto M, and Peter M. "Schmahmann's Syndrome - Identification of the Third Cornerstone of Clinical Ataxiology." Cerebellum & Ataxias 2 (2015): 2. PMC. Web. 18 Sept. 2018.
60. Lawrenson C, Bares M, Kamondi A, Kovács A, Lumb B, Apps R, Filip P, and Manto M "The Mystery of the Cerebellum: Clues from Experimental and Clinical Observations." Cerebellum & Ataxias 5 (2018): 8. PMC. Web. 18 Sept. 2018
61. Groenewegen HJ. The Basal Ganglia and Motor Control and The Basal Ganglia and Learning Functions; Neural Plasticity, Vol. 10, No. 1-2, 2003.
62. Albin RL, Young AB, Penney JB. The functional anatomy of basal ganglia disorders. Trends Neurosci. 1989 Oct;12(10):366-75.
63. Deng YP, Albin RL, Penney JB. Differential loss of striatal projection systems in Huntington's disease: a quantitative immunochemical study. J Chem Neuroanst 2004;27:143-164.
64. Leisman G, Braun-Benjamin O, and Melillo R. Cognitive-motor interactions of the basal ganglia in development. Front Syst Neurosci. 2014; 8: 16.
65. Ziller K and Amunts K. Centenary of Brodmann's Map—conception and fate. Nature Review/Neuroscience. Vol. 11 Feb 2010 p139-45.
66. Byrne H. Chapter 7: Learning and Memory, Neuroscience Online Neuroscience. uth.tmc.edu. Department of Neurobiology and Anatomy, The UT Medical School at Houston. Ed., John H. Byrne.1997.
67. Moscovitch M, Rosenbaum SR, Gilboa A, Addis DR, Westmacott R, Grady C, McAndrews MP, Levine B, Black S, Winocur G and Nadel L. Functional neuroanatomy of remote episodic, semantic and spatial memory: a unified account based on multiple trace theory. J Anat (2005) 207, pp 35-66.
68. Bruner, Emiliano. "Language, Paleoneurology, and the Fronto-Parietal System." Frontiers in Human Neuroscience 11 (2017): 349. PMC. Web. 2 Oct. 2018.
69. Kreisler A, Godefroy O, Delmaire C, Debachy B, Leclercq M, Pruvo JP and Leys D. The anatomy of aphasia revisited. NEUROLOGY 2000;54:1117–1123.
70. Anderson JM, Gilmore R, Roper S, Crosson B, Bauer RM, Nadeau S, Beversdorf DQ, Cibula J, Rogish M, Kortenkamp S, Hughes JD, Gonzalez Rothi LJ, Heilman KM. Conduction aphasia and the arcuate fasciculus: A reexamination of the Wernicke-Geschwind model. Brain Lang. 1999 Oct 15;70(1):1-12.

71. Shaywitz SE, Mody M, Shaywitz BA. Neural Mechanisms in Dyslexia. Current Directions in Psychological Science Vol 15 No.6. Home / Current Directions in Psychological Science, Volume 15, Number 6, December 2006 pp. 278-281(4)
72. Brownsett SLE and Wise RJS. "The Contribution of the Parietal Lobes to Speaking and Writing." Cerebral Cortex (New York, NY) 20.3 (2010): 517–523. PMC. Web. 2 Oct. 2018.
73. Cappelletti M, Lee H, Freeman E, Price C. THE ROLE OF THE RIGHT AND LEFT PARIETAL LOBES IN THE CONCEPTUAL PROCESSING OF NUMBERS. Journal of cognitive neuroscience. 2010;22(2):331-346. doi:10.1162/jocn.2009.21246.
74. Huff T, Dulebohn SC. Neuroanatomy, Visual Cortex. [Updated 2018 Apr 15]. In: StatPearls [Internet]. Treasure Island (FL): StatPearls Publishing; 2018 Jan-. Available from: https://www.ncbi.nlm.nih.gov/books/NBK482504/
75. Gruter T, Gruter M, Carbon CC: Neural and genetic foundations of face recognition and prosopagnosia. J Neuropsychol 2:79-97, 2008.
76. Wright A, Chapter 8: Higher Cortical Functions: Language. Neuroscience Online neuroscience.uth.tmc.edu. Department of Neurobiology and Anatomy, The UT Medical School at Houston. Ed., John H. Byrne.1997
77. Wright A, Chapter 9: Higher Cortical Functions: Association and Executive Processing. Neuroscience Online neuroscience.uth.tmc.edu. Department of Neurobiology and Anatomy, The UT Medical School at Houston. Ed., John H. Byrne.1997
78. Hathaway WR, Newton BW. Neuroanatomy, Prefrontal Cortex. [Updated 2018 Apr 25]. In: StatPearls [Internet]. Treasure Island (FL): StatPearls Publishing; 2018 Jan-. Available from: https://www.ncbi.nlm.nih.gov/books/NBK499919/
79. Folstein MF, Folstein SE, and Mchugh PR. "Mini-Mental State," A Practical Method for Grading the Cognitive State of Patients for the Clinician. J. Psychiat. Res., 1975, pp 189-198. Peramon Press. Printed in Great Britain.
80. Nasreddine ZS, Phillips NA, Bédirian V, Charbonneau S, Whitehead V, Collin I, Cummings JL, Chertkow H. The Montreal Cognitive Assessment (MoCA): A Brief Screening Tool For Mild Cognitive Impairment. Journal of the American Geriatrics Society 53:695-699, 2005.
81. Ledesma LK, Diputado BV, Orteza GO and Santillan CE. De-Westernization of a Dementia Screening Scale: The Philippine Experience. Philippine Journal of Psychology. Vol. 26, No.2: 30-38, 1993.
82. Stevens MS, Normal Sleep, Sleep Physiology, and Sleep Deprivation: Normal https://emedicine.medscape.com/article/1188226-overview Dec 3, 2015 Medscape. Chief Editor: Selim R Benbadis.

83. Cooper JM, Halter KA and Prosser A. Neurobiology of Sleep and Circadian Rhythms Volume 5, June 2018, Pages 15-36 open access Neurobiology of Sleep and Circadian Rhythms. https://www.sciencedirect.com/science/article/pii/S2451994417300342
84. Institute of Medicine (US) Committee on Sleep Medicine and Research; Colten HR, Altevogt BM, editors. Sleep Disorders and Sleep Deprivation: An Unmet Public Health Problem. Washington (DC): National Academies The Role of the Right and Left Parietal Lobes in the Conceptual Processing Press (US); 2006. 2, Sleep Physiology. Available from: http://www.ncbi.nlm.nih.gov/books/NBK19956/
85. Noirhomme Q, Soddu A, Vanhaudenhuyse A, Lehembre R, Bruno M-A, Gosseries O, Demertzi A, Maudoux A, Schnakers C, Boveroux P, Boly M, Laureys S. Functional neuroimaging approaches to the changing borders of consciousness. Journal of Psychophysiology, Vol 24(2), 2010, 68-75.
86. Laureys S, Berre J, and Goldman S. Cerebral Function in Coma, Vegetative State, Minimally Conscious State, Locked-in Syndrome and Brain Death. 2001 Yearbook of Intensive Care and Emergency Medicine J-L Vincent (Ed.). Springer, Berlin, pp. 386-396.
87. Dietrich A. Functional neuroanatomy of altered states of consciousness: The transient hypofrontality hypothesis. Consciousness and Cognition 12(2003)231-256.
88. Kotchoubey B, Pavlov YG. A Systematic Review and Meta-Analysis of the Relationship Between Brain Data and the Outcome in Disorders of Consciousness. Frontiers in Neurology. 2018;9:315. doi:10.3389/fneur.2018.00315.
89. Walker MC, O'Brien D. Neurological examination of the unconscious patient. J R Soc Med 1999;92:353-355
90. Shuaib A, Butcher K, Mohammad AA, Saqqur M, Liebeskind DS.Collateral blood vessels in acute ischaemic stroke: a potential therapeutic target.Lancet Neurol.2011;*10*:909–921.doi:10.1016/S1474-4422(11)70195-8
91. Østergaard L, Jespersen SN, Mouridsen K, et al. The role of the cerebral capillaries in acute ischemic stroke: the extended penumbra model. J Cereb Blood Flow Metab. 2013;33(5):635-48.
92. Plum and Posner's Diagnosis of Stupor and Coma. 4th Edition. Eds: Posner, J., Saper, C.B., Schiff, N.D. and Plum, F. Publisher: Oxford University Press. 2007.
93. Teasdale G. and Jennett B. Assessment of coma and impaired consciousness. A practical scale. 1974 Lancet 2(7872): 81-4

94. Fischer M, Rfuegg S, Czaplinski A, Strohmeier M, Lehmann A, Tschan F, Hunziker PR, and Marsch SC. Inter-rater reliability of the Full Outline of UnResponsiveness score and the Glasgow Coma Scale in critically ill patients: a prospective observational study. smarsch@uhbs.ch Critical Care 2010, 14:R64 doi:10.1186/cc8963
95. Wijdicks EF, Bamlet WR, Maramattom BV, Manno EM, McClelland RL: Validation of a new coma scale: the FOUR score. Ann Neurol 2005, 58:585-593
96. Ledoux D, Bruno M, Jonlet S, Choi P, Schnakers C, Damas F, Lambermont B, Damas P and Laurey S. Full Outline of Unresponsiveness compared with Glasgow coma scale assessment and outcome prediction in coma. in coma. Critical Care 2009, 13(Suppl 1):P107. http://ccforum.com/content/13/S1/P107
97. National Institute of Health, National Institute of Neurological Disorders and Stroke. Stroke Scale. http://www.ninds.nih.gov/doctors/NIH_Stroke_Scale.pdf
98. Herbowski L. Review Article: The Maze of the Cerebrospinal Fluid Discovery. Anatomy Research International, Volume 2013 (2013), Article ID 596027, 8 pages. http://dx.doi.org/10.1155/2013/596027
99. Greitz D. Cerebrospinal fluid circulation and associated intracranial dynamics. A radiologic investigation using MR imaging and radionuclide cisternography. Department of Neuroradiology, Karolinska Hospital, Stockholm, Sweden.Acta Radiologica. Supplementum 1993, 386:1-23
100. Khasawneh AH, Garling RJ, and Harris CA. Cerebrospinal fluid circulation: What do we know and how do we know it? Brain Circ. 2018 Jan-Mar; 4(1): 14–18.Published online 2018 Apr 18. doi: [10.4103/bc.bc_3_18]PMCID: PMC6057699 PMID: 30276331
101. Tyrrell PJ. Apraxia of gait or higher level gait disorders: review and description of two cases or progressive gait disturbance due to frontal lobe degeneration. J of the Royal Soc of Med. Vol 87. August 1994; pp 454-456.
102. Rengachary SS, Xavier A, Manjila S, Smerdon U, Parker B, Hadwan S, Guthikonda M. The legendary contributions of Thomas Willis (1621-1675): the arterial circle and beyond. J Neurosurg. 2008 Oct;109(4):765-75. doi: 10.3171/JNS/2008/109/10/0765.
103. Sinha KK. Brain Stem Infarction: Clinical Clues to Localise Them. Journal, Indian Academy of Clinical Medicine Vol. 1, No. 3 October-December 2000.
104. Caplan LR, Chung CS, Wityk RJ, Glass TA, Tapia J, Pazdera L, Chang HM, Dashe JF, Chaves CJ, Vemmos K, Leary M, Dewitt LD, and Pessin MS. New England Medical Center Posterior Circulation Stroke Registry: I. Methods, Data Base, Distribution of Brain Lesions, Stroke Mechanisms, and Outcomes.

J Clin Neurol. Apr 2005; 1(1): 14–30.Published online Apr 30, 2005. doi: 10.3988/jcn.2005.1.1.14
105. Balami JS, Chen, RL, and Buchanan, AM: Stroke syndromes and clinical management. QJMed 2013; 106-615.
106. Lees KR, Bluhmki E, von Kummer R, et. al. Time to treatment with intravenous alteplase and outcome in stroke: an updated pooled analysis of ECASS, ATLANTIS, NINDS, and EPITHET trials. Lancet. 2010;375(9727):169
107. Elzamly, K., Nobleza, C., Parker, E., & Sugg, R. (2018). Unilateral Upper Cervical Posterior Spinal Cord Infarction after a Neuroendovascular Intervention: A Case Report. *Case reports in neurological medicine, 2018*, 5070712. doi:10.1155/2018/5070712
108. Martirosyan NL, Feuerstein JS, Theodore BAN, Cavalcanti DD, Spetzler RF, and Preul MD. Vascular supply and vascular reactivity of the spinal cord under normal and pathologic conditions. J Neurosurg Spine 15:238-251, 2011
109. Kiliç T, Akakin A. The Cerebrospinal Venous System: Anatomy, Physiology, and Clinical Implications Anatomy of cerebral veins and sinuses. Medscape General Medicine > MedGenMed Neurology & Neurosurgery.
110. Ruiz DSM, Gailloud P, Rufenacht DA, et.al. The Craniocervical Venous System in Relation to Cerebral Venous Drainage. AJND Am J neuroradiol 23:1500-1508, Oct 2002.: Special issue on Chronic cerebro-spinal venous insufficiency.
111. Beggs CB. Cerebral Venous Outflow and Cerebrospinal Fluid Dynamics. Veins and Lymphatics. Vol. 3, No. 3 (2014):Special issue on chronic cerebro-spinal venous insuffieciency.
112. Pearce JMS. The Craniospinal Venous System. Eur Neurol. 2006;56:136-38.
113. Netter FH, Craig JA, Perkins J. (Illustrators), Hansen J, Koeppen BM. (Text). Atlas of Neuroanatomy and Neurophysiology. Selection from the Netter Collection of Medical Illustrations. Icon Custom Communications, 2002.

INDEX

A

Accomodation, 72–73, 75
Abdominal Reflex, 167
Accomodation reflex test, 80
A-delta fibers, 27–28, 178
Afferent, Efferent nerve, 4–5, 94, 117, 123, 126, 163, 174, 178
Alpha fibers, 163
   Cuneatus, nucleus, 36
   Cuneatus, fasciculus, 36–37, 171
   Gracilis fasciculus, 36–38, 152, 171
   Gracilis nucleus, 36, 153, 171
Amaurosis Fugax, 266, 272
Anisocoria, 74–75, 77–78, 119
Ankle reflex, 167
Anterior circulation strokes, 271–73
Anterior communicating artery aneurysm, 265
Anterior horn of the spinal cord, 19
Anterolateral spinothalamic tract, 25, 28–29
Apoplexy, 255
Arachnoid granulation, 253
Arterial collaterals, 232
Autoregulatory mechanism, 232
Arterial supply to the spinal cord

Anterior Spinal artery syndrome, 277
Pelvic or hypogastric arteries, 277
Artery to artery embolism, 266
Aspiration Pneumonia, 120, 130
Audiometer, 105
Auditory agnosia, 104–5, 216
Auditory evoked potential, 105
Auditory hallucination, 104
Auricular nerves, 125
Autonomic nerve affectation, 171
Autonomic Nervous System (ANS), 152, 173
   ANS fibers
      Afferent A delta fibers, 178
      Efferent Beta 1 fibers, 178
      Post Ganglionic fibers, C fibers, 27, 153, 178
   ANS neurotransmitters
      Acetyl Choline, 177
      Nitrous Oxide (NO), 178
      Nor-epinephrine (NE), 177
   Central Nervous Components (CNS), 174
      Brainstem centers of the ANS, 174
      Cortical & Subcortical ANS participants, 14, 174
      Preganglionic Parasympathetic

neurons (PSNS), 175
Spinal Cord ANS participants, 174
Intermediate gray horn at S2-S4 (PSNS), 155
Intermediate gray horn at T1-L2 (SNS), 155
Preganglionic neurons, 155, 174–76
Peripheral Nervous System (PNS)
Bernard-Horner's Syndrome, 176
Hemi-anhydrosis, 176
Pancoast-Tobias Syndrome, 177
Post-ganglionic neurons, 174
Mesenteric ganglia, 177
Paravertebral Cervical Sympathetic Ganglia (SNS), 156
Walls of large intestines and GU (PSNS), 176
Vagal efferent receptors, 127
Axons, 9

B

Babinski sign, 22–24, 50, 92, 138, 161, 165, 167, 170
Back bones, 142, 144
Baroreceptors, 116, 120, 126–27
Basal Ganglia, 13, 133, 195–96, 198, 200, 202
Dopamine striatal neurons, D1 & D2, *197*
Dopamine transmitter, 197
Excitatory glutaminergic transmitter, 197
Globus Pallidus, 197
Neostriatum or Striatum
Caudate nucleus, 197
Putamen
Substancia Nigra, Compacta, 196–97
Substancia Nigra, Reticulata, 197
Subthalamic nucleus, 197
GABA transmitter, 197
Basilar membrane, varying thickness and stiffness, 101
Bell's Palsy, 90, 93–94, 98
Benign Paroxysmal Postural Vertigo (BPPV), 110–11
Blink Reflex Electromyography, 84
Brain death, 113
Brain Death Criteria, 86

C

Cacosmia, 52
Caloric Test, 112–13
Ice caloric test, 113, 129, 246
Cardiac, esophageal and pulmonary plexuses, 126
Cardio-embolic stroke, 258
Carotid Sinus and Carotid Body Reflex, 120
Cavernous hemangioma, 78
Central Aqueduct, 252
Cerebellar functional system
Cortico-cerebellar cognitive/affective system, 191
Cortico-cerebellar sensory/motor system, 191
Vestibulo-cerebellar oculo-spinal system, 110–11
Cerebellar herniation, 130
Cerebellar Layers
Climbing fibers, 188
Inner layer and granule cells, 189
Middle layer and Purkinje cells, 188, 190
Mossy fibers, 188

Cerebellar Nuclei
  Dentate Nucleus, 189
  Fastigial Nucleus, 190
  Interposed Nucleus, 190
Cerebellar Peduncles
  Inferior cerebellar peduncle
    (restiform body), 189
  Middle cerebellar peduncle
    (brachium pontis), 189
  Superior cerebellar peduncle
    (brachium conjunctivum, 189
Cerebrospinal Fluid (CSF) volume, 13
C-fibers, 27–28, 178
Chemoreceptors, 116, 120, 126–27
Circle of Willis, 43
Cisterna magna, 252
Clonus, 24, 164, 167
CN II Optic Nerve, 53, 55–57, 174
CN I Olfactory Nerve anatomy,
  46, 115
CN IX Afferent taste sensation
  posterior 1/3 of the tongue., 125
CN IX Glossopharyngeal Nerve
  parasympathetic, 96
CN VII Facial Nerve
  Facial nerve motor, 84, 92
    Lower facial motor weakness,
      crossed innervation, 92
    Upper facial motor neuron, bilateral
      innervation, 92
  Nervus Intermedius, 91, 93–94,
    96–97
  Chorda tympani, 91, 94, 96–98
  Parasympathetic nucleus of the
    Salivatory Nucleus (SN), 94
  Pterygopalatine ganglia supply, 94
  Submandibular and Sublingual
    glands, 91

CN VIII Components
  Cochlear Nerves, 99
  Vestibular Nerves, 99
CN XII Tongue homunculus
  Axon decussates, 135
  Hypoglossal nerve stimulation, 137
  Hypoglossal neurons during REM
    sleep, 137
  Tongue fasciculation and atrophy,
    137, 139
CN XI Origin of Accessory Nerve
  Nucleus Ambiguus (NA), 116–17,
    126, 131–32, 174–75
  Spinal Accessory N., 131
CN X Vagus nerve
  Hering-Breuer Reflex
  Apneutic center of the pons
    (AC), 127
  Inspiratory Center of the Medulla
    (IC), 127–28
  Nucleus Solitarius, 128
Cochlear Reflex, 101
Cognitive function of the
  cerebellum, 191
Collateral vessels, 258
Color blindness, 57
Color light bands, 55
Conjugate eye movements, 72
Consciousness, 229
  Arousal & awareness, 229
  Reticular Activating System, 129
Corneal reflex, 84, 86, 94, 245
  absence of corneal reflex, 84
Cortico-spinal tract, 147
Cover of the brain
  Arachnoid mater, subarachnoid
    space, 55
  Epineurium, 13

Meninges, subdural space, 13
Pia mater, 13
Cover-uncover test, 79
Cranial Nerve I neurological examination, 52
Cranial Nerve Nuclei, 6, 45–46, 109, 119
Cranial Nerves, 44–45
Cranial Nerves to extra ocular muscles
  CN III Occulomotor nerve, 68–69, 74
    Edinger-Westphal Nucleus (EWN), 70, 73, 175
    Parasympathetic nerve (PN) pupiloconstrictor muscles, 175
  CN VI Abducens nerve, 69, 78, 92
    Superior oblique muscles, 68–69
  CN VII Trochlear nerve, 68, 76
    Lateral rectus muscles, 68
Cremasteric reflex, 167
Cribriform plate, 49
Crossed deficits, 119
CSF circulation, fig.54, *251*
  CSF in infections of the brain, 252
  Choroid plexus, 252
  CSF Rhinorrhea, 49, 52

D

Deafness types
  Conduction deafness, 104–5
  Sensory-neural deafness, 105
Demyelinating Diseases, 11
Dendrites, 9
Dendritic receptors, 9
Dermatomal distribution, 39, 83
Descending modulators, non-pain group, 26, 28

Periaqueductal Gray Neurons (PAG), 29
Rostral Ventral Medullary Neurons (RVM), 29
Direct light reflex test, 79
Direct Pathway, 196, 198
Discriminatory sensation, 35–36
Discriminatory sensations
  Graphesthesia, 36
  Proprioception, 35–36, 106, 152–53, 171
  Stereognosis, 36
  Test, 173
  Vibratory Sensation, 35–36, 38, 171
Distal, 5, 185
Doll's head maneuver, 77
Dominant Brain, concept, 205 Dorsal Cochlear Nuclei (DCN), 102–3 Dorsal Motor Nucleus, 126, 175 Duret hemorrhages, 75
Dysmetria, 193, 274
Dysosmia, 52

E

Electrical neural conduction
  Action potential, depolarization, 8, 10, 171
  Gates, 9–10
  Gradient, 9
  hyperpolarized state, 10
  Ion transfer, passive active, 9, 11
  Resting state, 9
  Self-propagating, 10
  Transmission, 9
  voltage gated calcium, 10
  Voltage Shifts, 10
Electro-mechanical transduction, 102

Electromyography tests, 157
Epiglottis and base of tongue taste sensation, 123
Eustachian tubes, 101, 104
Evaluation of the ANS functions, 152
Explosive speech, 139, 274

F

Finger-to-nose test, 192
Flocculonodular lobes, 189
Focal lesions, 21
Focal seizure, 7–8, 11, 22, 27
   Partial Seizure, 51
   Temporal lobe seizure, 51
Foramen of Lushka, 252
Foramen of Magendie, 252
Foramen of Munroe, 252
Fourth ventricle, 252
From Nucleus Ambiguus, 132
Frontal lobe, anatomy, 217–22

   Amygdala, cingulate cortex, 219
   Cingulate gyrus, 49, 219
   Conjugate deviation, 72, 270
   De-westernization of Dementia Screening Scale, 221
   Dorsal gyrus, 219
   Executive functions, 219
   Frontal Gaze Center, 69, 72
   Frontal release signs, 219
   Functional disorders or psychiatric disorders, 221
   Medial gyrus, 219
   Mini Mental Status Examination (MMSE), 220–21
   Montreal Cognitive Assessment (MOCA), 221

Orbito frontal cortex, 219
Precentral gyrus, 72
Sucking and grasp reflex, 273
Frontal lobe signs, 267

G

GABA interneurons, 28
Ganglia
   Cranial nerve ganglia, 5–6, 43–44, 46, 67, 92, 117, 138, 163, 175
   Dorsal ganglia, 5, 15, 27–28, 32–33, 83, 142, 144, 151, 157, 171, 178
   Pseudo-bipolar neuron, 27, 83
   Sympathetic Ganglia, 5, 155, 174, 176, 180
Gastro-esophageal peristalsis, 129
Gate control theory, 28
General Classification of Pain
   Neuropathic pain, 85, 156
   Somatic pain, 32
   Visceral pain, 32
   Referred pain, 32
Generalized seizures, 22
Golden period in stroke, 270
G protein-coupled receptors (GPCRs), 11
G protein, 11
Gray matter, spinal cord, 13, 15, 17, 19, 131, 145, 163, 276
   Anterior horn, 19–20, 59, 145, 148
   Intermediate zone, 145
   Posterior horn, 27, 145
   Ten functional neuronal groups, 145

300　INDEX

H

Hemiparesis/hemiplegia, 21, 24, 185, 270, 281
Herpes Simplex Encephalitis, 50
Homunculus or Little man, 17
Horizontal Gaze mechanism, 72–73
　Frontal Gaze Centers (FGC), 72
　Medial longitudinal fasciculus (MLF), 70, 72
　Pontine Gaze Center (PGC), 69, 72
Hypoglycemic encephalopathy, 21
Hyposmia, 52
Hypothalamus, xxi, 5–6, 49, 58–59, 96, 115, 119, 121, 129, 155, 174

I

Imbalance or Dizziness, 110
Indirect light reflex test, 79
Indirect Pathway, 196, 198
Inferior Colliculi (IC), 102
Inferior Glossopharyngeal ganglia (IGG), 117
　Nucleus Solitarius and CN V, 117–18
Inferior Laryngeal Nerve or Recurrent Laryngeal Nerve, 126
Inner hair cells, 102
Internal acoustic canal, 93–94, 98, 102
Internal capsule, 19, 21, 86, 92–93, 135, 138, 271
Intracranial pressure, normal, 55, 75
　Communicating hydrocephalus, 253
　　Bladder and bowel incontinence, 267
　　Gait apraxia of Bruns, 254
　　Papilledema, 254
　　Primitive reflexes, 253
　　Sunset sign, 77–78, 254
　Non-communicating or obstructive hydrocephalus, 253
　Spinal manometer, 250

L

Laminae, 5
Lateral Geniculate Ganglia, 59, 70, 73
Lateral Lemniscus Nuclei (LLEN), 102–3
Lateral medullary syndrome, 119–20, 274
Lateral ventricles, 13
Lenticulo striae vessels, 268
　Internal capsule infarct, 268
Ligand-gated channel
　Gamma-aminobutyric acid ligand-gated channel, 10
　Glutamine neurotransmitters, 10
Light reflex, 4, 73, 77, 79
Limbic system, 1, 27, 30, 49, 51, 70
Long loop reflex, 29
Lower Motor Neuron Signs, 165, 170
Lumbar puncture, 250

M

MCA syndromes, 270
Mechanical ventilators, 128
Medial Geniculate Ganglia, 103
Medial Lemniscus, 30, 36–37, 96, 125
Meniere's Disease, 111
Meningeal artery, 266
Meyer's loop, 59
Middle ear infection and internal acoustic nerve, 94, 104
Middle ears, 91, 94, 100, 104

Mitral neurons, 47–49
  Tufted cells, 47
Monochromatic, 57
Motor examination, 167
Motor Neuron Disease, 87, 134, 139
  Amyotrophic lateral sclerosis, 134
Movement Disorder, 133
  Cervical Dystonia, 133
  Spasmodic Torticollis, 133
MS plaques, 170
Muller's muscle of the upper lid, 119
Multiple Sclerosis, 38, 73, 170
Muscle of Mastication CN V supply, 86–87
Muscle receptors
  Myasthenia Gravis (MG), 20, 78–79, 161–62
  Neuromuscular Junction (NMJ), 10, 18, 20, 78, 161
Myasthenia Gravis, 161

N

Negative Manifestations, 22
Negative Movement Disorders, 200
Neostriatum or Striatum, 196, 198
Nerve Conduction Velocity (NCV) Studies, 157
Neuroanatomy, anatomic landmarks
  Anterior, 4, 13, 41, 49–51, 94, 96, 98, 109, 117, 125, 145, 150, 164, 276
  Anterolateral, 25, 28–29, 145
  Lateral, 4, 13, 22
  Medial, 4, 36, 49, 51, 57, 69, 109, 115, 145, 176, 204
  Posterior, 4, 13, 29, 38–39, 96, 116–18, 125, 143, 145, 213

Spinothalamic Tract, 25, 28
Neurological Examination, Unconscious
  Conjugate eye deviation, 72, 270
  Corneal reflex examination, 245
  Full Outline of Unresponsiveness Score (FOUR), 242
  Glasgow coma scale (GCS) table V., 242
  Graded stimulus and describing response, 233, 239
  Midriasis and Miosis, 243
  Modified Rankin Scale, 243
  National Institute of Health Stroke Scale (NIHS), 242
  Ocular bobbing, 77, 237
  Patterns of respiration
    Apneustic breathing, 235
    Ataxic or Biot's respiration, 235
    Central Neurogenic Hyperventilation, 233
    Cheyne-Stokes respiration, 233
Neurological examination for pain sensation, 33
Neurology, definition, 1
Neurophobia, xx
Nigrostriatal Pathway, 198
Parkinson's Disease, 51, 199
Nociceptive fibers and noxious stimuli, 27, 30
Nodes of Ranvier, 7–8, 11, 22, 27
Non-convulsive seizures 233
Non-valvular atrial fibrillation, 259
Nuclear groups of the CN VII
  Motor neurons, 84, 86, 91–92

Nucleus Solitarius (NS), 96, 118, 126–27
Superior salivatory nucleus., 96
Nucleus Ambiguus (NA)
  Stylopharyngeal muscle for swallowing, 116
Nucleus Tractus Solitarius (NTS), 125, 174
Nystagmus, 112

O

Occipital lobe, anatomy, 216–18
  Apperceptive Agnosia, 218
  Associative Agnosia, 218
  Contralateral Neglect, 218
  Cortical blindness, 216
  Hemianopsia, 216
  Prosopagnosia, 218
  Visual Agnosia, 38, 63, 78, 216, 219
Olfactory bulb, glomeruli, 47, 50, 174
Olfactory cortex, medial anterior temporal lobe, 49, 51
Olfactory Epithelium, 47
Olfactory receptors
  Odiferous substance, 47
Olfactory tract, 43, 49–50
Oligodendrocytes myelin formation, 11, 53
Optic chiasma, 57, 170
Optic cup or optic nerve head, 53, 57
Optic nerve, 59
Optic radiation, 59
Optic tract, 52, 57, 59, 61
Organ of Corti, 102
Ossicles, ears
  Malleus, 101
  Stapes, 101

Otic ganglia neurons, 115
  Parotid Gland, 116, 125, 175
  Tongue Mucus glands, 117
Outer hair cells, 102
Oval window, 100–101

P

Pain, 25–32
  International Association for the Studies of Pain (IASP), definition, 30
  Mycobacterium leprae, 27
  Pain as friend, 25
  Total Pain concept, 31–32
Palmo-mental reflex, 167
Paradoxical embolism, 260
Paresis, paralysis definition, 21, 167–68, 186
Parietal lobe, anatomy, 210–15
  Acalculia, 215, 264, 273–74
  Agraphia, 215, 265
  Alexia, 215
  Angular gyrus, 210, 215
  Aphasia, 212
    Different types of aphasia, table IV., 213
    Conduction aphasia, 214
    Dyslexia, 53, 63, 215
    Dysphasia, 212
    Expressive aphasia or Broca's aphasia, 214
    Global aphasia, 214
    Grammar, 212
    Interpretation of emotion and connotation, 214
    Phonemes, 212

Phonology, 212
Postcentral gyrus, 30, 83, 96, 111, 125, 147, 173
Prosody, 212
Syntax, 212
Transcortical motor aphasia, 214
Transcortical sensory aphasia, 214
Verbal execution of prosody, 214
Wernicke's aphasia, 213
Wernicke's area, 210
Parieto-insular Vestibular Cortex (PIVC), 111
Parosmia, 52
Peripheral Nerve ANS, 141
  Parasympathetic Nervous System (PSNS), 154, 173
  Reflex sympathetic dystrophy (RSD) or complex regional, 156
  Paravertebral sympathetic ganglia, 155
  Postganglionic sympathetic neurons, 176
  Preganglionic neurons of the SNS, 176
  Reflex sympathetic dystrophy (RSD) or complex regional
    Allodynia 156, 172
    Hyperalgesia, 27, 156
    Pain syndrome (CRPS), 156
  Smooth muscles, 127–28, 152, 157, 163, 175–77
  Sympathetic Nervous System: 154, 173, 176
  Peripheral Nervous System (PNS), 157–62
  Dorsal Ganglia, 157
  Acute Guillain-Barre Syndrome, Chronic polyradiculities, 157

Dorsal Ganglionitis, 157
Herpes Zoster Infection, 32, 157
Neuromuscular junction, 161–62
  Post synaptic receptor, 8
  Myasthenia Gravis, 161–62
  Pre-synaptic Terminal, 161
  Pre-synaptic Terminal, Botulinum toxicity, 161
  Pre-synaptic Terminal, Lambert-Eaton Disease, 161
Peripheral nerves, 5, 11, 13, 20–21, 27, 32, 53, 78, 134, 141–42, 148, 150–52, 156–58, 162–66, 174
  Median nerve palsy or "Benediction hand" or "ape hand," 159
  Carpal Tunnel Syndrome, 159
  Radial nerve palsy or "Wrist drop," 159
  Ulnar nerve palsy or "Benediction hand" "claw hand," 159
Plexuses, 157–58
  Brachial plexitis, 157
  Roots, 13, 145, 150, 157–58, 162
Pharyngeal mucosal and gastrointestinal glands, 123
Parasympathetic, 73, 125, 152, 174
Phonation and vocal cord paralysis, 123, 126, 135, 137, 139
Photoreceptors, 55
Photo receptors
  Cones, 55, 57
  Rods, 55, 57, 119
Positive Movement Disorders, 200
  Chorea, 201
Post-central gyrus and homunculus, 17–19, 33, 41, 86, 92, 96, 111, 136, 152, 188
Posterior circulation strokes, 273

Crossed signs, 273
Table VI, 261, 274
Posterior Circulation Vessel, 261–64
Posterior circulation vessels
   Anterior inferior cerebellar artery, 262, 274
      Finger agnosia, 264
      Internal auditory artery, 262
      Internuclear opthalmoplegia, 73
      One and a half syndrome, 264
      Right-left disorientation, 265
      Top of the basilar artery, 264
      Visual agnosia, 216
      Visual and Auditory hallucination, 265
      Weber's syndrome, 264
   Anterior spinal artery, 261
   Basilar artery, 261
   Lateral medullary syndrome, 262
   Posterior inferior cerebellar artery, 111, 119
   Vertebral artery, 261
Post-herpetic neuralgia, 33
Post-synapse receptors, 10
Precentral gyrus, 69, 72, 86, 92, 135
Pre-synapse, 20
Pretectile, 59
Primary gustatory cortex, 118
Prosody of Language, 205
Proximal, 5
Pure motor weakness, 138
Pure sensory deficit, 138
Pyramidal Neuron, 9, 17, 19, 21–22, 92

R

Rapid pronation - supination test, 193
Reading dyslexia, 63

Reflexes, 163
   Deep tendon reflexes (DTR), 138, 161–63, 166–67, 171
   myotatic reflex, 163
   Gamma motor neurons, 163
   Gamma fibers, 165
   Inhibitory interneurons, 163–64
   Knee jerk reflexes, 170
   Muscle Spindles, 36, 163–64
      Ia and II afferent nerves, 163
      Intrafusal fibers, 163
   Reflex arc, 163–64
Reflexes, grading
   Hyperreflexia, 22, 165, 167, 170
Reperfusion treatment, 232
      Thrombolytic, rTPA, 232, 259, 271
Retinal Cells, 55
   Amacrine cells, 57
   Bipolar cells, 57, 59
   Ganglion cells, 56–57, 59, 61, 70, 180
   Horizontal cells, 57
Retina
   "window to the brain", 53
   Demyelination, 11,55
   Pappiledema, 55
   Retinal pallor and hemorrhage, 55
   Swelling or pallor of optic disc, 55

Reverse transduction or Feedback transduction, 102
Rinne's test, 105
Romberg's test, 193
Round windows, 101

S

Salivatory Nucleus, Parotid Gland, 125

Salivatory Secretions, 96
Saltatory Conduction of impulses, 8, 27
Scala media, 101
Scala tympani, 101
Scala vestibuli, 101
Scent, 47, 49, 51, 115
Schwann cells myelin formation, 11
Secondary Auditory Cortex, 103
Seizures, 12, 51–52, 63, 73, 104
    Aura, 51, 104
    Temporal lobe seizures, partial complex seizure, 51
    Uncinate fit, 51–52
    Positive manifestation, 22, 52
Sensors, 25, 28
Sensory abnormalities
    Allodynia, 172
    Anesthesia, 27
    Hyperaesthesia, 172
    Hypoaesthesia, 172
Sensory receptors, 15, 83, 118, 170
    Bare ending, 171
    Golgi tendons, 170
    Pacinian corpuscles, 171
Sleep, 223–27
    Arousal Maintaining System (System C), 227
    Cyclic sleep pattern or circadian rhythm, 225
    Dopamine transmitter, 227
    Dorsal raphe, 227
    Sleep recording (fig.46), 224
    Hypocretin or orexin, excitatory, 227
        cataplexy, 227
        Narcolepsy, 227
    Histamine, 227
    Hypothalamus, lateral, 227
    Tegmental nucleus, lateral dorsal, 227
    Locus coeruleus, 227
    Monoamine transmitters, 227
    Non-rapid eye movement (NREM), 227
    Non-rapid eye movement (NREM) stages, 223
    Noradrenaline, 227
    Pedunculopontine tegmental nucleus, 227
    Pontine neuronal system, 225
    Hypothalamus, posterior lateral, 227
    Rapid eye movement (REM), 223
    Serotonine, 227
    Sleep Cycle Inducing System (System S), 227
    Tuberomammillary nucleus (TMN), 227
    Hypothalamus, Ventrolateral preoptic nucleus (VLPN), 227
    GABA, 227
    Galanin, 227
Sleep paralysis, 227
Spasticity, 22, 165
Spinal Cord
    Conus Medullaris Syndrome, 145
    Four functional segments, 144
    Lumbar tap procedures, 145
    Cauda Equina or Filum terminale, 142, 144–45
Spiral ganglion, 100, 102
Stapedius muscles, reflex, 90–91, 93–94, 98, 101
    Hyperacusis, 94, 98
    startle response, 103
Striatum three sectors
    Associative sectors, 199
    Limbic sectors, 199

Sensorymotor sectors, 192, 199, 225
Stroke, 255
Stylomastoid foramen, 93
Sub-acute combined degeneration, 38
Subarachnoid space-pia matter junction, 252
Subclavian steal syndrome, 260
Summary, 162
   Clinico-pathologic correlation, 282
   Differential diagnosis, 282
   Localization, 282
   Neurological examination, xx
   Neurophysiology, 282
   Pathophysiology, 282
Superior colliculi, 59, 150
Superior Laryngeal Nerve, 125–26
   External Laryngeal Nerve, 126
   Internal Laryngeal Nerve, 126
Superior Olivary Nuclei (SON), 102
Superior saggital sinus, 253
Superior Sagittal Sinus, 279
Swallowing and breathing synchrony, 123
Symmetric and proximal muscle weakness, 5, 162
Sympathetic nerve (SN), 73–74, 97, 120, 176
   Pupilodilator muscles, 176

T

Tabes Dorsalis, 38
Taste bud receptor channel, 96
   Anterior two-thirds of the tongue, 117
Taste sensation, five types, 96
Tears, 89, 97
Tectorial membrane, 100, 102
Temporal lobe, anatomy, 206–10
   Amnesia, retrograde & anterograde, 208
   Amygdala, 49, 96, 174, 209
   Auditory agnosia, 209
   Declarative type of memory, 207
   Hippocampus, 206–7
   Memory formation, 49
   Partial complex seizures, 209
   Primary Auditory Cortex, 100, 103
   Temporal lobe seizure, psychomotor seizure, 209
   Uncus, 49, 51, 74–75, 206
   Uncinate fit, 51–52, 209
Terminal "button," 9–10, 20–21
Third ventricle, 253
Thrombi or clots & emboli, 258
Thyrotoxic myopathies, 78, 162
Tic Duloreaux or Trigeminal Neuralgia, 85
   Trigger points, 85
Total Pain concept, 30
Tracts, 9, 15, 19, 119, 145, 153
Transverse myelitis, 162
   Trigeminal Divisions
   Tumor embolism, 259

U

Uncal herniation, 74–75
Upper Motor Neuron Signs, 23, 165, 170

V

Vagal nerve stimulation, 128
Venous Drainage of the CNS, 277–79
   Cavernous sinus, cranial nerves, 279

Cavernous sinus thrombosis, 78
Cerebral venous thrombosis, 280
Deep system, sigmoid sinus, 279
Jugular veins, 279
Spinal venous plexus, drainage, 277
Superficial system, superior saggital sinus, 279
Valveless spinal venous plexus, 277
Prostatic plexuses, 277
Ventral Cochlear Nuclei (VCN), 102
  Thalamus, Ventroposterio Intermedius (VPI), 111
  Thalamus, Ventroposterior medial (VPM), 118
  Thalamus, Ventroposterolateral (VPL), 6, 30, 37, 152
  Thalamus, Ventroposterorinferior (VPI), 30, 111
Vertebral Columns, 144
  Degenerative osteophytes, 144
  Disc herniation, 144
  Listhesis, 144
Vertical gaze control
  Interstitial Nucleus of Cajal (INC), 77
  Rostral interstitial longitudinal fasciculus (RILF), 77
  Localization
  Horizontal lines, 42
  Vertical Neuroanatomic lines, 42
Vertigo, 110–12, 273–74
Vestibular apparatus, 106
  Ampulla, 106–8
  Diaphragmatic membrane or copula, 106
  Crista Ampullaris, 108
  Hair Cells, 108, 111–12

Semicircular canal (SCC), 77, 99, 106–7, 111
  Endolymph, 106
  Perilymph, 101, 106
  Utricle and Saccule, 106
  Scarpas Ganglia, 108
  Hair cells in the macula, 108
  Otoconia, 107–8
  Otolithic membrane, 108
Vestibule-collic reflex (VCR), 106
Vestibule-ocular reflex (VOR), 106, 112
Vestibule-spinal reflex (VSR), 106, 109
Visual acuity, text, 63
Visual field, 52, 54–55, 59, 63, 65, 72
Visual Field Abnormalities
  Bitemporal hemianopsia, 61
  Superior quadrant anopsia, 59–60
Visual Field tests, perimetry
  Confrontation test, 63
  Visual threat, 65
Vital Signs, 231
  Blood Pressure, 231
  Heart rate, 233
  Respiratory rate, 128, 141, 173
  Temperature, 233

W

Walking in straight line test, 193
Weakness, grading, 22
Weber's test, 105
White matter
  Anterior cortico-spinal tract uncrossed, 147
  Descending Cortical and Brainstem Fibers, Table I., 147, 150

Fasciculus Gracelis and Cuneatus, 38, 152
  Alpha fibers, 151
  Golgi Tendon organs, 151
  Large myelinated IIb fibers, 151
Lateral cortico-spinal tract or pyramidal tract, 19, 147
  topographical arrangement, 146
Lateral Spino-thalamic tract, 153
  Bare ending receptors, 171
  Nociceptive fibers, 27–30, 33, 37, 85
Motor Neuron Axons Ventral Anterior Rami, 150
Myotomal Distribution, 150, 152, 162, 168
Ascending fibers, Others Table II., 152
Tracts or funiculae, 145

www.ingramcontent.com/pod-product-compliance
Lightning Source LLC
Chambersburg PA
CBHW020628220526
45464CB00001B/58